# PATHOLOGIC BASIS OF DISEASE:

# Self Assessment and Review

# PATHOLOGIC BASIS OF DISEASE:

# Self Assessment and Review

4th EDITION

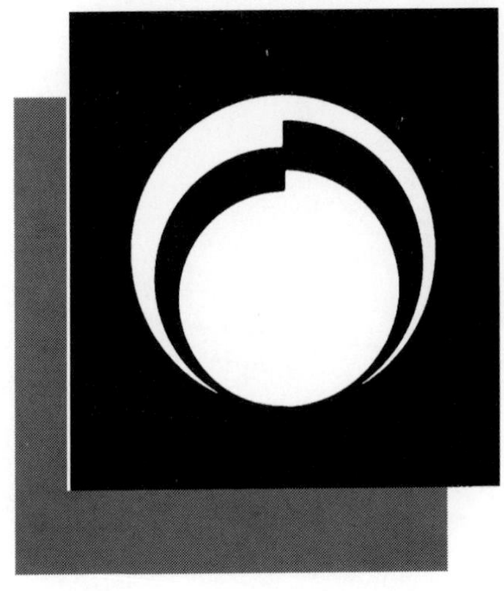

**CAROLYN COMPTON, M.D., Ph.D.**

Associate Professor of Pathology
Harvard Medical School
Associate Pathologist
Massachusetts General Hospital
Boston, Massachusetts

W. B. SAUNDERS COMPANY
*A Division of Harcourt Brace & Company*
Philadelphia, London, Toronto, Montreal, Sydney, Tokyo

**W. B. SAUNDERS COMPANY**
*A Division of Harcourt Brace & Company*

The Curtis Center
Independence Square West
Philadelphia, PA 19106

**Library of Congress Cataloging-in-Publication Data**

Compton, Carolyn C.
Pathologic basis of disease : self assessment and review / Carolyn C. Compton. — 4th ed.
p. cm.
ISBN 0-7216-4041-9
1. Pathology—Examinations, questions, etc. I. Title.
[DNLM: 1. Pathology—examination questions. QZ 18 C738p 1995]
RB119.C65 1995
616.07'076—dc20
DNLM/DLC 94–44208

International Edition ISBN 0–7216–6282–X
PATHOLOGIC BASIS OF DISEASE: Self-Assessment and Review ISBN 0–7216–4041–9



Printed in the United States of America.

Last digit is the print number: 9 8 7 6 5 4 3 2 1

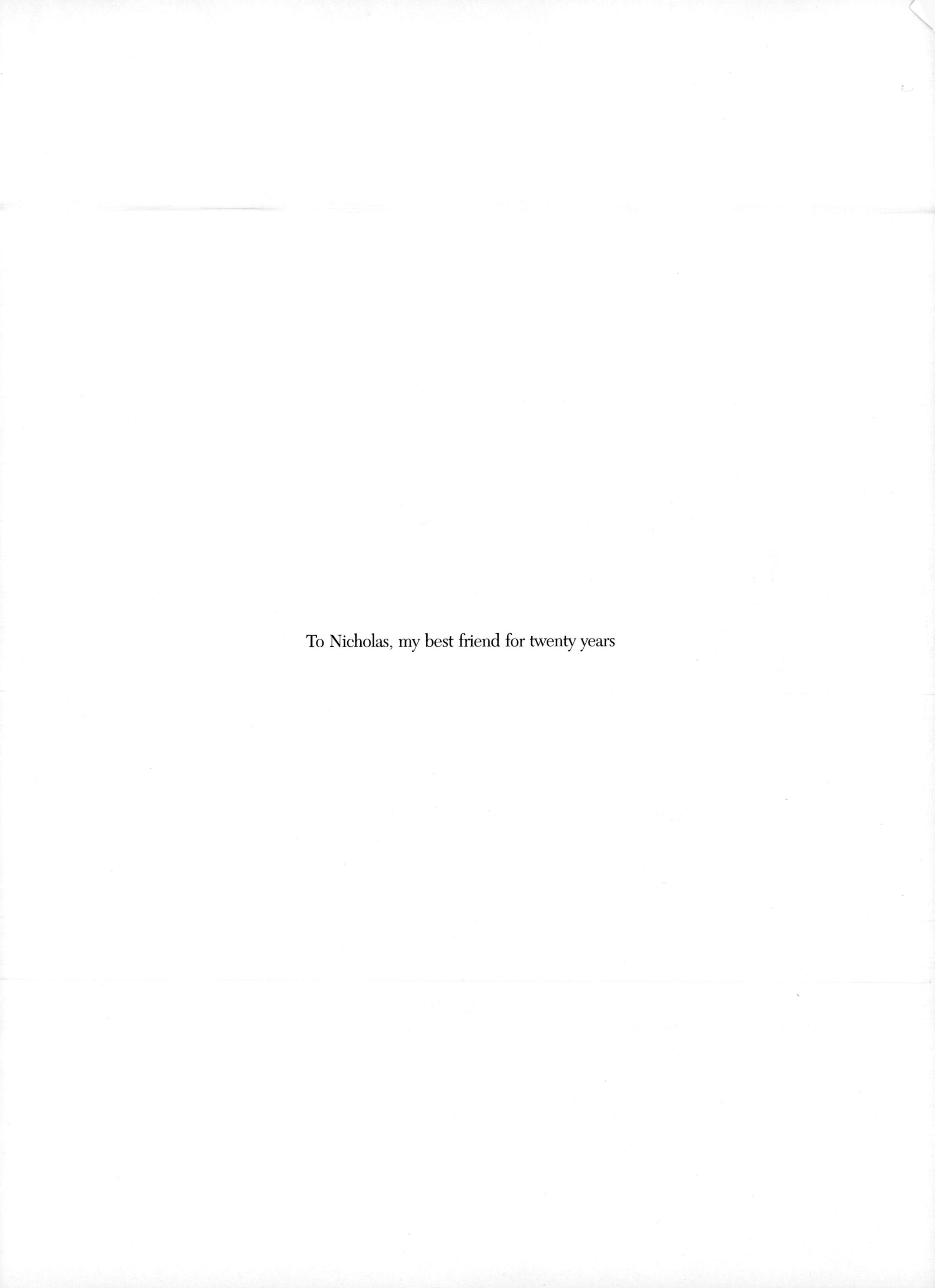

To Nicholas, my best friend for twenty years

# Preface

OK, here's the story, kids. This edition has been completely updated and almost entirely rewritten, but the biggest change from previous editions is that the dreaded K-type question has been banished. You know the one:

Medical school causes nervous breakdowns because:

1. Stratospheric tuition makes staggering student debt inevitable
2. The accompanying feelings of rampant incompetence and profuse inadequacy in the face of overwhelming numbers of facts to be learned and skills to be mastered could put a dent in even Bill Buckley's self-esteem
3. The reward for finishing is something even more stressful (internship)
4. It's hard to ignore the fact that business school is a lot shorter and leads to MUCH higher paying jobs

Answers:

A: 1, 2, and 3
B: 1 and 3
C: 2 and 4
D. 4 only
E. None of the above

So, you won't be tortured with these anymore. That's the good news.

As for the rest of the book, it is formulated on the traditional style of standardized examinations, which may help in preparation for quizzes, finals, or boards. The questions are not meant to be examples of actual test questions, however. The questions are meant to serve as tools for study and to stimulate critical thought about the topics covered. I hope you enjoy using it and learn some things in the process. I certainly had fun (and learned a lot) writing it. Don't be discouraged if you don't know ALL the answers. That's not really the point. Thinking about the information in a new way IS the point. If you actually know all the answers, you probably don't need this book anyway.

I have tried to cover major issues and important details (i.e., not trivia). The short explanations at the end of each chapter give concise answers to each question and expand on each answer choice. All information is based on the 5th Edition of *Robbins Pathological Basis of Disease.* The page numbers listed at the end of each answer refer to the places in the textbook to which you can refer for more information on the subjects discussed. You may want to consult the text for further study. Best wishes to you all and good luck on the boards.

# Acknowledgments

The author thanks

1. Nicholas and Dan, who provided both moral support and emergency computer consultations
2. Kath and Gret, who provided editorial support
3. Dr. Stanley Robbins and Dr. Ramzi Cotran, my much admired mentors
4. My students and residents, from whom I am always learning

Answer: All of the above.

# Contents

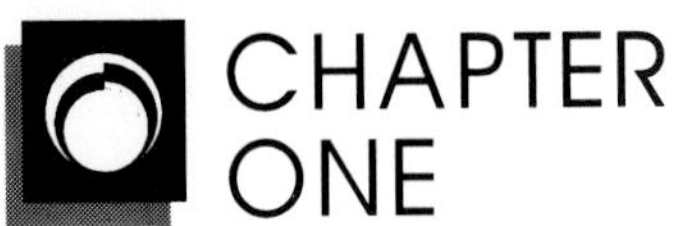

CHAPTER ONE

# General Pathology

**DIRECTIONS:** For Questions 1 through 45, choose the ONE BEST answer to each question.

**1.** Generalized edema results from all of the following disorders EXCEPT:

A. Systemic hypertension
B. Congestive heart failure
C. Cirrhosis
D. Nephrotic syndrome
E. Hyperaldosteronism

**2.** Disorders that predispose to thrombosis include all of the following EXCEPT:

A. Pancreatic carcinoma
B. Pregnancy
C. Vitamin K deficiency
D. Sickle cell anemia
E. Severe burns

**3.** Antithrombotic substances made by endothelial cells include all of the following EXCEPT:

A. Von Willebrand's factor
B. Nitric oxide
C. Prostacyclin (prostaglandin $I_2$)
D. Thrombomodulin
E. Tissue-type plasminogen activator

**4.** Markedly increased susceptibility to pyogenic infections occurs in all of the following conditions EXCEPT:

A. Deficiency of the third component of complement
B. Common variable immunodeficiency
C. Chronic granulomatous disease of childhood
D. DiGeorge's syndrome
E. Chédiak-Higashi syndrome

**5.** The feature most important in distinguishing a malignant from a benign tumor is:

A. Lack of encapsulation
B. High mitotic rate
C. Presence of necrosis
D. Presence of metastases
E. Nuclear pleomorphism (anaplasia)

**6.** In hypoxic cell injury, swelling of the cells occurs because:

A. Intracytoplasmic lipids accumulate
B. Intracytoplasmic proteins accumulate
C. Intracytoplasmic glycogen increases
D. Intracytoplasmic lipofuscin accumulates
E. Water enters the cell

**7.** Cell injury from chemically unstable molecules known as "free radicals" is a major consequence of each of the following pathologic processes EXCEPT:

A. Lead poisoning
B. Irradiation damage
C. Oxygen toxicity
D. Carbon tetrachloride poisoning
E. Bacterial infection

**8.** In an inflammatory response, neutrophils release molecules that produce all of the following effects EXCEPT:

A. Chemotaxis of monocytes
B. Chemotaxis of lymphocytes
C. Degranulation of mast cells
D. Increased vascular permeability independent of histamine release
E. Connective tissue digestion

**9.** In immunologic reactions, lymphocytes secrete factors (lymphokines) that are chemotactic for all of the following cells EXCEPT:

A. Neutrophils
B. Platelets
C. Eosinophils
D. Macrophages
E. Basophils

**10.** Mediators of increased vascular permeability in acute inflammatory responses include all of the following EXCEPT:

A. Leukotriene $E_4$
B. Complement complex C5b-9
C. Leukotriene $C_4$
D. Bradykinin
E. Platelet-activating factor

**11.** The most reliable histopathologic evidence of chronicity in an inflammatory process in the liver (hepatitis) is the presence of:

A. Lymphocytic infiltrates
B. Bile duct destruction
C. Councilman bodies
D. Fibrosis
E. Plasmacytic infiltrates

**12.** A large aggregate of epithelioid histiocytes is seen in a microscopic section of an ovary removed at surgery. Your diagnosis is:

A. Granulation tissue
B. Granuloma pyogenicum
C. Granulosa cell tumor
D. Granuloma
E. Granulocytosis

**13.** All of the following neoplasms are malignant EXCEPT:

A. Glomus tumor
B. Carcinoid tumor
C. Wilms' tumor
D. Seminoma
E. Acute disseminated Langerhans' cell histiocytosis

**14.** Hereditary conditions that are associated with a high risk of malignancy include all of the following EXCEPT:

A. Von Hippel-Lindau disease
B. Li-Fraumeni syndrome
C. DiGeorge's syndrome
D. Fanconi's anemia
E. Ataxia-telangiectasia

**15.** Cytokines secreted by tumors that induce angiogenesis and assist the tumor in establishing its blood supply include all of the following EXCEPT:

A. Tumor necrosis factor
B. Fibroblast growth factor
C. Transforming growth factor-$\alpha$
D. Transforming growth factor-$\beta$
E. Platelet-derived growth factor

**16.** The cell surface antigen detected by monoclonal antibodies and known as CD7 is a marker for:

A. T cells
B. B cells
C. Monocytes and granulocytes
D. Myeloid stem cells
E. Natural killer cells

**17.** Mast cell granules contain all of the following substances EXCEPT:

A. Leukotriene $D_4$
B. Prostaglandin $D_2$
C. Histamine-releasing factor
D. Platelet-activating factor
E. Interleukin-1

**18.** In myocardial ischemia, irreversibly injured myofibers are distinguishable by:

A. Cytoplasmic fatty change
B. Glycogen depletion of the cytoplasm
C. Cellular swelling
D. Clumping of nuclear chromatin
E. Contraction bands in the cytoplasm

**19.** Generation of free radicals is a major mechanism of membrane damage associated with all of the following processes EXCEPT:

A. Oxygen toxicity
B. Radiation injury
C. Carbon tetrachloride poisoning
D. Acute ischemia
E. Acute inflammation

**20.** All of the following factors delay wound healing EXCEPT:

A. Stasis in the venous system draining the wound
B. Systemic antibiotic administration
C. Increased systemic glucocorticoid levels
D. Thrombocytopenia
E. Systemic deficiency of vitamin C

**21.** Autoantibodies play a major role in the pathogenesis of all of the following disorders EXCEPT:

A. Graft-versus-host disease
B. Myasthenia gravis
C. Systemic lupus erythematosus
D. Atrophic gastritis associated with pernicious anemia
E. Type I (insulin-dependent) diabetes mellitus

**22.** Reactive systemic amyloidosis (secondary amyloidosis) is associated with all of the following diseases EXCEPT:

A. Ulcerative colitis
B. Rheumatoid arthritis
C. Multiple myeloma
D. Renal cell carcinoma
E. Chronic bronchitis

**23.** All of the following statements correctly describe amyloid EXCEPT:

A. It is digested by amylase.
B. It is stained on histologic sections by Congo red.
C. It is sometimes generated from $\beta_2$-microglobulin.
D. It is sometimes generated from transthyretin.
E. It is sometimes generated from atrial natriuretic factor.

**24.** Activation of Hageman factor (factor XII) leads to activation of all of the following catalytic systems EXCEPT:

A. The complement system
B. The (P-450) mixed-function oxidase system
C. The kinin system
D. The fibrinolytic system
E. The coagulation system

**25.** Red infarctions are produced by all of the following events EXCEPT:

A. Coronary artery thrombosis
B. Pulmonary embolism
C. Torsion of the testis
D. Superior mesenteric artery atheroembolism
E. Portal vein thrombosis

**26.** Shock is commonly associated with all of the following conditions EXCEPT:

A. *Escherichia coli* sepsis
B. Myocardial infarction
C. Cholera
D. Acute pancreatitis
E. Cerebral infarction

**27.** Ionizing radiation is causally linked to all of the following human malignancies EXCEPT:

A. Acute leukemia
B. Thyroid carcinoma
C. Hepatocellular carcinoma (hepatoma)
D. Lung cancer
E. Osteosarcoma

**28.** All of the following genes (known as "tumor suppressor genes") provide negative control over cell proliferation EXCEPT:

A. The *p53* gene
B. The *DCC* ("Deleted in Colon Cancer") gene
C. The *Rb* gene
D. The *WT-1* gene
E. The *bcl*-2 gene

**29.** Which of the following factors is assessed in the grading of a malignant tumor?

A. The number of lymph node metastases
B. The size (diameter) of the primary tumor
C. The extent of invasion of the primary tumor into surrounding structures
D. The degree of cytologic differentiation of the primary tumor
E. The presence or absence of liver metastases

**30.** All of the following complications of large burn injuries produce shock EXCEPT:

A. Disseminated intravascular coagulation from massive tissue destruction
B. Endotoxemia from *Pseudomonas* sepsis
C. Fluid losses from the wound surface
D. Pulmonary embolism from prolonged immobilization
E. Anaphylaxis from smoke inhalation

**31.** All of the following statements correctly describe oncogenes EXCEPT:

A. Oncogenes are derived from viral DNA that has been incorporated into the genome.
B. Oncogenes encode proteins that resemble the products of normal genes.
C. Some oncogene products are growth factors.
D. Some oncogene products are growth factor receptors.
E. Some oncogene products activate nuclear transcription.

**32.** An immunoperoxidase stain of an anaplastic tumor demonstrates the presence of desmin in the tumor cell cytoplasm. This finding is compatible with a diagnosis of:

A. Malignant schwannoma
B. Squamous cell carcinoma
C. Rhabdosarcoma
D. Lymphoma
E. Mesothelioma

**33.** Cellular proteins that are important to a carcinoma's ability to invade the surrounding extracellular matrix include all of the following EXCEPT:

A. CD44 adhesion molecule
B. Laminin receptor
C. Fibronectin receptor
D. Type IV collagenase
E. Cathepsin D

**34.** Pathologic forms of hyperplasia that are associated with an increased risk of malignancy in the tissue of origin include all of the following EXCEPT:

A. Atypical hyperplasia of the endometrium
B. Atypical lobular hyperplasia of the breast
C. Hyperplasia of the gastric pits (Ménétrier's disease)
D. Nodular hyperplasia of the prostate
E. Myelodysplasia (myelodysplastic syndrome) of the bone marrow

**35.** A sequence of metaplasia-dysplasia-neoplasia typically occurs in the oncogenesis of all of the following cancers EXCEPT:

A. Squamous cell carcinoma of the bladder
B. Carcinoid tumor of the small bowel
C. Squamous cell carcinoma of the lung
D. Adenocarcinoma of the esophagus
E. Squamous cell carcinoma of the endocervix

**36.** All of the following types of molecules function in the control of cell growth EXCEPT:

A. Cyclins
B. *Ras* proteins
C. G proteins
D. Mitogen-activated protein kinases
E. Selectins

**37.** All of the following factors promote neutrophil emigration into tissues during acute inflammatory responses EXCEPT:

A. Leukotriene $B_4$
B. Nitric oxide
C. Intercellular adhesion molecule-1
D. Complement fragment C5a
E. Platelet-activating factor

**38.** All of the following statements correctly describe transforming growth factor-β EXCEPT:

A. It promotes monocyte migration.
B. It promotes fibroblast migration.
C. It promotes fibroblast proliferation.
D. It promotes collagen synthesis by fibroblasts.
E. It promotes collagen breakdown (turnover) by fibroblasts.

**39.** Factors that are important in protecting normal cells from potential injury from free radicals generated in the course of an inflammatory response include all of the following EXCEPT:

A. Glutathione peroxidase
B. Ceruloplasmin
C. Catalase
D. $\alpha_2$-Macroglobulin
E. Transferrin

**40.** Pathologic lesions produced by vascular congestion include all of the following EXCEPT:

A. Nutmeg liver
B. Brown induration of the lung
C. Gandy-Gamna bodies of the spleen
D. Strawberry gallbladder
E. Stasis dermatitis of the legs

**41.** In which of the following conditions does amyloid of the AA type (having fibrils composed of amyloid-associated [AA] protein) occur?

A. Type II diabetes mellitus
B. Alzheimer's disease
C. Medullary carcinoma of the thyroid
D. Chronic renal failure
E. Ulcerative colitis

**42.** A tumor that tends to spread over the surfaces of viscera or body cavities rather than metastasizing via blood vessels or lymphatics is:

A. Colon carcinoma
B. Gastric carcinoma
C. Mesothelioma
D. Renal cell carcinoma
E. Hepatocellular carcinoma (hepatoma)

**43.** The greatest number of cancer deaths in females in the United States is caused by:

A. Pancreatic cancer
B. Colon cancer
C. Ovarian cancer
D. Breast cancer
E. Lung cancer

**44.** The tumor that occurs with the highest incidence in males in the United States is:

A. Pancreatic cancer
B. Colon cancer
C. Prostate cancer
D. Esophageal cancer
E. Lung cancer

**45.** All of the following viruses are capable of producing malignancies in human beings EXCEPT:

A. Human papillomavirus
B. Cytomegalovirus
C. Epstein-Barr virus
D. Hepatitis B virus
E. Hepatitis C virus

**DIRECTIONS:** For Questions 46 through 71, you are to decide whether EACH choice is TRUE or FALSE.

For each of the following statements about histocompatibility antigens (also known as HLAs or human leukocyte antigens), decide whether it is TRUE or FALSE.

**46.** Histocompatibility (HLA) molecules bind fragments of foreign proteins for presentation to antigen-specific T cells.
**47.** Class II HLAs (HLA-D) are found on the cell surface of all normal nucleated cells.
**48.** Class I HLAs (HLA-A, HLA-B, HLA-C) interact only with CD4+ T cells.
**49.** The chance that two siblings will be HLA identical is 50%.
**50.** The genes that encode the components of the complement system are located within the HLA gene complex.
**51.** Recognition of a virally infected cell by a T lymphocyte is dependent on the presence of HLA-D on the infected cells.
**52.** Individuals who possess the HLA-B27 haplotype are nearly 100 times more likely to get ankylosing spondylitis than those who lack HLA-B27.

For each of the following statements about tissue atrophy, decide whether it is TRUE or FALSE.

**53.** Atrophic cells contain fewer than normal numbers of cytoplasmic organelles (mitochondria, endoplasmic reticulum, etc.).
**54.** Atrophy occurs in otherwise normal tissues if their workload is decreased.
**55.** Atrophy occurs in otherwise normal tissues if the blood supply is decreased.
**56.** The appearance of autophagic vacuoles in cells undergoing atrophy signals irreversible cell injury and impending cell death.
**57.** Atrophy begins to occur in most tissues immediately after death of the individual.

For each of the following statements about the acquired immunodeficiency syndrome (AIDS), decide whether it is TRUE or FALSE.

**58.** AIDS is caused by a double-stranded DNA virus.
**59.** The CD4 molecule on T cells is a high-affinity receptor for the AIDS virus.
**60.** The AIDS virus is capable of producing neoplastic transformation of infected cells.
**61.** Monocytes in the peripheral blood constitute a major reservoir of the virus in infected individuals.
**62.** Humoral (B-cell) immune responses to new antigens are unimpaired in AIDS patients.
**63.** Lymphomas of B cells are more common than T-cell lymphomas in AIDS patients.
**64.** Hemophiliacs are at high risk of developing AIDS.

For each of the following statements about general tumor biology, decide whether it is TRUE or FALSE.

**65.** Most tumors are clones derived from a single transformed cell.
**66.** Most benign tumors resemble normal tissues, both morphologically and functionally.
**67.** Malignant tumors typically grow more rapidly than benign tumors.
**68.** Only malignant tumors are capable of metastasizing.
**69.** Malignant tumors typically penetrate and destroy surrounding normal tissues.
**70.** Initial dissemination of metastases from carcinomas usually occurs via hematogenous routes.
**71.** Enlargement of lymph nodes in the region around a tumor reliably indicates the presence of metastatic disease.

**DIRECTIONS:** For Questions 72 through 77, the set of lettered headings is followed by a list of numbered words or phrases. For each numbered word or phrase choose:

A—if the item is associated with (A) only
B—if the item is associated with (B) only
C—if the item is associated with *both* (A) and (B)
D—if the item is associated with *neither* (A) nor (B)

For each process or lesion listed below, choose whether it is characterized primarily by an inflammatory response, an immunologic response, both, or neither.

A. Inflammatory response
B. Immunologic response
C. Both
D. Neither

**72.** Suture granuloma
**73.** Marantic endocarditis
**74.** Streptococcal pneumonia
**75.** Sunburn
**76.** Hashimoto's thyroiditis
**77.** Lead poisoning

**DIRECTIONS:** Questions 78 to 115 are matching questions. For each numbered item, choose the most likely associated lettered item from those provided. Each numbered item has ONLY ONE answer. Within each group, each lettered item may be the answer to one, more than one, or none of the numbered items

For each of the biologic properties of mast cell mediators of type I (anaphylactic type) hypersensitivity reactions listed below, decide whether it is produced by leukotriene $C_4$, histamine, prostaglandin $D_2$, all of these, or none of these.

A. Leukotriene $C_4$
B. Histamine
C. Prostaglandin $D_2$
D. All of these
E. None of these

**78.** Is stored in granules in mast cell cytoplasm
**79.** Causes smooth muscle spasm
**80.** Attracts eosinophils
**81.** Increases vascular permeability
**82.** Causes platelet aggregation
**83.** Attracts neutrophils

For each of the autoantibodies listed below, choose the autoimmune disease with which it is linked most strongly.

A. Grave's disease
B. Sjögren's syndrome
C. Systemic lupus erythematosus
D. Systemic sclerosis (scleroderma)
E. Primary biliary cirrhosis
F. Goodpasture's syndrome
G. Myasthenia gravis
H. Atrophic fundal gastritis associated with pernicious anemia

**84.** Anti-double-stranded DNA
**85.** Scl-70 (anti-DNA topoisomerase I)
**86.** Anti-basement membrane
**87.** SS-B (La) (antiribonucleoprotein)
**88.** Anticentromere (anticentromeric proteins)
**89.** Anti-intrinsic factor
**90.** Anti-mitochondria
**91.** Anti-histone
**92.** Anti-acetylcholine receptor
**93.** Anti-thyroid-stimulating hormone receptor

For each of the biologic properties described below, decide whether it is characteristic of epidermal cells, fibroblasts, both, or neither.

A. Epidermal cells (keratinocytes)
B. Fibroblasts
C. Both
D. Neither

**94.** Under physiologic conditions, they undergo continuous proliferation throughout life
**95.** They respond so rapidly to surgical skin incisions that migration across the wound is complete within 24 to 48 hours
**96.** They produce type IV collagen
**97.** They produce type II collagen
**98.** They synthesize fibronectin
**99.** They are induced to migrate by fibronectin
**100.** They are induced to divide by transforming growth factor-β
**101.** They are induced to divide by transforming growth factor-α
**102.** They are induced to divide by platelet-derived growth factor
**103.** They are induced to divide by interleukin-1

For each of the conditions listed below, decide whether it is causally related to cigarette smoking, alcohol abuse, both, or neither.

A. Cigarette smoking
B. Alcohol abuse
C. Both
D. Neither

**104.** Esophageal carcinoma
**105.** Acute esophagitis
**106.** Pancreatic carcinoma
**107.** Acute pancreatitis
**108.** Gastric carcinoma
**109.** Acute gastritis
**110.** Renal cell carcinoma
**111.** Bladder carcinoma
**112.** Pharyngeal carcinoma
**113.** Hodgkin's disease
**114.** Breast carcinoma
**115.** Ovarian carcinoma

**DIRECTIONS:** Questions 116 through 282 are matching questions. For each numbered item, choose the most likely associated lettered item from those provided. Each numbered item has ONLY ONE answer. Within each group, each lettered item may be the answer to one, more than one, or none of the numbered items.

For each of the causes of fatty liver listed below, decide whether it increases free fatty acid entry into liver cells, decreases fatty acid oxidation, increases triglyceride formation, decreases apoprotein synthesis, or does all of these.

A. Increases free fatty acid entry into liver cells
B. Decreases fatty acid oxidation
C. Increases triglyceride formation
D. Decreases apoprotein synthesis
E. All of these

**116.** Alcohol ingestion
**117.** Protein malnutrition
**118.** Carbon tetrachloride poisoning
**119.** Corticosteroid therapy
**120.** Starvation

For each of the descriptions of intracellular pigment accumulation listed below, decide whether it refers to lipofuscin, melanin, hemosiderin, or none of these.

A. Lipofuscin
B. Melanin
C. Hemosiderin
D. None of these

**121.** Accumulates in the cartilage of patients with ochronosis
**122.** Accumulates in the lungs of patients with mitral stenosis
**123.** Accumulates in the lungs of coal miners
**124.** Accumulates in the synovium of patients with pigmented villonodular synovitis
**125.** Accumulates in the colonic mucosa of some laxative abusers

For each of the cellular responses listed below, decide whether it describes a typical example of hypertrophy, hyperplasia, metaplasia, dysplasia, or none of these.

A. Hypertrophy
B. Hyperplasia
C. Metaplasia
D. Dysplasia
E. None of these

**126.** The response of cardiac muscle to systemic hypertension
**127.** The response of bronchiolar epithelium in chronic bronchitis
**128.** The response of adrenocortical cells to a pituitary adenoma producing adrenocorticotrophic hormone
**129.** The response of prostatic stroma in benign prostatic hypertrophy
**130.** The response of colonic epithelium in long-standing ulcerative colitis

For each of the statements about autoimmune disease listed below, decide whether it describes systemic lupus erythematosus, Sjögren's syndrome, systemic sclerosis (scleroderma), all of these, or none of these.

A. Systemic lupus erythematosus
B. Sjögren's syndrome
C. Systemic sclerosis (scleroderma)
D. All of these
E. None of these

**131.** It occurs with increased incidence in those with hereditary deficiency of the second component of complement.
**132.** It is associated with a 40-fold increased risk of lymphoid malignancy.
**133.** It is associated with dermatomyositis.
**134.** It is associated with an increased risk of epithelial malignancy (carcinoma).
**135.** It typically produces arthritis.
**136.** Anti-centromere antibodies are characteristically produced.
**137.** Glomerular lesions are extremely rare.
**138.** Renal failure is the most common cause of death.
**139.** Immunoglobulin deposition is found in normal-appearing skin.
**140.** Response to corticosteroids is excellent.

For each of the characteristics of immunodeficiency disease listed below, decide whether it describes X-linked agammaglobulinemia of Bruton, common variable immunodeficiency, DiGeorge's syndrome, or none of these.

A. X-linked agammaglobulinemia of Bruton
B. Common variable immunodeficiency
C. DiGeorge's syndrome
D. None of these

**141.** Is characterized by a failure of pre-B cells to mature into B cells
**142.** Is caused by a defect in lymphoid stem cells
**143.** Is associated with tetany
**144.** Is associated with a high incidence of systemic lupus erythematosus
**145.** Often is associated with deletions of the C4A (complement) gene
**146.** Is associated with an increased incidence of lymphoid malignancy
**147.** Is *not* associated with persistent *Giardia lamblia* infection and malabsorption

For each of the conditions listed below, decide whether the major pathogenetic mechanism of the associated tissue edema and/or ascites is related to:

A. Decreased plasma oncotic pressure
B. Increased hydrostatic pressure
C. Increased endothelial permeability
D. Lymphatic obstruction
E. None of these

**148.** Nephrotic syndrome
**149.** Congestive heart failure
**150.** Cirrhosis
**151.** Thermal burn
**152.** Kwashiorkor
**153.** Bee sting
**154.** Pregnancy
**155.** Excessive salt intake
**156.** Hydrops fetalis
**157.** Constrictive pericarditis
**158.** Metastatic carcinoma
**159.** Ménétrier's disease

For each of the conditions listed below, decide whether it most commonly produces coagulation necrosis, liquefaction necrosis, enzymatic fat necrosis, caseous necrosis, or none of these.

A. Coagulation necrosis
B. Liquefaction necrosis
C. Enzymatic fat necrosis
D. Caseous necrosis
E. None of these

**160.** Cholera
**161.** Myocardial infarction
**162.** Pott's disease
**163.** Tuberculoid leprosy of skin
**164.** Acute pancreatitis
**165.** Wet gangrene of the great toe
**166.** Giardiasis (small bowel)
**167.** Cerebral infarction
**168.** Acute tubular necrosis (kidney)

For each of the conditions listed below, decide whether it is an example of an immunologically mediated disorder of the anaphylactic type (type I), cytotoxic type (type II), immune complex type (type III), cell-mediated type (type IV), or whether it is not an immunologically mediated disorder at all.

A. Type I, anaphylactic-type immune response
B. Type II, cytotoxic-type immune response
C. Type III, immune complex disorder
D. Type IV, cell-mediated hypersensitivity response
E. Not an immunologically mediated disorder

**169.** Erythroblastosis fetalis
**170.** Poison ivy dermatitis
**171.** Hay fever
**172.** Polyarteritis nodosa
**173.** Acute poststreptococcal glomerulonephritis
**174.** Graft-versus-host disease
**175.** Dopamine-induced hemolytic anemia
**176.** Penicillin-induced urticaria
**177.** Cyclosporine-induced renal injury
**178.** Chlorpromazine-induced cholestatic jaundice
**179.** Pulmonary asbestosis
**180.** Chronic berylliosis

For each of the biologic characteristics listed below, decide whether it describes T cells, B cells, macrophages/monocytes, all of these cell types, or none of these.

A. T cells
B. B cells
C. Macrophages/monocytes
D. All of these
E. None of these

**181.** Are found in the circulating blood
**182.** Are found in the cortex of lymph nodes
**183.** Display immunoglobulin G on their cell surface
**184.** Do not usually display class II histocompatibility antigens (HLA-D) on their cell surface
**185.** Do not have cell surface receptors for complement
**186.** Are able to lyse antibody-coated target cells by means of a nonphagocytic mechanism
**187.** Function in the negative regulation (turning off) of the immune response
**188.** Are capable of lysing tumor cells without previous sensitization
**189.** Initiate delayed-type cell-mediated (type IV) hypersensitivity responses
**190.** Produce leukotriene mediators of anaphylaxis
**191.** Respond chemotactically to leukotriene $B_4$
**192.** Arise from stem cells in the bone marrow

For each of the situations listed below, decide whether bilirubin, hemosiderin, ceroid, lipofuscin, or none of these pigmentations would be expected to be seen.

A. Bilirubin
B. Hemosiderin
C. Ceroid
D. Lipofuscin
E. None of these

**193.** Myocytes in an elderly, malnourished individual
**194.** Hepatocytes in an elderly, malnourished individual
**195.** Kupffer's cells in a patient recovering from hepatitis
**196.** Sinus histiocytes in the peribronchial lymph nodes of a smoker
**197.** Skin keratinocytes in Addison's disease
**198.** Kupffer's cells in an individual with hereditary spherocytosis
**199.** Kupffer's cells in bile duct obstruction
**200.** Splenic phagocytes in malaria
**201.** Splenic phagocytes after a hemolytic transfusion reaction
**202.** Dermal macrophages of tatooed skin

For each of the conditions listed below, decide whether the associated inflammatory cell infiltrate is composed predominantly of neutrophils, monocytes/macrophages, eosinophils, plasma cells, or lymphocytes.

A. Neutrophils
B. Monocytes/macrophages
C. Eosinophils
D. Plasma cells
E. Lymphocytes

**203.** Acute myocardial infarction (2 to 3 days in age)
**204.** Acute hepatitis B
**205.** Sarcoidosis
**206.** Primary tuberculosis
**207.** Polyarteritis nodosa
**208.** Reflux esophagitis
**209.** Primary syphilis
**210.** Löffler's syndrome
**211.** Filariasis
**212.** Bronchial asthma

For each of the biologic effects listed below, decide whether it is produced by one of the following cytokines, all of them, or none of them:

A. Interleukin-1
B. Interleukin-2
C. Tumor necrosis factor-α
D. γ-Interferon
E. All of the above
F. None of the above

**213.** Made by virtually any cell
**214.** Activate(s) macrophages
**215.** Made only by activated T cells
**216.** Stimulate(s) natural killer cell growth
**217.** Induce(s) expression of human leukocyte antigen class II molecules in many cells
**218.** Directly kill(s) bacteria
**219.** Stimulate(s) hematopoiesis
**220.** Prevent(s) viral replication

For each of the properties listed below, decide whether it is characteristic of CD4+ helper T cells, natural killer cells, CD8+ cytotoxic T cells, all of these, or none of these.

A. CD4+ helper T cells
B. Natural killer cells
C. CD8+ cytotoxic T cells
D. All of these
E. None of these

**221.** Lack the ability to destroy tumor cells
**222.** Are not phagocytic
**223.** Contain granules in their cytoplasm
**224.** Are capable of lysing only antibody-coated cells
**225.** Possess cell surface receptors for the Fc fragment of immunoglobulin G
**226.** Recognize antigens only in association with class I human leukocyte antigens
**227.** Recognize antigens only in association with class II human leukocyte antigens

For each of the conditions listed below, decide whether it is characterized by inflammation of the serous, fibrinous, suppurative, granulomatous, or mononuclear cell (predominantly lymphocytic and monocytic) type.

A. Serous inflammation
B. Fibrinous inflammation
C. Suppurative inflammation
D. Granulomatous inflammation
E. Mononuclear cell (predominantly lymphocytic and monocytic) inflammation

**228.** Cat scratch disease
**229.** Acute viral pneumonia
**230.** Acute appendicitis
**231.** Rheumatic pericarditis
**232.** Schistosomiasis
**233.** Adult hyaline membrane disease
**234.** Second-degree thermal burns
**235.** Friction blisters
**236.** Acute viral hepatitis
**237.** Acute ascending cholangitis
**238.** Initial stage of primary biliary cirrhosis
**239.** Uremic pericarditis

For each of the cellular events listed below, which occur in acute inflammatory reactions to bacterial infection, decide whether it is mediated by interleukin-1, intercellular adhesion molecule-1, complement fragment C5a, complement fragment C3b, protein kinase C, nicotinamide-adenine dinucleotide phosphate oxidase, or none of these molecules.

A. Interleukin-1
B. Intercellular adhesion molecule-1
C. Complement fragment C5a
D. Complement fragment C3b
E. Protein kinase C
F. Nicotinamide-adenine dinucleotide phosphate oxidase
G. None of these

**240.** Induction of endothelial cell expression of adhesion molecules for neutrophils
**241.** Increasing the binding avidity of neutrophil receptors for endothelial adhesion molecules
**242.** Attachment of neutrophils to endothelium (via binding to leukocyte surface integrins)
**243.** Chemotactic attraction of neutrophils
**244.** Opsonization of bacteria for phagocytosis
**245.** Killing of bacteria
**246.** Production of arachidonic acid metabolites from phospholipids

For each of the tumor types listed below, decide which (if any) of the following substances typically would likely be found in the tumor cells by immunohistochemical stains, helping to identify the tumor.

A. α-Fetoprotein
B. Carcinoembryonic antigen
C. Desmin
D. Human chorionic gonadotropin
E. None of these

**247.** Lymphoma
**248.** Neuroblastoma
**249.** Hepatoma
**250.** Colonic carcinoma
**251.** Choriocarcinoma
**252.** Medullary carcinoma of the thyroid
**253.** Rhabdosarcoma

For each of the neoplasms listed below, decide if Epstein-Barr virus, human papillomavirus, herpes simplex type 1, hepatitis B virus, or none of these viruses is thought to be causally related to at least some tumors of that type.

A. Epstein-Barr virus
B. Human papillomavirus
C. Herpes simplex type 1
D. Hepatitis B virus
E. None of these

**254.** Cervical carcinoma
**255.** Breast carcinoma
**256.** Nasopharyngeal carcinoma
**257.** Burkitt's lymphoma
**258.** Cutaneous squamous cell carcinoma
**259.** Fibrosarcoma
**260.** Adult T-cell lymphoma/leukemia
**261.** Cholangiocarcinoma
**262.** Hepatoma
**263.** Angiosarcoma of the liver

For each of the paraneoplastic syndromes listed below, decide whether it is strongly associated with bronchogenic carcinoma, pancreatic carcinoma, renal cell carcinoma, prostatic carcinoma, or none of these tumor types.

A. Bronchogenic carcinoma
B. Pancreatic carcinoma
C. Renal cell carcinoma
D. Prostatic carcinoma
E. None of these

**264.** Malignant form of acanthosis nigricans
**265.** Hypercalcemia
**266.** Cancer-associated dermatomyositis
**267.** Hypertrophic osteoarthropathy
**268.** Hyponatremia
**269.** Polycythemia
**270.** Nephrotic syndrome
**271.** Anemia (nonmyelophthisic)
**272.** Malignancy-associated myasthenia gravis
**273.** Peripheral neuropathy

For each of the descriptions of molecular complexes found on the surfaces of cells of the immune system listed below, decide whether it characterizes CD3, CD4, CD8, all of these, or none of these.

A. CD3
B. CD4
C. CD8
D. All of these
E. None of these

**274.** Serves as a receptor for class I histocompatibility molecules
**275.** Serves as a receptor for class II histocompatibility molecules
**276.** Serves as a receptor for interleukin-2
**277.** Serves as a receptor for complement
**278.** Serves as a receptor for the Fc portion of immunoglobulin G
**279.** Is part of the class I histocompatibility molecular complex
**280.** Is part of the class II histocompatibility molecular complex
**281.** Is part of the T-cell antigen receptor complex
**282.** Is part of the B-cell antigen receptor

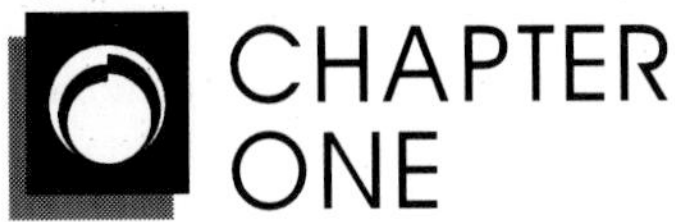

# General Pathology

## ANSWERS

**1. (A)** Generalized noninflammatory edema is produced when the factors that determine body fluid compartmentalization are altered to favor the entry of fluid into the extravascular compartment. Common causes of such imbalances include increases in intravascular hydrostatic pressure (e.g., in congestive heart failure or in cirrhosis with portal hypertension) and reduced plasma oncotic pressure, resulting either from inadequate synthesis (e.g., in cirrhosis) or increased loss of albumin (e.g., with the nephrotic syndrome). Increased osmotic pressure in the interstitial fluid related to sodium retention, such as occurs in the presence of increased aldosterone, is another primary cause of generalized edema.

Generalized edema occurs only in the presence of increased hydrostatic pressure in the venous or lymphatic systems, the sites of resorption of extravascular interstitial fluid. Systemic hypertension in the arterial system does not result in edema. *(pp. 93–95)*

**2. (C)** A number of clinical situations are associated with an increased incidence of thrombosis and are known as hypercoagulable states. Some hypercoagulable states are due to primary genetic defects in anticoagulant factors (e.g., deficiencies of antithrombin III, protein C, protein S, or fibrinolytic proteins), and the pathogenesis is a straightforward reflection of the deficiency of the antithrombotic agent. However, most hypercoagulable states are acquired, secondary processes that occur in association with a wide variety of clinical conditions, and, overall, the specific mechanisms involved in their pathogenesis are less well understood.

In general, cancers (especially adenocarcinomas) greatly increase the risk of secondary hypercoagulable states. For example, about 10% of patients with pancreatic carcinoma develop migratory thrombophlebitis, a condition known as Trousseau's syndrome. The thrombotic tendency is believed to be related to the release of platelet aggregating factors and procoagulants from the tumor cells.

Pregnancy, especially the late pregnancy and early postpartum periods, also increases the risk of thrombosis, but the relative risk is lower compared to that associated with cancer. The pathogenesis of the hypercoagulable state in pregnancy is poorly understood but may be related to the influence of the altered hormonal environment on production of coagulation factors or to vascular stasis secondary to venous compression by the distended uterus. In the postpartum period, thrombogenic substances released from the placenta at delivery may be important.

In sickle cell anemia, intravascular stasis underlies the predisposition to thrombosis for which this condition is notorious (see Chapter 7, Question 13).

Severe tissue injury, such as that incurred in severe burns or trauma, causes release of "tissue factor" (a cellular lipoprotein released from damaged tissues or expressed on the surface of activated monocytes, endothelial cells, and other cells that converts coagulation factor VII to VIIa during the first step of the "extrinsic" coagulation pathway) and predisposes to thrombosis. Other factors contributing to hypercoagulability in burns and trauma include direct endothelial injury and immobilization with vascular stasis.

Vitamin K deficiency, in contrast, predisposes to bleeding rather than to thrombosis. Vitamin K is essential to the biosynthesis of prothrombin and coagulation factors VII, IX, and X. Thus, vitamin K deficiency results in depletion of these factors, the consequence of which is a coagulopathy and bleeding diathesis (see Chapter 3, Question 14). *(pp. 103–106; 907)*

**3. (A)** Endothelial cells are largely responsible for maintaining the normal intravascular antithrombotic environment. They elaborate a number of substances that act via both independent and interrelated mechanisms to inhibit thrombosis under homeostatic conditions. Antithrombotic substances produced by endothelial cells include nitric oxide (NO), prostacyclin (prostaglandin $I_2$: $PGI_2$), thrombomodulin, and tissue-type plasminogen activator (t-PA).

The antithrombotic activity of NO and $PGI_2$ are due to their antiplatelet effects. They are both powerful inhibitors of platelet aggregation. The antithrombotic activity of thrombomodulin is due to its (indirect) anticoagulant effects. Thrombomodulin coverts thrombin from a procoagulant to an anticoagulant. When complexed with thrombomodulin, thrombin activates protein C (a potent anticoagulant), which, in turn, cleaves coagulation factors Va and VIIIa. In contrast to the aforementioned, the antithrombotic activity of t-PA is due to fibrinolysis. It promotes degradation and removal of fibrin deposits from the endothelial surface.

Von Willebrand's factor is indeed an endothelial product, but it is a prothrombotic agent. It stimulates both aggregation of platelets and platelet adhesion to endothelial surfaces. *(pp. 100–101)*

**4. (D)** The most important defense mechanisms against pyogenic infections are humoral immune responses (antibacterial antibody production) and inflammatory reactions with phagocytosis and killing of bacteria by neutrophils. Thus, disorders that affect either of these processes are associated with increased susceptibility to pyogenic infection.

The third component of complement (cleavage fragment C3b, in specific) plays a critical role as an opsonin in inflammatory responses to pyogenic bacteria, so C3 deficiencies increase susceptibility to infection by these organisms. Common variable immunodeficiency (CVI) represents a heterogeneous group of disorders that result in hypogammaglobulinemia (generally affecting all the antibody classes, but sometimes only immunoglobulin G). The defect in humoral immunity occurring in CVI results in increased susceptibility to pyogenic infection. Both chronic granulomatous disease of childhood and the Chédiak-Higashi syndrome are disorders of leukocyte function that predispose to pyogenic infection. In chronic granulomatous disease of childhood, $H_2O_2$ production by neutrophils is deficient, leading to a defect in the myeloperoxidase-$H_2O_2$ halide bactericidal system (see Question 245) and susceptibility to catalase-producing bacteria. In the Chédiak-Higashi syndrome, a number of defects in phagocyte function are present, including impaired chemotactic responses and deficient degranulation.

DiGeorge's syndrome is a disorder of the cellular immune system only. Inflammatory mechanisms and humoral immunity are unimpaired in patients with DiGeorge's syndrome. Thus, susceptibility to pyogenic infection is not increased. *(pp. 64; 216–218)*

**5. (D)** Although a number of pathologic features (such as high proliferation [mitotic] rate, cellular anaplasia with nuclear pleomorphism, lack of encapsulation, and the presence of necrosis and hemorrhage) are typically associated with malignant tumors, benign tumors may occasionally display one or more of these features as well. Therefore, the only feature that is absolutely diagnostic of malignancy is metastasis. Although so-called benign tumors are capable of producing considerable morbidity and even mortality through local compressive effects or secretion of systemically active substances such as hormones, benign tumors never metastasize. *(pp. 245–250)*

**6. (E)** Hypoxia is the most common cause of cell injury. It usually is caused by ischemia (decreased blood flow) to the tissue, but depletion of the oxygen-carrying capacity of the blood or toxic injury to intracellular oxidative enzymes also may cause hypoxic injury. One of the most common histologic hallmarks of hypoxic cell injury, especially in cells with a high rate of aerobic metabolism, is acute cellular swelling (cellular edema). Cellular swelling occurs with sodium influx into the cell (accompanied by influx of an iso-osmotic quantity of water). Sodium influx is a consequence of the loss of function of the membrane pumps that normally maintain low intracellular concentrations of sodium (compared with the extracellular fluid). These membrane-associated ion pumps require ATP as their energy source, and they cease to function as oxygen tension within the cell decreases, oxidative phosphorylation by mitochondria ceases, and glycogen (a temporary source of ATP generated from anaerobic glycolysis) is depleted. In short, the biochemical means to produce ATP are lost.

Although intracytoplasmic accumulations of abnormal amounts of lipid, protein, glycogen, or lipofuscin may occur in some forms of cell injury, they usually do not occur with hypoxia. Moreover, although accumulation of any of these substances may cause affected cells to increase in size, the process would not be known as "cellular swelling." This term applies exclusively to intracellular edema (see Questions 18 and 116). *(pp. 7; 25–28)*

**7. (A)** Free radicals are chemically unstable, highly reactive molecules that are generated in many types of chemical and toxic pathologic processes. They are capable of profound cellular injury, chiefly through their ability to damage unsaturated fatty acids in cell membranes. The generation of free radicals requires either a powerful outside energy source (e.g., ionizing radiation) or oxidation-reduction reactions that add single extra electrons to molecules capable of accepting them (such as oxygen). Molecules having an odd number of electrons are formed, and the unpaired electrons are free to participate in chemical bond formation (e.g., lipid peroxidation, which causes cell membrane damage). Alternatively, free radicals may donate their extra electrons to yet another molecule that, in turn, becomes a free radical.

In radiation damage, free radical formation usually is mediated through the radiolysis of water, leading to the formation of hydroxyl radicals, which are highly injurious to the cell. In oxygen toxicity, oxygen acts as an electron acceptor to form the highly reactive free radical superoxide. In carbon tetrachloride ($CCl_4$) poisoning, $CCl_4$ itself acts as the electron acceptor and becomes a free radical. In bacterial infection, reactive oxygen metabolites (superoxides) are elaborated within the lysosomes of neutrophils and macrophages following phagocytosis of bacterial organisms (see Question 245). Although free radicals are essential to the bactericidal function of phagocytes, they may cause damage to surrounding tissues when released from the cytoplasm of activated and/or dying neutrophils.

Unlike the above forms of injury, which are mediated by free radicals, lead poisoning is caused by direct toxic damage to cells. Lead binds to sulfhydryl groups on cell membranes, causing increased membrane permeability and inhibition of ATPase-dependent membrane transport. Furthermore, it binds to and denatures proteins, cleaves transfer ribonucleic acid (tRNA), and causes functional derangement of phosphokinase C (part of the second messenger system in brain cells). However, none of its many toxic activities is dependent on metabolic conversion or free radical formation. *(pp. 11–14; 391)*

**8. (B)** The "azurophilic granules" found in the cytoplasm of neutrophils are specialized lysosomes that contain myeloperoxidase, lysozyme, acid hydrolases, elastase, collagenase, defensins, phospholipase $A_2$, bacterial permeability–increasing protein, cathepsin G, and cationic proteins. The latter include a chemotactic factor for monocytes, factors that increases vascular permeability directly or by releasing histamine from mast cells, and factors that inhibit movement of other neutrophils and eosinophils. The neutral proteases of azurophilic granules are capable of connective tissue destruction via digestion of collagen, elastin, and cartilage. In addition, the "specific granules" of neutrophils contain type IV collagenase capable of digesting basement membranes.

Although activated lymphocytes release molecules (lymphokines) that are chemotactic for neutrophils, the reverse is not true. Neutrophils do not produce chemoattractants for lymphocytes. *(pp. 72–73; 174)*

**9. (B)** Besides the ability to initiate, carry out, and terminate immune responses, lymphocytes also are able to produce acute inflammatory responses through their ability to recruit a variety of inflammatory cell types. Activated T cells manufacture and release a variety of biologically active molecules called lymphokines (cytokines produced by lymphocytes). A number of lymphokines are chemotactic agents for neutrophils, eosinophils, monocytes/macrophages, and basophils as well as other lymphocytes.

Platelets do not respond with chemotactic movement to any known substance. Like the erythrocyte (the other blood-borne cell lacking a nucleus), the platelet appears incapable of directed cell movement toward a chemoattractant. However, platelets can be activated by molecules secreted by other cells, such as platelet-activating factor derived from basophils, neutrophils, endothelial cells, and macrophages. "Activation" of platelets causes them to aggregate and to release their active agents, such as histamine and serotonin, but it does not involve chemotaxis. *(pp. 65; 77; 102; 70; 174–175)*

**10. (B)** Increased permeability leading to tissue edema is one of the hallmarks of acute inflammation. Vascular leakiness is produced by a number of chemical mediators that act directly on blood vessels to increase permeability. Perhaps the best known among these mediators is histamine, an amine released from mast cells and platelets in response to various forms of tissue injury. Platelet-activating factor (PAF), a phospholipid-derived mediator elaborated by basophils, neutrophils, monocytes, and endothelial cells, causes platelet aggregation and release of histamine. In addition, PAF itself is a potent, direct mediator of vascular permeability. In extremely low concentrations, PAF induces vasodilation and increases vascular permeability with a potency of 100 to 10,000 times greater than that of histamine.

Bradykinin, a potent vasoactive peptide generated during activation of the kinin system following tissue injury, not only increases vascular permeability but causes contraction of smooth muscle, blood vessel dilation, and pain. Bradykinin is produced when coagulation factor XII (Hageman factor) is activated through contact with collagen, basement membrane material, cartilage, or endotoxin. Activated factor XII converts the blood-borne factor prekallikrein to kallikrein, which, in turn, enzymatically mediates the conversion of kininogen to bradykinin.

Leukotrienes are metabolic products of arachidonic acid, a 20-carbon polyunsaturated fatty acid that is derived either from the diet or from linoleic acid metabolism. They are produced by leukocytes via a metabolic pathway initiated by lipoxygenase that converts arachidonic acid to 5-HETE, the precursor of all leukotriene molecules. Leukotrienes $C_4$, $D_4$, and $E_4$ all cause intense vasoconstriction and bronchospasm and are at least 1000 times as potent as histamine in increasing venular permeability.

The complement system consists of 20 component plasma proteases (together with their cleavage products) that are activated in inflammatory and immune responses. The end result of complement activation is production of the C5b-9 complex ("membrane attack complex"), which produces membrane lysis (of a microbial agent, it is hoped, although parenchymal cells also may be injured) but has no permeability effect. During activation of the cascade, cleavage products are produced that have numerous biologic activities. Among those that produce increased vascular permeability are C3a and C5a, the latter being the more potent. *(pp. 66–70)*

**11. (D)** In general, tissue infiltration by mononuclear cells, principally lymphocytes, plasma cells, and macrophages, is considered one of the histologic hallmarks of chronic inflammation. However, in immunologically mediated forms of inflammation, such as acute viral hepatitis, inflammatory infiltrates consist primarily of mononuclear cells regardless of the stage of the disease and, therefore, are not reliable indicators of the chronicity of the process. Bile duct destruction and Councilman body formation (hepatocellular apoptosis) both can be seen in either acute or chronic phases of numerous inflammatory conditions of the liver. Bile duct proliferation or hepatocellular regeneration accompanied by ceroid (lipofuscin) deposition (a sign of previous hepatocellular destruction with uptake and metabolism of cell debris by phagocytic Kupffer's cells) would be indicative of an inflammatory process of longer duration.

Fibrosis is by far the most reliable indicator of chronicity in any inflammatory process, including that of the liver. Thus, a special stain for collagen often is performed routinely on liver biopsies to estimate the duration, degree of destruction, and amount of subsequent scarring (indicative of irreversible damage) produced by inflammatory processes in the liver. *(pp. 18; 75–76; 79–80; 850–852)*

**12. (D)** A granuloma is an aggregate of epithelioid histiocytes (macrophages). Granulomas may form either as a nonspecific inflammatory response to foreign bodies or as part of a type IV (cell-mediated or "delayed") hypersensitivity response initiated by specifically sensitized T lymphocytes. A variety of microorganisms, including mycobacteria as well as some bacteria, viruses, fungi, protozoa, and parasites, typically elicit immunologic responses of the delayed hypersensitivity type, the hallmark of which is granuloma formation. Unfortunately, there are a number of nongranulomatous lesions with "sound-alike" names that easily may be confused with "granuloma" but are neither pathogenetically nor histopathologically related to granulomas.

Granulation tissue is newly forming, immature connective tissue that represents the first step in scar formation occurring during wound repair. It consists of activated fibroblasts, collagen-poor extracellular matrix composed predominantly of proteoglycans, and proliferating capillaries. As more fibrillar collagen is deposited, granulation tissue matures into scar.

Granulation tissue-type proliferations of blood vessels developing as polypoid lesions following trauma to the skin or oral mucosa have, unfortunately, been given the highly misleading (and, strictly speaking, incorrect) name of "granuloma" pyogenicum. Such proliferations occurring in the mouths of pregnant women specifically are called "granuloma" gravidarum. However, neither of these lesions is a granuloma. They are both lesions composed of granulation tissue.

Granulosa cell tumors are ovarian stromal tumors derived from the granulosa cells of the ovarian follicle. Like the cells from which they arise, some of these tumors secrete estrogens.

Granulocytosis refers to increased numbers of circulating neutrophils, a hallmark of acute inflammatory conditions such as infection. *(pp. 80–82; 85–87; 506–507; 631; 1074)*

**13. (A)** Unfortunately for oncologists, surgeons, and pathologists alike, names of tumors do not always correspond to the rules of nomenclature that are meant to indicate whether the tumor is benign or malignant. For example, a tumor name composed of the word root for the tissue of origin plus the suffix "-oma" denotes a benign neoplasm of that tissue. Designations for malignant tumors are usually compound names: the tissue of origin plus "sarcoma" (if of connective tissue origin) or "carcinoma" (if of epithelial origin). However, according to accepted nomenclature, it is impossible to know from the names of certain tumors whether they are benign or malignant. In these cases the information simply must be memorized (unpleasant though this suggestion may be). *(pp. 242–244)*

Glomus tumors are completely benign neoplasms that arise from the modified smooth muscle cells of glomus bodies in arterioles with arteriovenous anastomoses. They usually occur in the distal portions of the fingers and toes, where glomus bodies are most commonly found. Simple surgical excision is completely curative (both for the tumor and for the considerable pain they produce). *(p. 507)*

Carcinoid tumors are malignant neoplasms of neuroendocrine cells that occur most commonly in the gastrointestinal tract and lung. They vary in their biologic aggressiveness, and it is impossible to predict their behavior from their histopathologic appearance (nearly all of them look "benign" in that they are extremely well differentiated). Although most carcinoid tumors exhibit slow growth, they are locally invasive and potentially are capable of metastasizing. *(pp. 726; 818)*

Wilms' tumor, a tumor that occurs predominantly in the pediatric age group, is a malignant neoplasm of renal origin. It is composed of a number of different cell types, all derived from the mesonephric mesoderm. Like Ewing's sarcoma, the vastly improved long-term survival now associated with these neoplasms represents a triumph of aggressive combined-modality oncologic therapy. When treated with chemotherapy, radiation, and surgery, long-term survival is achieved in 90% of cases. Even recurrences can be treated successfully. *(pp. 464–465)*

Although they vary in their biologic behavior, all germ cell tumors of the testis are malignant neoplasms. Seminoma, the most common testicular germ cell tumor, is composed of uniform, undifferentiated cells thought to be derived from primary germ cells. Seminomas are extremely radiosensitive and tend to remain localized for long periods of time. Thus they have the best prognosis among the testicular germ cell neoplasms. More than 90% of seminomas that are confined to the testis (stage I) or that have spread only to the lymph nodes below the diaphragm (stage II) can be cured. *(pp. 1016; 1021)*

Acute disseminated Langerhans' cell histiocytosis is a neoplastic proliferative disorder of Langerhans' cells or their bone marrow precursors. Also known as Letterer-Siwe disease, it usually occurs in infants and children and is a rapidly progressive, lethal disease unless treated with intensive chemotherapy. With treatment, 50% of patients survive 5 years. *(p. 726)*

**14. (C)** For many types of cancer, it is now well established that heredity plays a role, be it major or minor, in predisposing an individual to the development of malignancy. Some of the most striking and obvious associations between heredity and tumor risk are exemplified by genetic syndromes.

Von Hippel-Lindau (VHL) disease is a rare autosomal dominant disorder that is characterized by a strong predisposition to the development of a variety of benign and malignant tumors throughout the body. Among these, the most characteristic are retinal hemangioblastoma, hemangioblastoma of the cerebellum, and renal cell carcinoma. The disease is caused by mutation in a tumor suppressor gene (the VHL gene) located on chromosome 3 that encodes a protein involved in signal transduction or cell adhesion. *(pp. 268t; 986; 1354)*

The Li-Fraumeni syndrome is an inherited germline mutation of the *p53* tumor suppressor gene. The defect predisposes affected individuals to the development of a wide range of malignancies including breast cancer, sarcomas (e.g., "hereditary osteosarcomas"), and brain tumors. *(pp. 266; 1235)*

Fanconi's anemia is an autosomal recessive form of aplastic anemia. In addition to profound marrow hypofunction, affected individuals are at increased risk of developing leukemia or lymphoma. This disease is characterized by cellular sensitivity to DNA cross-linking agents, a defect which is presumed to be related to a deficiency of endonucleases that eliminate interstrand cross links. The result is a high level of chromosomal instability and breakage. *(pp. 153; 286; 614)*

Like Fanconi's anemia, ataxia-telangiectasia is a "chromosomal breakage syndrome." It is an autosomal recessive neurocutaneous disorder characterized by prominent vascular (capillary) dilations of the head and neck along with cerebellar ataxia and nystagmus. There is neuronal loss in the cerebellum, medulla, spinal cord, and spinal ganglia. The thymus is either absent or poorly developed, and both cellular and humoral immune deficiencies result. This disorder is also associated with defective repair of chromosomal damage induced by ionizing radiation and a greatly increased risk of developing lymphoid malignancies. *(pp. 153; 286; 1335)*

DiGeorge's syndrome is a congenital immunodeficiency disorder characterized by developmental failure of the third and fourth pharyngeal pouches, with absence or hypoplasia of the thyroid and a selective T-cell deficiency. It is neither genetically determined nor associated with an increased risk of malignancy. *(pp. 217–218)*

**15. (A)** In order to obtain the nutrients necessary to sustain continued growth, tumors must establish their own blood supply. The induction of a blood supply is accomplished via secretions of cytokines that promote endothelial cell migration and proliferation. Under the inductive influence of these cytokines, new vessels bud from the blood supply of the surrounding tissues and grow into the tumor, a process known as tumor angiogenesis. These newly formed collateral vessels also provide the tumor with direct access to the systemic circulation, a situation that is optimal for hematogenous metastatic spread.

Fibroblast growth factor, transforming growth factor-α, transforming growth factor-β, and platelet-derived growth factor are all cytokines that (despite the specific functional implications of their names) have angiogenic activity as well as other growth-inductive effects. The secretion of these cytokines by tumors induces the growth of endothelial sprouts from surrounding vessels and the vascularization of their stroma. Some of these cytokines interact in a synergistic fashion, resulting in brisk vascular proliferation. These cytokines also are produced by normal cells and are critical to repair functions (wound healing) requiring the regeneration of a blood supply within the injured tissue.

Tumor necrosis factor (TNF) is not an angiogenic cytokine, and it may or may not be secreted by tumors. It is a cytokine that is produced primarily by activated macrophages and mediates many of the systemic ("acute-phase") reactions and local tissue responses occurring with inflammation and repair. It is suspected that TNF production by tumor cells (or macrophages reacting to the tumor) may be responsible for cancer cachexia, the wasting syndrome characterized by progressive loss of body fat and muscle that occurs in cancer patients. *(pp. 70–71; 275; 295)*

**16. (A)** With the microscope alone, it is not possible to differentiate one kind of small lymphocyte from another. With the development of monoclonal antibodies to distinctive cell surface antigens and their use in immunohistochemistry, it has become possible to positively identify individual immune cells of any type and to further delineate functionally distinct subsets among cells of a given type. Tumors of these cell types can be similarly identified. These distinguishing antigens are cell surface glycoproteins, some of which have known receptor functions. The antigens recognized by well-defined monoclonal antibodies have been cataloged numerically by international convention and are now known by their CD ("cluster designation") number.

CD7, for example, is an antigen present on all T lymphocytes, both intrathymic and peripheral. Other markers for T cells include CD3 (associated with the T-cell antigen receptor) and CD5 (also expressed in a small subset of B cells). Functional T-cell subsets such as helper/inducer cells and cytotoxic/suppressor cells can be recognized by their expression of CD4 and CD8, respectively.

B cells can be recognized by their specific CD10, CD19, CD20, CD21, and CD22 antigens. Both monocytes and granulocytes express CD13, whereas CD14 is expressed only on monocytes, and CD15 only on granulocytes. Myeloid stem cells are identified by their expression of CD34. Natural killer cells express both CD16 and CD5, but both of these antigens also may be found on other cells. *(pp. 172–174; 637)*

**17. (C)** Mast cell degranulation is a key initial event in type I (hypersensitivity or anaphylactic type) immune reactions. It is mediated by binding of antigen to antigen-specific immunoglobulin E (IgE) molecules that have become affixed to mast cells. Cellular attachment of IgE occurs with binding of the Fc portion of the molecule to specific IgE receptors (FcRϵ) on the mast cell surface. This reaction occurs only in previously "sensitized" individuals. "Sensitization" connotes the occurrence of an earlier immune response to the antigen, one that has been mediated by $T_H2$ helper/inducer cells (the specific subset of CD4+ helper cells required for IgE-producing B-cell stimulation) and has resulted in IgE production.

Mast cell granules represent an arsenal of powerful agents that mediate the early events in a type I immune response, such as bronchoconstriction, edema, mucus secretion, flushing, and (in severe cases) hypotension. The specific contents (and their respective effects) of mast cell granules include: (1) histamine (bronchospasm, increased vascular permeability, cholinergic nerve stimulation, and stimulation of bronchial mucus secretion); (2) leukotriene $B_4$ (chemotaxis of eosinophils and neutrophils); (3) leukotrienes $C_4$, $D_4$, and $E_4$ (prolonged bronchospasm, increased vascular permeability, and stimulation of bronchial mucus secretion); (4) platelet-activating factor (platelet aggregation and degranulation); (5) cytokines such as interleukin-1, tumor necrosis factor, and interleukin-6 (stimulatory effects on endothelial cells, leukocytes, and fibroblasts); and (6) proteases (local tissue damage and disruption of tissue structure).

Histamine-releasing factor, which induces the release of histamine from basophils, is not a product of mast cells. It is made by a variety of inflammatory cell types that are recruited by mast cells during the acute phase of a type I immune response. Thus, histamine-releasing factor is one of the mediators of the "late-phase reaction" of a type I response in which intense inflammation and tissue injury occur (without additional exposure to the antigen) hours after the acute response has subsided. *(pp. 70–71; 177–182; 690–692)*

**18. (E)** The morphologic changes associated with nonlethal (reversible) ischemic injury to myocardial cells typically include cytoplasmic fatty change, cellular swelling, nuclear swelling, and glycogen depletion of the cytoplasm. Cellular swelling results when the generation of ATP from aerobic metabolism slows or ceases in the oxygen-starved cell. Without ATP, membrane sodium pumps cannot be maintained, intracellular sodium accumulates, and water is drawn into the cell osmotically, causing the cell to swell (see Question 6). Fatty change results from alterations of fatty acid metabolism in the injured cell that cause lipids to accumulate in the cytoplasm. With decreased aerobic metabolism, ATP is generated from anaerobic glycolysis of glycogen (until glycogen stores are depleted), which generates lactic acid. The drop in intracellular pH caused by the accumulation of lactic acid in the cell leads to clumping of nuclear chromatin.

In general, irreversible cell injury can be recognized only after the overt morphologic features of necrosis develop, usually hours after the biologic death of the tissue. The most common of these features are cytoplasmic eosinophilia (a result of depletion of basophilic ribonucleic protein in the cytoplasm) and nuclear shrinkage (pyknosis) or degradation (karyorrhexis or karyolysis). A microscopic feature unique to necrotic cardiac muscle cells is the presence of contraction bands (broad eosinophilic cross-striations caused by myofilament overlap) in the cytoplasm ("contraction band necrosis"). These occur as a result of calcium influx into the dying cell (having lost the function of its membrane ion pumps), stimulating hypercontraction of the cytoplasmic myofibrillar elements. *(pp. 4–9; 14–15; 533; 536)*

**19. (D)** Free radicals are chemically unstable, highly reactive molecules that are capable of profound biologic injury, mediated, in part, by peroxidation of cell membrane lipids. Generation of free radicals in cells is usually the result of oxidation-reduction reactions yielding a free electron. Molecules that absorb the free electron become unstable free radicals (see Question 7). Oxygen frequently acts as an acceptor of free electrons and forms superoxide, a highly reactive free radical. Thus, free radical generation is a major pathogenetic mechanism in oxygen toxicity. Exogenous drugs or chemicals such as carbon tetrachloride also can act as electron-absorbing molecules productive of injurious free radicals.

One of the major mechanisms by which leukocytes are able to kill ingested microorganisms is through the generation of toxic free radicals within their phagolysosomes. Unfortunately, however, free radicals may be released extracellularly from leukocytes when activated by chemotactic agents, immune complexes, or phagocytic challenge, and damage to the surrounding tissue results.

Ionizing radiation also initiates free radical formation but does so principally through radiolysis of water. The resultant hydroxyl radicals are particularly damaging to cells.

In contrast to chemical and toxic types of cell injury, which often involve free radical formation, ischemic and hypoxic injuries have a different pathogenetic basis: namely, termination of aerobic metabolism. Loss of oxidative phosphorylation leads to depletion of cellular ATP. Concomitantly, lactic acid accumulates from anaerobic glycolysis, and cellular pH decreases. Depletion of ATP produces mitochondrial dysfunction, and oxygen deprivation with cellular acidosis produces both lysosomal and plasma membrane injury. *(pp. 6–14; 73)*

**20. (B)** Repair of tissue injury is a complex process involving the growth of cells and the synthesis and remodeling of extracellular matrix. Numerous factors contribute to the well-orchestrated biologic events in wound healing, and the process may be delayed if any of these critical factors is altered. Some "inflammation" is necessary for normal wound healing, because the cytokines and degradative enzymes produced by macrophages and neutrophils make critical contributions. However, too much inflammation can be detrimental to wound repair. For example, the increased inflammation and continuing tissue injury caused by wound infection greatly slows the entire reparative process. In fact, infection is the single most common cause of delayed wound healing. Thus, systemic administration of antibiotics would be expected to irradicate wound infection and, thereby, eliminate any wound healing delays that infection might cause.

Inadequate blood supply, on the basis of either arterial insufficiency or venous stasis, is well known to retard wound healing. Increased systemic levels of corticosteroids also have inhibitory effects on the wound healing process, probably the result of both their anti-inflammatory action and their ability to suppress collagen synthesis directly. Thrombocytopenia also may interfere with wound healing because: (1) excessive amounts of extravasated blood tend to accumulate in the wound site and serve as a medium for bacterial growth; and (2) platelets are a major source of platelet-derived growth factor, a mitogen for fibroblasts and smooth muscle cells important in the normal progression of fibroplasia at wound sites. Vitamin C is critical to the hydroxylation of proline in the biosynthesis of collagen, so deficiency of this vitamin, known as scurvy, produces profound defects in wound healing. *(p. 89)*

**21. (A)** Graft-versus-host disease is not an autoimmune process. It results from histocompatibility antigen (human leukocyte antigen) mismatch between a transplanted tissue (usually bone marrow) containing immunocompetent cells and host tissues. Thus, the T cells of the allograft react appropriately to the foreign tissue antigens of the immunoincompetent recipient. The resultant immune response is primarily cellular rather than humoral in type.

Myasthenia gravis, systemic lupus erythematosus, atrophic gastritis associated with pernicious anemia, and type I (insulin-dependent) diabetes mellitus are all examples of immunologically mediated diseases in which autoantibodies (rather than cellular cytotoxicity) produce the major mediators of disease. In myasthenia gravis, autoantibodies to the acetylcholinesterase receptors block normal transmission of impulses at the neuromuscular junction and produce profound muscle dysfunction (weakness). In systemic lupus erythematosus, a host of autoantibodies to various components of normal cells (especially nuclear constituents) mediate systemic cellular injury. Atrophic gastritis associated with pernicious anemia is an autoimmune disease characterized by autoantibodies directed against gastric parietal cells and intrinsic factors (one of their products). The result of this targeted injury is achlorhydria and vitamin $B_{12}$ deficiency (vitamin $B_{12}$ uptake is dependent on intrinsic factor) secondary to parietal cell depletion. Insulin-dependent diabetes mellitus (IDDM) is a complex process including both humoral and cellular autoimmune responses. Autoantibodies are highly characteristic of IDDM. Some of these antibodies may appear in the circulation before the development of symptomatic disease and may serve to predict impending IDDM. Over 90% of patients with IDDM have circulating islet cell antibodies directed against a variety of islet cell antigens. *(pp. 194; 200; 606–607; 913)*

**22. (C)** Amyloidosis occurring in association with an underlying chronic inflammatory condition is usually diffuse in distribution. Thus, it is known as reactive systemic amyloidosis or secondary amyloidosis. Rheumatoid arthritis is the disorder most frequently associated with reactive systemic amyloidosis. Other commonly associated conditions include ankylosing spondylitis and inflammatory bowel disease (both Crohn's disease and ulcerative colitis). Chronic infectious diseases like tuberculosis, chronic bronchitis, and osteomyelitis were once the conditions most frequently linked with secondary amyloidosis and, even at present, still may develop this complication if they go untreated. Reactive systemic amyloidosis also may occur in association with non–immunocyte-derived tumors such as renal cell carcinoma and Hodgkin's disease. In reactive systemic amyloidosis, the amyloid fibrils are composed of AA (amyloid-associated) protein. AA protein is a unique nonimmunoglobulin protein. It is derived from a circulating precursor known as serum amyloid-associated protein (SAA), which is made by the liver.

Amyloidosis that occurs as a result of unregulated immunoglobulin secretion by a malignancy of B cells or plasma cells, such as multiple myeloma, is categorized as "immunocyte-derived" or primary amyloidosis. In this condition, the amyloid fibrils are composed of immunoglobulin light chains (the products of the cells of the immunocyte dyscrasia). *(pp. 231–234)*

**23. (A)** Despite its name, amyloid is not biochemically related to starch and is not digested by amylase. Rather, amyloid is a fibrillar protein that (regardless of its chemical composition; see here and Question 22) has a characteristic cross β-pleated sheet conformation. Amyloid commonly is identified in histologic section by the Congo Red stain, which stains amyloid of any type a bright pink-red color. The dye molecules bind to the amyloid oriented in a single plane (a phenomenon related to the strict parallel alignment of protein chains in β-pleated sheet configurations), which makes them birefringeant under polarized light (the pink-red becomes apple green). Oil Red O is a dye used for staining neutral lipids.

The composition of amyloid differs according to the underlying disease with which it is associated. In immunocyte-derived (primary) amyloidosis, amyloid is generated from immunoglobulin light chains. In reactive systemic (secondary) amyloidosis associated with chronic inflammatory conditions of various types, the amyloid is derived from a circulating nonimmunoglobulin (serum amyloid-associated) protein, which is made by the liver (see Question 22 above). In amyloidosis complicating hemodialysis in patients with chronic renal failure, the amyloid is generated from $\beta_2$-microglobulin, a normal serum protein and a component of class I major histocompatibility complex molecules. In senile cardiac amyloidosis, as well as in familial amyloidotic neuropathies, the normal plasma protein transthyretin (previously known as "prealbumin"), which binds and transports thyroxine and retinol in the blood, is the major protein constituent of the amyloid fibrils. In isolated atrial amyloidosis, the amyloid protein is derived from atrial natriuretic factor. *(pp. 231–233)*

**24. (B)** Hageman factor is a circulating proenzyme (coagulation factor XII) that, when activated during tissue injury, initiates the activation of proteolytic cascades that yield the major chemical mediators of inflammation and hemostasis. Hageman factor is activated via contact with collagen or injured endothelium following vascular disruption. Activated Hageman factor, in turn, activates the complement system, the kinin system, the fibrinolytic system, and the coagulation system. The complement system is a series of 20 serum proteins (enzymes) that form a catalytic cascade. The end product of the complement cascade is a protein capable of lysing the cell (e.g., bacterium) to which it is attached ("membrane attack complex"). Furthermore, the split products of the intermediate reactions in the cascade are themselves powerful mediators of vascular and cellular events in acute inflammation. Activated Hageman factor also activates the kinin system, which leads to the generation of bradykinin, a potent vasoactive agent. Perhaps most importantly, Hageman factor plays the schizophrenic role of activating both the thrombogenic and anticlotting mechanisms. Plasminogen is proteolytically converted to (the thrombolytic enzyme) plasmin by activated factor XII. Simultaneously, activated Hageman factor initiates thrombosis through the intrinsic coagulation pathway.

The (P-450) mixed-function oxidase system is a series of enzymes contained in the endoplasmic reticulum of hepatocytes and other cells. In the liver, this enzyme system is important to the metabolism of drugs and toxins. Its activation, however, is unrelated to Hageman factor. *(pp. 13; 65–68; 104)*

**25. (A)** Red infarctions are named for their hemorrhagic quality (i.e., the infarcted tissue characteristically contains large amounts of extravasated blood). They usually are encountered in tissues with a double circulation, in loose tissues, or in tissues previously congested. In other tissues, they typically are associated with venous occlusion. Infarction of the lung from pulmonary embolism is a classic example of a red infarction in an organ with a dual blood supply. Testicular torsion (twisting of the vascular pedicle of the testis) leads to red infarction because the constricting pressure on the vessels produces occlusion of the venous outflow sooner than occlusion of the arterial inflow (blood comes in but cannot get out). Whether caused by venous (portal vein) or arterial (mesenteric artery) occlusion, infarction of the small intestine, with its loose submucosal connective tissue, is typically hemorrhagic. In contrast, coronary artery thrombosis is an example of arterial occlusion in a solid tissue with a single blood supply. Thus, it typically produces a white (nonhemorrhagic) infarct. *(pp. 114–115)*

**26. (E)** Shock is a state of inadequate perfusion of all body tissues that results in hypoxic injury to cells. Initially, the injury is reversible, but, if shock is sufficiently prolonged, irreversible organ damage or even death of the patient may ensue. A number of disorders of diverse etiology may produce hemodynamic or vascular collapse and shock (see Question 30). Among the most common are bacterial infections producing so-called septic shock, the result of pooling of blood in the peripheral circulation. Septic shock is usually associated with gram-negative bacteria (such as *Escherichia coli*) that release endotoxin, a lipopolysaccharide component of their cell wall.

Macrophages, which are activated by endotoxin, produce both interleukin-1 and tumor necrosis factor, which, in turn, mediate the systemic hemodynamic (and inflammatory) effects of septic shock. Cardiogenic shock, the result of reduced cardiac output, is most commonly caused by myocardial infarction. The characteristically profuse watery diarrhea of cholera leads to massive fluid losses and a reduction of the effective circulating blood volume, causing hypovolemic shock. Hypovolemic shock also may occur in acute pancreatitis, which causes excessive transudation and exudation of fluid from the site of inflammation into the peritoneal cavity.

A cerebral infarction commonly is known as a "stroke" (not to be confused with shock). Shock may lead to a stroke, especially in an individual with underlying atherosclerotic vascular disease involving the cerebral vessels and a precarious cerebral perfusion status to begin with. However, stroke seldom leads to shock unless an autonomic center has been infarcted. *(pp. 70; 117; 318)*

**27. (C)** Ionizing radiation, whether in the form of electromagnetic (e.g., x-rays) or particulate (e.g., α particles, β particles, protons, or neutrons) radiation, is carcinogenic. Thus, ironically, even the iatrogenic use of radiation for cancer treatment may itself cause cancer. For example, long-term survivors of Hodgkin's disease may develop acute leukemia or lung cancer as a consequence of their (otherwise successful) radiation therapy. Head and neck irradiation in infants and children has resulted in the development of thyroid cancer later in life in 9% of those exposed. Osteosarcoma has been a common consequence of exposure to radium among watch dial painters. Lung cancer occurs with a 10-fold increased frequency among miners of ores containing radioactive elements.

In humans, there is a spectrum of vulnerability of different tissues to the transforming effects of radiation. Some tissues, such as skin, bone, and the gastrointestinal tract, are relatively resistant to radiation-induced neoplasia. For example, although hepatocellular carcinoma (hepatoma) has been linked causally with both chemical (aflatoxin B1 from *Aspergillus flavus*) and viral (the hepatitis B virus and, probably, the hepatitis C virus as well) carcinogenic agents, this tumor is not induced by radiation. *(pp. 284–285; 289; 648; 879)*

**28. (E)** The uncontrolled proliferation of malignant tumors is related to mutations in genes that encode proteins which regulate growth of normal cells. At least two important classes of such genes have been identified (i.e., genes that exert either positive or negative growth control). Genes that encode growth-stimulatory proteins are known as "oncogenes," whereas genes that encode growth-suppressing proteins are known as "tumor suppressor genes." Thus, uncontrolled growth may result from either too much positive stimulation of proliferation, too little negative control over proliferation, or both. The *p53* gene, the *DCC* ("Deleted in Colon Cancer") gene, the *Rb* gene, and the *WT-1* gene are all examples of tumor suppressor genes. The *p53* gene encodes a nuclear phosphoprotein that regulates DNA replication, cell proliferation, and cell death. The *Rb* gene also encodes a nuclear phosphoprotein that regulates the cell cycle and serves as a brake on the progression of cells from the $G_0/G_1$ to the S phase of the cell cycle. Likewise, the *WT-1* ("Wilm's tumor"-1) gene product is localized to the cell nucleus and encodes a nuclear transcription factor. The *DCC* gene encodes a transmembrane protein (an adhesion protein–like molecule) likely to be involved in the transduction of negative growth signals (such as contact inhibition) into the cell.

In addition to oncogenes and tumor suppressor genes, a third class of genes important in the development of tumors has been defined more recently. These genes do not regulate cell proliferation. They regulate programmed cell death. Although genes that induce programmed cell death as well as genes that prevent it have been defined in mammals, only the latter have identified (so far) in humans. *Bcl*-2 is the prototype gene of this category. It prevents programmed cell death, so its overexpression in tumors is associated with extended cell survival (perhaps even immortalization). *(pp. 265–270; 464)*

**29. (D)** The grading of a malignant neoplasm is based on the degree of cytologic differentiation of tumor cells (how closely they resemble their normal cellular counterparts in their tissue of origin) and the number of mitoses (proliferation rate). "Low-grade" tumors are better differentiated than "high-grade" tumors. In general, there is an inverse correlation between the differentiation of a tumor and its biologic aggressiveness. In contrast to grading, staging of a tumor involves assessment of the extent of progression of the tumor at the time of its discovery. The stage of the tumor is determined by the size of the primary lesion, the extent of local infiltration, the number of regional lymph nodes involved by metastatic tumor, and the presence or absence of blood-borne metastases. Staging often determines the therapeutic approach to the tumor (e.g., whether surgical resection will be employed or not, or whether adjuvant chemotherapy or radiation therapy will be necessary following surgical excision). Often, tumor stage is also the most accurate predictor of survival (i.e., it determines the prognosis for many tumors). In general, the higher the stage of the tumor, the worse the prognosis. *(p. 297)*

**30. (E)** Hemodynamic or vascular collapse causing inadequate perfusion of tissues is known as shock (see Question 26). The major categories of shock include: (1) cardiogenic shock (reduced cardiac output from any cause); (2) hypovolemic shock (massive loss of blood or fluid from the intravascular compartment); (3) septic shock (infection by organisms causing peripheral vasodilation, endothelial damage, and/or disseminated intravascular coagulation [DIC]); (4) neurogenic shock (central nervous system injury with reflex peripheral vasodilation and pooling of blood in the peripheral vasculature); and (5) anaphylactic shock (systemic circulatory collapse from a generalized type 1 hypersensitivity immune response). In addition, disorders other than sepsis that produce DIC (e.g., via endothelial injury and/or release of tissue factor) also may generate shock via this mechanism.

Severe thermal burns may produce shock via several different mechanisms. With massive tissue injury, large amounts of tissue factor are released into the circulation and precipitate DIC by activating the extrinsic pathway of the coagulation system. Widespread vascular injury leads to progressive loss of fluid from burn wounds, producing hypovolemia and reduced circulating blood volume. Burn wound infection and systemic dissemination of organisms may produce septic shock, especially if the organisms involved are gram-negative bacteria (such as *Pseudomonas* species) that produce endotoxin (which mediates "endotoxic shock"; see Questions 10 and 26). Pulmonary embolism (and subsequent reduction in cardiac output) may complicate prolonged immobilization of bedridden burn patients (thus the importance of early institution of physical therapy).

Although smoke inhalation may cause severe pulmonary complications, including the adult respiratory distress syndrome (diffuse alveolar damage), it does not cause anaphylaxis or shock. *(pp. 117–118; 624–626)*

**31. (A)** Oncogenes encode proteins ("oncoproteins") resembling normal gene ("proto-oncogene") products that play various roles in the activation of cell proliferation. However, because they lack important regulatory elements, oncoproteins differ significantly from their normal counterparts. In other words, mutations of normal genes involved in cell proliferation that lead to loss of regulatory control of their activity render them oncogenic. Some proto-oncogenes encode growth factors (c-*sis*, *hst*-1, and *int*-2 genes), some encode proteins that regulate expression of normal growth factor genes *(ras* genes), and others encode growth factor receptors *(erb*-B and *fms* genes). Still others encode proteins that affect cell proliferation by activating nuclear transcription *(myc* genes) or mediating the transduction of stimulating signals received at the cell surface through the cell cytoplasm and into the nucleus *(ras* and *abl* genes).

Although proto-oncogenes first were discovered as "passenger genes" within the genome of acute transforming retroviruses (which cause rapid induction of tumors in animals and transformation of cells *in vitro*), they are not of viral origin. Viral oncogenes are actually cellular genes that are believed to have been "captured" (during evolution) by these viruses from cells they were infecting. The analogue of a given proto-oncogene within a viral genome is designated as "v-*oncogene*." *(pp. 259–265)*

**32. (C)** The cytoskeletal intermediate filaments of different classes of cells can be separated biochemically and immunochemically into at least five distinctive types: keratin filaments, desmin, vimentin, glial filaments, and neurofilaments. Although vimentin is produced by a wide variety of cells, including all mesenchymal cells and many types of epithelial cells, the other intermediate filaments are more limited and specific in their distribution. Keratins are made almost exclusively by epithelial cells. Glial filaments and neurofilaments are formed only by glial cells and neurons, respectively. Desmin is produced only by skeletal muscle cells.

Because of their cell-type specificity, intermediate filaments can be helpful in tumor diagnosis. The presence of desmin in an anaplastic tumor, for example, would support a diagnosis of rhabdosarcoma, because desmin is unique to muscle cells (smooth or striated). Analogously, keratin is the intermediate filament that one would expect to be expressed in a squamous cell carcinoma. Lymphomas and malignant schwannomas may express vimentin, but the finding is nonspecific because vimentin is produced by a wide variety of cells. Lymphoma is identified best by surface markers that are specific for lymphocytes rather than by intermediate filament expression (see Question 16). Schwannomas can be recognized by their production of S100 protein (also made by melanomas), a protein expressed by cells of neural origin. *(pp. 299; 1351)*

**33. (A)** The penetration of carcinomas through the basement membrane of the epithelium in which they arise, their subsequent infiltration of surrounding tissues, and, ultimately, lymphatic and blood vessel invasion with metastatic spread all involve interaction of tumor cells with extracellular matrix (ECM) proteins. Molecules produced by carcinomas that mediate their invasion of ECM include type IV collagenase, both laminin and fibronectin receptors, and cathepsin D. Type IV collagenase degrades the major structural component of surrounding basement membranes (permitting progression from "*in situ*" to "infiltrating" malignancy). Expression of integrins, which function as receptors for ECM components such as laminin, fibronectin, collagen, and vitronectin, allows the tumor to attach to the matrix and move through it as it simultaneously secretes proteases that degrade the ECM for easier passage through the tissue. Cathepsin D is a cysteine protease that is an important ECM degradative enzyme. It acts on a large number of ECM substrates, including fibronectin, laminin, and proteoglycans.

CD44 adhesion molecules are cell surface adhesion molecules that mediate implantation of tumor metastases in lymph nodes (possibly through interaction with the endothelium of venules in lymph nodes). Tumors with high levels of CD44 are especially adept at extravascular dissemination. However, CD44 does not mediate tumor invasion of the surrounding extracellular matrix. *(pp. 276–278)*

**34. (D)** Hyperplasia refers to an increase in the number of cells in an organ or tissue. Thus, it can occur only in those tissues which are composed of cells capable of mitotic activity. In some circumstances, hyperplasia represents a normal physiologic response and is beneficial. Compensatory hyperplasia, such as occurs in the remaining kidney after unilateral nephrectomy, and hormonally induced functional hyperplasia, such as that which occurs in the endometrium during the proliferative phase of the menstrual cycle, are examples of physiologic hyperplasia.

Atypical (or "adenomatous") hyperplasia of the endometrium, however, constitutes a pathologic form of hyperplasia that is associated with increased risk of malignant transformation. It occurs in postmenopausal women in whom an abnormally high, prolonged level of estrogenic stimulation is unaccompanied by progestational activity. Atypical hyperplasia of the endometrium is considered a premalignant lesion that has been shown to progress to endometrial carcinoma in about 25% of cases, with or without progestin therapy. Similarly, atypical hyperplasias of the breast (either ductal or lobular in type) are considered premalignant lesions. The more severe and atypical the hyperplasia, the greater the risk of malignancy.

Ménétrier's disease is also an example of pathologic epithelial hyperplasia. In this condition (etiology unknown), hyperplasia of the gastric surface mucosal glands occurs and, in a subset of cases, undergoes evolution to dysplasia and carcinoma. However, malignant transformation occurs much less commonly in Ménétrier's disease than in the previously mentioned examples of atypical endometrial hyperplasia or atypical hyperplasias of the breast.

Myelodysplasia of the bone marrow refers to a group of clonal stem cell disorders (myelodysplastic syndromes) characterized by maturation defects, ineffective hematopoiesis and increased risk of malignant transformation to acute myeloblastic leukemia. Thus, the bone marrow is usually hypercellular (hyperplastic) and crowded with cells that are cytologically atypical, but the peripheral blood is pancytopenic.

In contrast, nodular hyperplasia of the prostate is not considered to be a premalignant lesion. It is so common in elderly men (it occurs in more than 90% of men over the age of 70) that it arguably may be considered to be a normal aging process. Merely because it is extremely common, nodular hyperplasia often is found in prostates containing carcinoma, but the two processes are not related causally. *(pp. 654; 778; 1026; 1058; 1094–1095)*

**35. (B)** Metaplasia is a reversible change in which the normal cells of a tissue or tissue layer are replaced by other normal but inappropriate (for the location) cell types. Metaplasia results from altered differentiation of stem cells occurring as an adaptive response to chronic injury. Metaplasia itself is a benign process, but malignant change can develop in metaplastic tissue when the injury continues unabated over long periods of time. Tissues in which the development of carcinoma is typically preceded by progression through metaplasia and dysplasia include the endocervix and the lung. The normal endocervix and lung contain no squamous epithelium, and yet the most common type of carcinoma occurring in these tissues is squamous cell carcinoma. The cancers arise from a glandular epithelium that first undergoes squamous metaplasia, becomes progressively more dysplastic, and finally becomes cancerous. Although far less common than these examples, squamous cell carcinoma of the bladder is another example of malignant transformation of metaplastic squamous epithelium.

As a rule, metaplasias in human tissues represent grandular-to-squamous transitions. The single most notable exception to this rule is the squamous-to-glandular metaplastic transition of the esophageal mucosa that occurs in response to chronic reflux of gastric contents and is known as Barrett's esophagus. In about 10% of individuals with Barrett's esophagus, progressive dysplasia of the glandular epithelium ultimately results in the development of adenocarcinoma.

Carcinoid tumors of the small bowel apparently arise *de novo* from neoplastic transformation of intestinal epithelial stem cells, which have the potential to differentiate along neuroendocrine lines. Intestinal carcinoid tumors are not associated with either metaplastic or dysplastic precursor lesions. *(pp. 45; 48–49; 257; 723; 763; 1000; 1046–1049)*

**36. (E)** Cyclins, *ras* proteins, glutamyl transpeptidase (GTP)-binding proteins, and mitogen-activated protein kinases (MAPKs) are all molecules that function in the control of cell growth. Cyclins are a group of proteins that, when they bind to constitutive protein kinases within the cell, form complexes that catalyze the formation of proteins involved in DNA replication, spindle formation, and other key events in cell division. *Ras* proteins and G proteins are both GTP-binding proteins that function by coupling extracellular mitogenic signals to effector molecules within the cell. When the *ras*-GTP complex becomes bound to the phosphorylated signal receptor (a tyrosine kinase), *ras* becomes activated and phosphorylates a cascade of cytoplasmic enzymes known as the mitogen-activated protein kinases. The MAPKs, in turn, mediate activation of transcription factors necessary for cell division.

Selectins are nonimmunoglobulin adhesion molecules that are expressed on the surfaces of endothelial cells (and some other cell types). Endothelial selectins bind to specific oligosaccharides on the membranes of leukocytes, an interaction that mediates the adhesion of leukocytes to endothelial surfaces. Selectin expression on the endothelial cells of vessels at the site of an acute inflammatory process plays a key role in mediating leukocyte transmigration into the target tissue (see Question 37). Selectins, however, do not function in cell growth regulation. *(pp. 38–39; 57–58)*

**37. (B)** One of the hallmarks of an acute inflammatory response is neutrophilic infiltration. Drawn to the site of inflammation by chemotactic substances, migrating neutrophils first marginate to the periphery of vessels in the region of inflammation, stick to the endothelium, and then emigrate through the vessel wall to invade the tissue, where their phagocytic talents may be needed. Although small numbers of neutrophils may transiently marginate and stick to vascular endothelium under normal circumstances, these processes are markedly amplified in acute inflammation. Increased leukocyte adhesion is mainly the result of specific interactions between complementary "adhesion molecules" present on leukocyte and endothelial surfaces.

Several factors are known to promote endothelium-leukocyte adhesion through the modulation of adhesion molecules on endothelial cells and/or leukocytes. Interleukin-1 and tumor necrosis factor both stimulate expression of the immunoglobulin-type adhesion molecules intercellular adhesion molecule-1 (ICAM-1) and vascular adhesion molecule-1 (VCAM-1) on endothelial cells. ICAM-1 binds to specific $\beta_2$ integrin receptors (LFA-1 and MAC-1) on leukocytes, and VCAM-1 to the leukocyte surface $\beta_1$ integrin VLA-4. Activation of neutrophils by inflammatory mediators such as complement fragment C5a and leukotriene $B_4$ (which also promote neutrophil emigration by chemoattraction) increases the avidity of binding of their surface LFA-1 integrin molecules to ICAM-1 ligands on endothelial cells and promotes neutrophil-endothelium adhesion. Platelet-activating factor stimulates leukocyte adhesion by modulating expression of selectins (nonimmunoglobulin adhesion molecules) on endothelial cells that bind to specific oligosaccharides on leukocyte surfaces.

Nitric oxide is a short-acting inflammatory mediator produced by macrophages and endothelial cells. Its actions include relaxation of smooth muscle (producing vascular dilation), reduction of platelet aggregation and adhesion, and free radical formation. However, it does not mediate or promote neutrophil emigration into tissues. *(pp. 57–60; 70–72; 73–74)*

**38. (E)** Transforming growth factor-β (TGF-β) is a growth factor that plays several key roles in wound repair. It is a fibrogenic cytokine that is produced by a wide variety of cells, including platelets, activated macrophages, and epithelial cells. It is chemotactic for monocytes, and it stimulates both fibroblast migration and proliferation. TGF-β also stimulates fibroblasts to increase their production of collagen and extracellular matrix proteins and to decrease their degradation of these proteins. The end result is an increase in fibrous tissue (scar production), which is the basis of the nonspecific mechanism of repair following injury of nonregenerating tissues or chronic destructive inflammation of any tissue. *(pp. 80–81)*

**39. (D)** To protect themselves from the harmful effects of free radicals generated in inflammatory responses, normal tissues possess several endogenous antioxidant systems. Serum proteins such as ceruloplasmin, transferrin, and albumin are important circulating antioxidants. Other endogenous antioxidants include vitamin E and sulfhydryl-containing compounds such as cysteine and glutathione. These molecules are all nonenzymatic antioxidants that serve either to bind ions that catalyze the formation of free radicals (and thereby prevent free radical generation altogether) or to "scavenge" (bind and inactivate) free radicals that have already been generated. Enzymatic antioxidant systems include superoxide dismutase, which can inactivate superoxide, as well as catalase and glutathione peroxidase, both of which are capable of detoxifying hydrogen peroxide. Ultimately, limitation of tissue injury during acute inflammatory processes depends on the ability of these systems to control the destructive potential of free radicals.

$\alpha_2$-Macroglobulin is an antiprotease found in serum and various secretions. Although it is important in protecting normal tissues from the harmful effects of lysosomal proteases released from leukocytes during inflammatory reactions, it has no effect on free radicals. *(pp. 12–13; 73)*

**40. (D)** Congestion is a general term referring to increased blood volume in tissue caused by reduced venous drainage. Congestion may occur as a systemic phenomenon (e.g., congestive heart failure) or a local process (e.g., involving one organ or part of an organ). Passive congestion of the liver produces a mottled pattern of tissue discoloration known as "nutmeg liver" because it visually resembles the cut surface of a nutmeg. The appearance is created by deeply reddened congested centrilobular zones surrounded by pale, yellow-to-brown zones of liver at the lobule periphery. Hypoperfusion of the centrilobular zone with ischemic necrosis also contributes to the injury when nutmeg river occurs in association with heart failure. Chronic passive congestion of the lungs produces a lesion known as "brown induration." The lung tissue is brown as a result of hemosiderin deposition, and it is indurated (hard) as a result of collagen deposition in the chronically edematous alveolar septa. In the spleen, chronic passive congestion produces small fibrous nodules with hemosiderin deposition known as Gandy-Gamna bodies. They occur with increased portal pressure, which causes deposition of collagen in the basement membrane of the splenic sinusoids. As the name loudly announces (this one is a give-away), stasis dermatitis of the legs occurs as a result of impaired venous return and chronic congestion of the extremities.

Strawberry gallbladder refers to the gross appearance of the mucosa in gallbladders with cholesterolosis. In this innocuous disorder, the focal accumulations of lipid-laden macrophages in the mucosal lamina propria are seen as yellow flecks resembling the seeds on the surface of a strawberry. *(pp. 27; 97–98; 504–505; 670)*

**41. (E)** Amyloid of the AA type is derived from a circulating precursor protein made by the liver known as serum amyloid-associated protein. This type of amyloid characteristically occurs in two basic categories of disease: reactive systemic amyloidosis occurring in association with malignant tumors or chronic inflammatory conditions (e.g., ulcerative colitis) and the form of hereditary amyloidosis known as familial Mediterranean fever.

In type II diabetes mellitus, the amyloid that sometimes can be found in the pancreatic islets of Langerhans is derived from islet amyloid polypeptide, a unique protein made by the islet cells. In Alzheimer's disease, the amyloid is derived from $\beta_2$-amyloid protein (A$\beta_2$), which is derived from a much larger transmembrane precursor glycoprotein known as amyloid precursor protein. In medullary carcinoma of the thyroid, the amyloid that is characteristically present in the tumor stroma is derived from calcitonin, the polypeptide hormone product of the tumor cells. In chronic renal failure, the amyloidosis that complicates long-term hemodialysis derives from $\beta_2$-microglobulin (not to be confused with the $\beta_2$-amyloid protein of Alzheimer's disease), a normal serum protein that is a component of class I histocompatibility molecules. *(pp. 231–234)*

**42. (C)** Most malignant tumors tend to metastasize via the lymphatic or blood vessels. Only a few tumor types, such as mesotheliomas, deviate from these patterns and tend to spread over the surfaces of viscera or body cavities. This pattern of spread is so distinctive that mesothelioma often can be diagnosed radiologically by the thick rind of tumor tissue it characteristically produces over the surface of an involved lung.

Colon carcinoma is a classic example of a malignant tumor that initially metastasizes via the lymphatic system to local pericolonic lymph nodes and subsequently metastasizes to the liver via hematogenous routes. Renal cell carcinoma and hepatocellular carcinoma, in contrast, are common examples of tumors that typically spread by hematogenous routes from the outset. Gastric carcinoma utilizes both lymphatic and hematogenous routes of metastatic dissemination and may "seed" the peritoneum as well. However, none of these tumors is characterized by spreading over body cavities or organ surfaces as a preferential pattern of growth. *(pp. 250–251; 731; 817; 880; 987)*

**43. (E)** In the United States, lung cancer causes more deaths than any other form of malignancy. The overall death rate from cancer appears to be increasing in males, whereas, in females, it is decreasing slightly. The steady increase in the cancer death rate among males can be ascribed mainly to lung cancer. *(p. 253)*

**44. (C)** Prostate cancer occurs more frequently than lung cancer in males, and breast cancer occurs more frequently than lung cancer in females. However, neither of these tumors causes as many deaths as lung cancer (see Question 43). *(p. 253)*

**45. (B)** In humans, several different types of malignancies are related causally to infection by DNA viruses. Cervical carcinoma is linked with human papillomavirus infection. Burkitt's lymphoma is linked with Epstein-Barr virus infection. Hepatocellular carcinoma (hepatoma) is well known to be related etiologically to hepatitis B viral infection, and it is now becoming clear that hepatitis C viral infection is also an independent causal factor. Interestingly, human malignancy caused by RNA virus (retrovirus) infection is far less common. The single example known at present is a form of T cell leukemia/lymphoma caused by human T-cell leukemia virus type I.

Cytomegalovirus is a DNA virus of the herpes family that is a common opportunistic pathogen in immunosuppressed individuals, but it is not known to be oncogenic. *(pp. 286–289; 352; 879)*

**46. (True); 47. (False); 48. (False); 49. (False); 50. (True); 51. (False); 52. (True)**

**(46)** Histocompatibility antigens (human leukocyte antigens or HLAs) are cell surface antigens that are extremely important in the induction and regulation of immune responses (they also have some immunologic functions). They are encoded by a set of closely linked genes on chromosome 6 (called the major histocompatibility complex, or MHC) that usually are inherited *en bloc*. The major function of histocompatibility molecules is to bind peptide fragments of foreign proteins for presentation to antigen-specific T cells.

**(47)** Two major classes of HLA antigens have been defined. Class I antigens are glycoproteins encoded by HLA-A, -B, and -C loci, each representing a separate gene within the MHC. Class I antigens are present on virtually all nucleated cells. Class II antigens are those encoded by the HLA-D locus (containing three subregions: DP, DQ, and DR) of the MHC. Although the term HLA refers to "human leukocyte antigens," it is only the HLA-D antigens that are expressed exclusively on leukocytes (all macrophages, most B cells, and some T cells). Other cell types such as fibroblasts, endothelial cells, renal tubular cells, and epidermal keratinocytes can be induced to express HLA-D antigens (e.g., by γ-interferon) but do not express them constitutively.

**(48)** Class I HLA (HLA-A, HLA-B, and HLA-C) antigens interact only with CD8+ cytotoxic T cells. CD4+ T cells can recognize foreign antigens only in association with HLA-D molecules and therefore are referred to "class II restricted" T cells.

**(49)** The genes that code for both classes of HLA antigens are highly polymorphic. The set of subtypes of each class I and class II antigen are inherited as a unit that constitutes a haplotype. One set or haplotype is inherited from each parent. According to the laws of Mendelian genetics, siblings can have only four possible combinations of haplotypes. There is only a 25% chance that two siblings will be HLA identical. The odds are 50% that two siblings will share one haplotype and 25% that they will not share any haplotype. The concept of haplotype sharing becomes important when genetically related or genetically identical organ transplant donors are sought. The histocompatibility molecules are the antigens that evoke rejection of allogeneic (genetically nonidentical) organs which have been transplanted to immunocompetent hosts (allograft rejection). Conversely, they also may mediate immune attack of the host by the graft (graft-versus-host disease) if the transplanted allogeneic tissue contains immunocompetent cells and the recipient is immunologically impaired.

**(50)** Both the genes that encode the components of the complement system and the genes that encode tumor necrosis factor (α and β) are located within the MHC. These genes are situated between the genes encoding the class I and class II HLA molecules.

**(51)** Recognition of a virally infected cell by a T lymphocyte is dependent on the coincident presence of class I HLA molecules on the surface of the infected cell. Viral antigens are bound to newly synthesized class I heavy chains within the infected cell. The viral peptide–class I complex then associates with $\beta_2$-microglobulin to form a stable trimer that is transported to the cell surface. Antigen-specific CD8+ cytotoxic T cells "recognize" the viral antigen when associated with the class I molecule, and proceed to destroy the cell displaying the complex. In this way, virally infected cells are eliminated. Class II HLA antigens do not play a role in this response.

**(52)** A variety of diseases are strongly associated with specific HLA subtypes. Perhaps the best known and strongest association is that between ankylosing spondylitis and HLA-B27. Individuals who possess the HLA-B27 antigen have a 90-fold greater chance of developing ankylosing spondylitis than those who are negative for HLA-B27. *(pp. 175–177; 193–194)*

**53. (True); 54. (True); 55. (True); 56. (False); 57. (False)**

**(53 through 55)** "Atrophy" refers to diminished size resulting from loss of anatomic substance that is often accompanied by diminished function. The term may refer to changes in individual cells, in portions of tissues, or in entire organs. Atrophy represents an adaptive response of otherwise normal tissue to reductions in normal functional stimuli and/or to impairments in physiologic support systems. Thus, atrophy may occur as a result of diminished workload, innervation, blood supply, nutrition, or endocrine stimulation. It also may occur with aging. On an elemental level, atrophy is due to a reduction in the structural components of cells, including decreases in cytoplasmic organelles and cytostructural elements. Although decreased cell function may occur as a consequence, atrophy does not imply that the affected cells are dead or even moribund.

**(56)** Although autophagic vacuoles often form within cells undergoing atrophy, they are not a sign of irreversible cell injury. Autophagy is a mechanism by which injured or effete organelles are eliminated from living cells. **(57)** Both atrophy and autophagy are to be distinguished from autolysis, the process by which dead tissues are digested enzymatically by lysosomal enzymes released from necrotic cells. *(pp. 15; 47–48)*

**58. (False); 59. (True); 60. (False); 61. (False); 62. (False); 63. (True); 64. (False)**

**(58)** Since the first cases of the acquired immunodeficiency syndrome (AIDS) were reported in 1981, this devastating and lethal disease has been the subject of intensive research and enormous public concern. AIDS is an infectious disease that is transmitted sexually (either homosexually or heterosexually) or parenterally (e.g., via blood transfusions or intravenous drug use). The causative agent is a single-stranded RNA retrovirus belonging to the lentivirus family known as human immunodeficiency virus (HIV). Infection is characterized by a long incubation period followed by a slowly progressive immunosuppressive disease with an inevitably fatal outcome (usually from overwhelming infection). There are two known types of HIV (HIV-1 and HIV-2), both of which cause AIDS. HIV-1 is the most common type associated with AIDS in the United States, Europe, and Central Africa, whereas HIV-2 is prevalent in West Africa.

**(59)** The CD4 molecule is a high-affinity receptor for the "gp120" surface glycoprotein of HIV. Thus, helper T cells, which have high densities of CD4 on their surfaces, are the major target of HIV infection. The internalized virus undergoes reverse transcription to form cDNA that becomes incorporated into the host cell genome when the cell divides. On future stimulation by cytokines or antigen exposure and initiation of DNA transcription, the infected cell transcribes the integrated proviral DNA, and complete viral particles are formed (an event known as "productive infection"). The extensive viral budding that occurs during productive infection leads to the lysis of the host cell. This destruction of HIV-infected CD4+ T cells results in a profound deficiency of cell-mediated immunity, which is the hallmark of AIDS. In contrast to the circulating T-cell populations of normal individuals, in which the ratio of helper (CD4+) to suppressor (CD8+) cells is approximately 2:1, the CD4+:CD8+ T-cell ratio is inverted in AIDS patients because of the severe deficiency of CD4+ cells. **(60)** Although HIV belongs to the family of retroviruses that includes human T-cell leukemia viruses (HTLV-1 and HTLV-II), HIV is nontransforming and does not cause leukemia or other malignancies. Both HIV and HTLV target CD4+ helper T cells. However, HIV causes impairment of function and destruction of helper T cells, whereas HTLV causes neoplastic transformation.

**(61)** Monocytes, macrophages, and follicular dendritic cells in lymphoid tissues (not in the peripheral blood) constitute a major reservoir of the HIV virus in infected individuals. These cells bear CD4 molecules on their surfaces (in lower densities compared to helper T cells) that may bind the virus, but they may also take up virus by direct phagocytosis or by binding of antibody-coated HIV particles to their cell surface Fc receptors. Infected macrophages typically contain large numbers of replicated viral particles within their cytoplasmic vacuoles but manifest little viral budding from their surface. Within the macrophage cytoplasm, the virus may escape host defense mechanisms, and the infected macrophages are able to transport the virus to various parts of the body with impunity. In particular, involvement of the central nervous system, which is a major target of HIV infection, most likely occurs via migration of infected monocytes into the brain.

**(62)** Abnormalities of B cell function also occur in AIDS. Paradoxically, immunoglobulin levels often are elevated in AIDS patients as a result of polyclonal B cell activation. B cell stimulation may occur in response either to infectious agents such as Epstein-Barr virus or cytomegalovirus, to HIV envelope glycoproteins, or to cytokines (especially interleukin-6) produced by HIV-infected macrophages. Despite elevated immunoglobulins and spontaneously activated B cells, AIDS patients cannot mount an antibody response to new antigens. With the onset of full-blown AIDS syndrome, B-cell proliferation subsides, and lymph nodes become depleted of B as well as T cells.

**(63)** Non-Hodgkin's lymphomas (primarily high-grade B-cell tumors, such as Burkitt's lymphoma or immunoblastic B-cell lymphoma) are second only to Kaposi's sarcoma as the most frequent neoplastic complication of AIDS. The genesis of these tumors is thought to be related to the long-term polyclonal B cell proliferation that occurs concomitantly with dwindling T-cell and macrophage function and multiple viral infections.

**(64)** AIDS can be transmitted by transfusion of whole blood or blood components such as platelets or plasma. Thus, hemophiliacs were formerly at very high risk of developing AIDS from transfused blood products. The risk was especially high for those who received factor VIII concentrates (which are produced by pooling blood obtained from several thousand blood donors) prior to 1985. In 1985, blood banks began to screen donors, to test donated blood for anti-HIV antibody, and to use viral-inactivating heat treatment for clotting factor concentrates. These measures have reduced (virtually eliminated) transfusion-associated HIV transmission dramatically, and hemophiliacs are no longer at high risk of contracting HIV. Transfusion of whole blood represents the only remaining iatrogenic risk. However, even the extremely small remaining risk of acquiring AIDS through transfusion with seronegative blood (containing virus but no anti-HIV antibodies) may potentially be eliminated via testing for the viral particles themselves (e.g., by polymerase chain reaction amplification). At present, parenteral transmission of AIDS is caused far more commonly by intravenous drug abuse than by blood transfusion. *(pp. 219–231)*

**65. (True); 66. (True); 67. (True); 68. (True); 69. (True); 70. (False); 71. (False)**

**(65)** Most human tumors are clonal. That is, they are derived from the proliferation of a single neoplastically transformed cell. Nevertheless, cellular heterogeneity within given tumors usually exists and may result from new mutations in the genetically unstable, evolving neoplasm or variable expression of genes in different subsets of tumor cells.

**(66)** Most benign tumors are well differentiated. That is, they closely resemble their normal tissues of origin, both morphologically and functionally. In contrast, malignant tumors vary widely in the extent to which they resemble their normal tissue counterparts. Some may be quite well differentiated and, in this regard, may be difficult to distinguish morphologically from benign tumors. Other malignancies may be wildly anaplastic, bearing little resemblance to their tissue of origin. It can be difficult merely to identify such tumors. The degree of differentiation manifested by most malignant tumors lies between these two extremes, however. Sometimes, the degree of differentiation of the malignant cells may vary from region to region within the same tumor.

**(67)** In general, the rate of growth of tumors is inversely related to their degree of differentiation: the more differentiated, the slower the growth. Thus, most malignant tumors grow faster than their benign counterparts.

**(68)** A few other key features distinguish malignant from benign neoplasms. The most important and incontrovertible is the ability of malignant tumors (but not benign tumors) to metastasize. No matter what its growth rate or degree of differentiation (or any other feature of the tumor), a neoplasm can be identified definitively as malignant if it metastasizes.

**(69)** Progressive infiltration and destruction of surrounding normal tissue structures is another highly characteristic feature of malignant tumors. However, this feature is less definitive than metastasis in identifying a tumor as malignant because some benign tumors may be locally invasive (yet never metastasize). Desmoid tumors are well known examples of locally aggressive tumors that do not metastasize.

**(70)** Carcinomas usually metastasize via lymphatics, whereas sarcomas typically metastasize via hematogenous routes. **(71)** Nevertheless, enlargement of lymph nodes in the region surrounding a carcinoma does not necessarily mean that metastatic tumor is present. Regional lymph node enlargement may represent reactive hyperplasia occurring as a consequence of stimulation by tumor antigens, necrotic cell debris, or superimposed infection of the devitalized tissues associated with the tumor. When metastatic involvement of enlarged regional lymph nodes is suspected, biopsy may be required to differentiate between reactive and tumorous nodes. This can be an essential step in accurately staging a malignant tumor, because most staging systems for carcinomas ("TNM" staging systems) are based on assessments of tumor size (T), nodal status (N), and extranodal metastases (M). *(pp. 242–251; 1265)*

**72. (A); 73. (D); 74. (C); 75. (A); 76. (B); 77. (D)**

Inflammation and immunologic responses are complex reactions that have evolved because of their overall benefit to the organism. However, these same reactions may also cause injury to the organism and, in doing so, form the bases of specific disease processes. In general, inflammation is characterized by a programmed response to injury of almost any cause (e.g., trauma, burns, infection) occurring in vascularized living tissue. The response is integrally related to repair of the injured tissue and is mediated primarily by granulocytes, macrophages, and chemical factors derived from plasma. Immune responses, in contrast, are the body's strategic defense system against invasion by pathogens. Immune reactions are characterized by highly specific offensive attacks directed against molecular substances known as antigens (belonging to the potential "invader") and are mediated by lymphocytes with the help of antigen-presenting cells (e.g., macrophages, dendritic cells, and Langerhans' cells). Inflammatory and immune responses overlap in two fundamental ways: (1) all immune reactions produce tissue injury and, thereby, cause inflammation, and (2) some cytokines produced by activated immune cells are actually mediators of inflammation (e.g., interleukin-1 and tumor necrosis factor) (see Questions 213 through 220). Thus, immune responses are one category of inflammation-provoking injury, but many inflammatory reactions do not involve immune responses.

**(72)** A granulomatous response to an inert foreign body such as surgical suture material is a type of inflammatory reaction and, in contrast to type IV hypersensitivity responses with granuloma formation, requires no participation of the immune system. *(p. 81)*

**(73)** In contrast to infectious endocarditis, which evokes an inflammatory response in the surrounding valvular tissue, nonbacterial thrombotic (marantic) endocarditis is characterized by the formation of bland fibrin thrombi on valve leaflets with no significant accompanying inflammatory reaction. Although its pathogenesis is uncertain, nonbacterial thrombotic endocarditis is thought to be related to hypercoagulability. *(pp. 554–555)*

**(74)** Streptococcal infection produces both an exuberant inflammatory reaction and an immunologic response to the organism. Both responses are important host defense mechanisms against pyogenic bacteria, so disorders that produce defects in either lead to increased susceptibility to staphylococcal and other pyogenic infections. *(pp. 53; 182–184; 320; 337–338)*

**(75)** Sunburn is a classic example of inflammation induced by cutaneous injury from the radiant energy of ultraviolet light. *(pp. 402–405)*

**(76)** Although the name implies an inflammatory response ("itis") in the thyroid, Hashimoto's thyroiditis is an autoimmune disorder mediated by both cellular and humoral immune responses to thyroidal antigens. *(pp. 1126–1127)*

**(77)** Lead poisoning is caused by the direct toxic effects of lead on the hematopoietic system, nervous system, gastrointestinal tract, and kidneys. Neither an inflammatory nor an immunologic response is evoked by this toxic process. Because of the insidious nature of the injury, the disease often goes unrecognized for long periods of time. *(pp. 390–392)*

**78. (B); 79. (D); 80. (E); 81. (D); 82. (E); 83. (E)**

**(78)** Mast cell mediators of anaphylaxis are of two types: (1) primary mediators that are preformed and stored in cytoplasmic granules; and (2) secondary mediators, including cytokines and substances derived from cell membrane phospholipids, that are synthesized *de novo* when mast cell degranulation is triggered. Primary mediators include biogenic amines (histamine and adenosine), chemotactic factors for eosinophils and neutrophils, heparin, and enzymes (e.g., chymase, tryptase, acid hydrolases). Secondary mediators include platelet-activating factor (PAF), products of arachidonic acid metabolism, including both leukotrienes ($B_4$, $C_4$, $D_4$, and $E_4$) and prostaglandins (principally $D_4$), and cytokines. Tumor necrosis factor-α (TNF-α), interleukins (IL-1, IL-3, IL-4, IL-5, IL-6), and granulocyte-macrophage colony stimulating factor are among the cytokines produced by mast cells.

**(79 and 81)** Vascular permeability is increased by histamine, leukotrienes $C_4$, $D_4$, and $E_4$, prostaglandin $D_2$, PAF, and complement-activating neutral proteases. Smooth muscle contraction is produced by all of these same substances, except for the neutral proteases. The leukotrienes and prostaglandin $D_2$ are far more powerful than histamine in inducing both these reactions, however.

**(80 and 83)** Mast cell granules contain both eosinophil chemotactic factor of anaphylaxis and neutrophil chemotactic factor of anaphylaxis. Leukotriene $B_4$ is also highly chemotactic for neutrophils, eosinophils, and monocytes, and PAF is chemotactic for neutrophils and eosinophils. Many of the mast cell cytokines are also chemoattractants for granulocytes. TNF-α attracts neutrophils and eosinophils, and IL-4 is important for the recruitment of eosinophils. However, histamine, prostaglandin $D_2$, and leukotrienes $C_4$, $D_4$, and $E_4$ are not chemotactic.

**(82)** Of all the mast cell mediators, only PAF causes platelet aggregation. It also causes platelets to degranulate and release histamine. Furthermore, PAF is a potent direct-acting effector of both bronchospasm and increased vascular permeability. *(pp. 178–182)*

**84. (C); 85. (D); 86. (F); 87. (B); 88. (D); 89. (H); 90. (E); 91. (C); 92. (G); 93. (A)**

In many systemic and organ-specific autoimmune diseases, distinctive autoantibodies are produced. Such antibodies may or may not be related clearly to the pathogenesis of the disease, do not occur in every case, and are almost never pathognomonic. Nevertheless, they are diagnostically useful markers and are frequently part of the clinical evaluation of patients with suspected autoimmune diseases.

**(84 and 91)** Antinuclear antibodies directed against a variety of nuclear antigens occur in many autoimmune diseases, including systemic lupus erythematosus (SLE), Sjögren's syndrome, and systemic sclerosis (scleroderma). However, autoantibodies to individual nuclear antigens may be linked more expressly to specific diseases. For example, antibodies to native double-stranded DNA are virtually diagnostic of SLE. They occur in only 40 to 60% of cases, however. Antihistone antibodies are also characteristic of SLE and occur in 50 to 70% of cases. They are especially common in drug-induced lupus, occurring in more than 95% of cases. *(pp. 200–201)*

**(85 and 88)** Two antinuclear antibodies that are more or less unique to systemic sclerosis have been identified: anti-Scl 70 and an anticentromere antibody. The antigen Scl-70 is associated with DNA topoisomerase I. Anti-Scl 70 is present in about 70% of patients with diffuse systemic sclerosis. The anticentromere antibody is present in only about 10% of those with diffuse systemic sclerosis but occurs in 80 to 90% of those with the more limited form of the disease (confined to fingers, forearms, and face) known as the CREST syndrome (*c*alcinosis, *r*aynaud's phenomenon, *e*sophageal dysmotility, *s*clerodactyly, and *t*elangiectasia). *(pp. 210–211)*

**(86)** Anti–basement membrane antibodies are the diagnostic feature of Goodpasture's disease, an archetypal example of a disease caused by autoantibodies. This disease causes rapidly progressive glomerulonephritis and hemorrhagic interstitial pneumonitis and, if untreated, is fatal. However, elimination of the autoantibodies effectively reverses the disease. Thus, Goodpasture's disease can be cured by simultaneous plasma exchange and immunosuppression in order to remove circulating antibodies and reduce further antibody production, respectively. *(pp. 717; 947)*

**(87)** Antibodies directed against two ribonucleoprotein antigens, designated as SS-A (Ro) and SS-B (La), are highly characteristic of Sjögren's syndrome and can be detected in up to 90% of patients. SS-B (La) is considered more specific than SS-A (Ro), because the latter also occurs in 30 to 50% of patients with SLE. (Remember, the "SS" stands for Sjögren's syndrome and not systemic sclerosis!). An antibody (anti-Sm) directed against a different antiribonucleoprotein known as the Smith antigen is highly specific for (virtually diagnostic of) SLE and is not seen in Sjögren's syndrome. *(pp. 201; 209)*

**(89)** Antibodies to intrinsic factor (IF) and gastric parietal cells are distinctive features of the atrophic fundal gastritis associated with pernicious anemia. The antibodies mediate immunologic destruction of gastrtic parietal cells, the cells that make both HCl and IF. Thus, hypo- or achlorhydria is produced, and about 10% of patients develop an overt megaloblastic (pernicious) anemia as a result of their inability to absorb vitamin $B_{12}$, a cofactor required for DNA synthesis. *(p. 607)*

**(90)** Antimitochondrial antibodies are seen in 95% of patients with primary biliary cirrhosis (PBC), a chronic destructive inflammatory condition of intrahepatic bile ducts. Although PBC is characterized by a number of immunologic abnormalities, direct proof that the duct destruction is immunologically mediated is still lacking. Why antibodies to mitochondria develop is also unclear, but the phenomenon is virtually diagnostic of PBC. *(p. 868)*

**(92)** Myasthenia gravis is an autoimmune disease caused by antibodies to acetylcholinesterase receptors (AChR) on postsynaptic membranes at neuromuscular junctions. Receptors are destroyed, and transmission of nerve impulses across neuromuscular junctions is lost, resulting in generalized loss of muscle function. Circulating anti-AChR autoantibodies are present in virtually all patients with myasthenia gravis, and they can transfer the disease passively to animals. *(p. 1292)*

**(93)** Grave's disease is autoimmune hyperthyroidism caused by antibodies to the thyroid-stimulating hormone (TSH) receptors on thyroid follicular cells that mimic the functions of TSH. These antibodies are thought to stimulate both thyroid hyperfunction and growth, producing both goiter and hyperthyroidism. *(p. 1129)*

**94. (A); 95. (A); 96. (A); 97. (D); 98. (C); 99. (C); 100. (D); 101. (C); 102. (B); 103. (B)**

During cutaneous wound healing, three diverse cell types—keratinocytes, fibroblasts, and endothelial cells—synchronously proliferate and interact to repair the defect.

**(94)** Unlike fibroblasts, which normally undergo proliferation only in response to tissue injury (a "stable" cell type), epidermal cells undergo continuous proliferation throughout life (a "labile" cell type). **(95)** Following a cutaneous wound such as a surgical incision, epidermal cells rapidly migrate across the wound, establishing epithelial continuity within 24 to 48 hours. This speedy response takes place long before the reparative response of the underlying connective tissue has begun to evolve. **(96)** The basal cells of the newly reformed epithelium lay down new basement membrane, the primary component of which is type IV collagen. **(97)** Fibroblasts produce both type I and type III collagen, but neither keratinocytes nor fibroblasts produce type II collagen, a type found only in cartilage, intervertebral discs, and the vitreous body.

**(98 and 99)** Fibroblasts are capable of abetting the process of epithelial cell migration across the wound surface through their production of fibronectin. This large glycoprotein promotes epithelial cell attachment and spreading upon the extracellular matrix (ECM) below. Fibronectin binds to a number of ECM proteins, including collagen, fibrin, heparin, and proteoglycans. It also binds to cells via specific integrin receptors (transmembrane glycoproteins that bind to the cell skeleton on the *inside* of the cell and to ECM elements on the *outside* of the cell). Thus, epithelial cell adhesion to the ECM is mediated through fibronectin binding. The interaction with fibronectin is a signal for epithelial cell migration, spreading, and, ultimately, permanent attachment to the ECM (via regeneration of the complex structures of the dermoepidermal junction). Keratinocytes can also synthesize fibronectin, so they are capable of aiding themselves in this process. Fibroblast migration across the healing wound is promoted by fibronectin through similar mechanisms, and in addition, fibronectin fragments are chemotactic for fibroblasts.

**(100)** Fibroblasts and epithelial cells are activated and induced to divide by growth factors present in healing wounds. Two of the most important growth factors (polypeptide cytokines that act locally as hormones to modulate cellular activity) involved in wound healing have been given the unfortunate and misleading names of "transforming" growth factors. These growth factors first were isolated from transformed cells and were believed to be involved in the transforming process. However, they now are known to be products of normal cells and to play key roles in regulating normal processes such as embryogenesis and wound healing by inducing cell growth and differentiation. Transforming growth factor-β (TGF-β) is produced by a wide variety of cell types, including macrophages, endothelial cells, platelets, T cells, and epithelial cells. It stimulates fibroblast chemotaxis, collagen production, and fibronectin expression and inhibits collagen breakdown by decreasing protease production and increasing protease inhibitor production. Thus, its net effect is fibrogenesis (scar formation). It is not directly mitogenic for either fibroblasts or epithelial cells. Indirectly, through stimulation of platelet-derived growth factor (which *is* mitogenic for fibroblasts), fibroblast proliferation may be increased in the presence of TGF-β in the right circumstances. However, TGF-β is a growth inhibitor for epithelial cells, and, at high concentrations, is growth inhibitory for fibroblasts as well.

**(101)** Transforming growth factor-α (TGF-α) is a polypeptide similar to epidermal growth factor (EGF), a factor named for its ability to enhance epidermal proliferation and keratinization. However, TGF-α is a mitogen for fibroblasts as well. TGF-α binds to EGF receptors on cells and produces the same biologic responses as EGF.

**(102 and 103)** Other factors that stimulate fibroblast activity and proliferation during the wound healing process are platelet-derived growth factor (PDGF) and interleukin-1 (IL-1). PDGF is a polypeptide stored in the α granules of platelets and released on platelet activation. It also is produced by macrophages, endothelial cells, smooth muscle cells, and epithelial cells. It is a powerful mitogen and chemotactic factor for fibroblasts, smooth muscle cells, and monocytes. IL-1 is a polypeptide that, besides stimulating proliferation of fibroblasts, stimulates both collagen and collagenase synthesis by fibroblasts. Many cells (e.g., monocytes, macrophages, endothelial cells, glial cells, and keratinocytes) produce IL-1. *(pp. 36–37; 40–42; 70; 85–89)*

**104. (C); 105. (C); 106. (A); 107. (B); 108. (B); 109. (C); 110. (A); 111. (A); 112. (C); 113. (D); 114. (D); 115. (D)**

Sadly, a great number of debilitating inflammatory conditions and human cancers are caused by the chronic use of two readily available but highly injurious substances, cigarettes and alcohol.

**(104, 105, and 109)** The esophagus and stomach are both highly susceptible to injury and neoplastic transformation by cigarettes and alcohol. Acute esophagitis, acute gastritis, and esophageal carcinoma are all related causally to both cigarettes and alcohol. **(108)** Chronic alcohol abuse is also associated with an increased risk of stomach cancer. *(pp. 381–383; 390; 761; 764; 771)*

**(112)** Pharyngeal carcinoma is linked closely with both cigarette smoke and alcohol. *(pp. 382; 390)*

**(106 and 107)** The pancreas responds somewhat differently to each of the two substances. Acute and chronic pancreatitis are linked to alcohol abuse, whereas pancreatic carcinoma is associated with cigarette smoking. *(pp. 382; 389; 901–902; 905)*

**(110 and 111)** Cancers of the gastrointestinal tract are not the only extrapulmonary malignancies linked to cigarette smoking, however. Transitional cell carcinoma of the bladder and renal cell carcinoma also occur with significantly greater frequency in cigarette smokers. Alcohol consumption does not appear to be linked causally to these malignancies. *(pp. 986; 1001)*

**(113, 114, and 115)** There is no significantly increased risk of developing Hodgkin's disease, ovarian carcinoma, or breast cancer with either cigarette smoking or alcohol abuse, but this is small consolation. *(pp. 647; 1101; 1065)*

**116. (E); 117. (D); 118. (D); 119. (A); 120. (A)**

Fatty change refers to intracellular accumulation of triglycerides (neutral lipids) within parenchymal cells produced by some imbalance in the cellular production, utilization, or mobilization of fat. It is usually the result of some form of nonlethal cell injury. Although it may occur in other organs (e.g., heart, skeletal muscle, kidney), fatty change is seen most frequently in the liver (the major site of fat metabolism).

**(116)** In the United States, alcohol is the most common cause of fatty liver. It has a variety of lipogenic effects, including increased free fatty acid mobilization and entry into liver cells, decreased fatty acid oxidation, increased esterification of fatty acids to triglycerides, and decreased production of apoprotein (the protein to which lipid must be coupled in order to export it from the cell).

**(117 and 118)** Both toxic exposure to carbon tetrachloride and protein malnutrition lead to lipid accumulation in liver cells by reducing apoprotein synthesis, which consequently decreases secretion of lipoprotein (the export form of lipid).

**(119 and 120)** Increased lipid mobilization from adipose tissue leading to excessive entry of free fatty acids into the liver is the major mechanisms of hepatic fatty change caused by corticosteroids or starvation. *(pp. 14; 25–26)*

**121. (D); 122. (C); 123. (D); 124. (C); 125. (A)**

**(121)** Although pigment accumulation is usually not harmful to cells, it can be a distinctive marker for specific pathologic processes. For example, in patients with alkaptonuria, a rare inherited metabolic disease, accumulation of the brown-black pigment homogentisic acid occurs in the skin, connective tissue, and cartilage. The pigmentation of tissues that occurs in alkaptonuria is known as ochronosis. *(p. 28)*

**(122)** Patients with mitral stenosis classically develop brown, indurated lungs. The brown color is due to hemosiderin accumulation secondary to chronic leakage of red blood cells from damaged pulmonary vessels (the damage results from chronic pulmonary hypertension). *(pp. 681–682)*

**(123)** The black color of the lungs in coal miners, however, is due to a marked accumulation of inhaled exogenous carbon pigment. To a lesser degree, this also occurs in the lungs of city dwellers as a result of urban air pollution. *(pp. 28; 706)*

**(124)** Pigmented villonodular synovitis is an unusual condition of unknown etiology characterized by neoplastic synovial overgrowth usually involving the knee or hip. Typically, the proliferating mass of synovium is variably pigmented by hemosiderin, presumably of traumatic origin. *(p. 1260)*

**(125)** In yet another bizarre condition called melanosis coli, the colonic mucosa becomes diffusely blackened by deposition of melanin-like pigment in mucosal macrophages. The pigment is derived from lipofuscin, polymers of lipid and phospholipid complexed with protein. These complexes result from lipid peroxidation of cellular membranes occurring during cell injury. In this case, the injury to colonic epithelial cells is produced by cathartics of the antracene (anthraquinone) type. *(p. 28)*

**126. (A); 127. (C); 128. (B); 129. (B); 130. (D)**

Hypertrophy, hyperplasia, and metaplasia are adaptive changes that cells may undergo in response to alterations in their environment. In brief, hypertrophy refers to increased cell size, hyperplasia to an increase in cell numbers, and metaplasia to a change in cell type occurring via altered cellular differentiation. Dysplasia, in contrast, is considered to be a pathologic rather than an adaptive response. Dysplasia refers to derangements in cellular responses that result in atypical development. In epithelial tissues, dysplasia is associated strongly with the development of carcinoma and often precedes the appearance of overt malignancy.

**(126)** The response of cardiac muscle to systemic hypertension is a classic example of cellular hypertrophy. Cardiac myocytes do not undergo cell division in postnatal life. Therefore, in the absence of the ability to proliferate, cardiac muscle cells respond to an increased work load by enlarging. Each cell becomes larger by increasing its cytoplasmic content of contractile elements. *(pp. 37; 46; 542)*

**(127)** One of the cardinal histopathologic features of chronic bronchitis is goblet cell metaplasia of the bronchiolar epithelium. In contrast to normal bronchioles, which are lined only by ciliated columnar cells and Clara cells, the bronchioles of the chronic bronchitic contain large numbers of mucin-producing goblet cells. These develop from the bronchiolar reserve cells as a result of chronic exposure to cigarette smoke or other noxious agents. Early in the course of the disease, the metaplastic change is an adaptive one and appears to be reversible. *(pp. 48; 689)*

**(128)** Prolonged increased stimulation by adrenocorticotrophic hormone (ACTH) typically induces adrenocortical hyperplasia. The hyperplasia may be nodular or diffuse, and its extent is a function of the duration and level of the ACTH excess. *(pp. 44; 1151–1152)*

**(129)** The "hypertrophy" referred to in the disorder known as benign prostatic hypertrophy is that of the entire gland, which undergoes diffuse nodular enlargement. On microscopic examination, however, it becomes obvious that the glandular enlargement is due to hyperplasia of both the stromal and glandular elements of the tissue. Thus, the disease is now more properly termed nodular hyperplasia of the prostate. *(pp. 1025–1026)*

**(130)** Perhaps the most important pathologic change associated with long-standing ulcerative colitis is dysplasia of the colonic epithelium. Patients with ulcerative colitis are at increased risk of developing colonic carcinoma, and epithelial dysplasia precedes the development of malignancy in these patients. Epithelial dysplasia therefore is considered a premalignant change. Surveillance biopsy procedures are performed in patients with long-standing disease with the goal of detecting high-grade dysplastic changes and performing prophylactic colectomy before overt malignancy develops. *(p. 806)*

**131. (A); 132. (B); 133. (D); 134. (E); 135. (A); 136. (C); 137. (B); 138. (A); 139. (A); 140. (E)**

As the name implies, autoimmune diseases are disorders caused by immunologic attack directed against constituents of the body's own tissues ("self-antigens"). Both systemic lupus erythematosus (SLE) and systemic sclerosis (scleroderma) are primary autoimmune disease processes involving multiple organ systems. Although Sjögren's syndrome may occur in primary form as an isolated disorder (known as the "sicca syndrome"), it is usually a secondary process occurring in association with other autoimmune diseases.

**(131)** SLE is believed to be caused by a fundamental defect in the immune system producing abnormalities of both B and T cells. The disorder has a genetic predisposition, but expression of the disease in predisposed individuals may be influenced by environmental factors. In 6% of cases, SLE is associated with an inherited deficiency of the second component of complement (C2), the genes for which are located within the major histocompatibility complex (MHC) along with the genes for the histocompatibility antigens (see Questions 46 and 50). Thus, the association of SLE and hereditary C2 deficiency may reflect genetic derangements in certain chromosomal regions governing the immune response. **(135)** Although SLE involves virtually every organ system, joint involvement with articular pain is the single most common clinical manifestation and must be differentiated from other forms of arthritis. **(138)** The most devastating manifestation, however, is kidney involvement. Lupus nephritis may lead to renal failure, the major cause of mortality in SLE. **(139)** As in many other autoimmune disorders, skin involvement is common in SLE. In contrast to the skin involvement in dermatomyositis, systemic sclerosis, and chronic discoid lupus erythematosus, immunoglobulin deposition is found along the dermoepidermal junction of normal-appearing as well as clinically involved skin in SLE.

**(132)** Sjögren's syndrome is an uncomfortable disorder characterized by dry eyes and dry mouth resulting from immunologically mediated destruction of lacrimal and salivary glands. It also has the unfortunate distinction of being associated with a 40-fold increased risk of developing a lymphoid malignancy. **(137)** Another feature of Sjögren's syndrome that distinguishes it from SLE and systemic sclerosis is the rarity of glomerular lesions, which are quite common in the latter two disorders. Instead of glomerular disease, renal involvement in Sjögren's syndrome takes the form of tubulointerstitial nephritis.

**(133)** Dermatomyositis, an "inflammatory" myopathy, is actually an autoimmune process. It may occur alone or in association with other autoimmune connective tissue disorders, including SLE, Sjögren's syndrome, and systemic sclerosis (the most commonly associated disease).

**(134)** Women with dermatomyositis have an increased risk of developing visceral cancers (lung, stomach, ovary), but neither SLE, Sjögren's syndrome, nor systemic sclerosis is known to increase the risk of visceral malignancy.

**(136)** Systemic sclerosis, a disorder characterized by excessive collagen synthesis with systemic fibrosis, shares a variety of serologic abnormalities with other autoimmune connective tissue disorders. Two autoantibodies more or less unique to systemic sclerosis are useful in establishing this diagnosis: an anticentromere antibody and an antibody directed against a nonhistone nuclear protein called Scl-70 (see Questions 85 and 88).

**(140)** Although immunosuppression with corticosteroids is of variable benefit in controlling the clinical manifestations of most autoimmune connective tissue disorders, a consistently excellent response to this mode of therapy is associated only with mixed connective tissue disease. *(pp. 199–215)*

**141. (A); 142. (D); 143. (C); 144. (A); 145. (B); 146. (B); 147. (C)**

In contrast to immunodeficiencies that arise as a secondary consequence of infection, malnutrition, aging, autoimmune disease, or exposure to immunosuppressive agents, primary immunodeficiency disorders are almost always genetic in origin.

**(141 and 144)** X-linked agammaglobulinemia of Bruton is the most common form of primary immunodeficiency disease. As the name denotes, it is an X-linked disorder, restricted to males. It is caused by a defect in pre–B cell maturation and is characterized by a virtual absence of immunoglobulin production. The gene responsible for X-linked agammaglobulinemia encodes a protein-tyrosine kinase (involved in signal transduction pathways) that is expressed in B cells but not in T cells. Indeed, T cells are unaffected in this disease. Because the defect abrogates humoral immune responses, patients are subject to recurrent bacterial infections. Somewhat paradoxically, however, affected individuals are at greatly increased risk of developing autoimmune diseases such as systemic lupus erythematosus, rheumatoid arthritis, and dermatomyositis. Although a high frequency of rheumatoid arthritis also is associated with common variable immunodeficiency (CVI), systemic lupus erythematosus is not particularly common in association with this disease as compared with X-linked agammaglobulinemia of Bruton.

**(142)** As in X-linked agammaglobulinemia of Bruton, CVI and DiGeorge's syndrome both are characterized by derangements in immunocyte maturation rather than an underlying defect in lymphoid stem cells. A stem cell defect produces deficiencies of both B and T cells and results in a much more serious disease known as severe combined immunodeficiency.

**(143)** DiGeorge's syndrome is a selective T cell deficiency. It is caused by a failure of development of the third and fourth pharyngeal pouches, the embryologic origin of both the thymus and the parathyroids. Thus, a total absence of cell-mediated immunity is accompanied by deranged serum calcium regulation and tetany in this disease. **(147)** Both Bruton's X-linked agammaglobulinemia and CVI are frequently complicated by persistent intestinal infection with *Giardia lamblia*, which produces chronic diarrhea and malabsorption. In contrast, this complication is not associated with DiGeorge's syndrome.

**(145 and 146)** CVI represents a heterogeneous group of disorders characterized by hypogammaglobulinemia (usually involving all antibody classes but sometimes limited to immunoglobulin G) related to abnormal immunoregulation and/or defective B cell differentiation. The underlying molecular defect varies from case to case and may involve either B cell or T cell function. It is a relatively common form of immunodeficiency and often is associated with specific changes in the complement genes, especially deletions of the C4A gene and rare alleles of the C2 gene. Of graver significance is the association of this disorder with the development of lymphoid malignancy, which sometimes develops late in the course of the disease. *(pp. 221–223)*

**148. (A); 149. (B); 150. (B); 151. (C); 152. (A); 153. (C); 154. (B); 155. (E); 156. (A); 157. (B); 158. (D); 159. (A)**

Edema is the term that refers to the accumulation of an abnormal amount of fluid in the interstitial tissue spaces or body cavities. Ascites is a localized form of edema in which edema fluid collects in the peritoneal cavity. Edema is the result of a disturbance in the balance of forces that normally keep about 75% of all the extracellular fluid within the intravascular compartment. The remaining 25% of body fluid is contained in the interstitium of tissues and is separated from the intravascular fluid by the semipermeable barrier provided by the endothelium and its basement membrane.

Maintenance of the balance between the interstitial and intravascular fluid compartments depends on several factors: (1) the intravascular hydrostatic pressure, (2) the oncotic pressure exerted by the plasma proteins, (3) the hydrostatic pressure of the interstitial fluid, (4) the lymphatic drainage of the interstitial tissue spaces, and (5) the integrity of the vascular endothelium. Disorders that promote edema either decrease plasma oncotic pressure, lymphatic drainage, or endothelial integrity, or they increase intravascular hydrostatic pressure or osmotic tension in the interstitial fluid (usually related to sodium retention). In some diseases, several of these alterations occur simultaneously.

**(148 and 159)** Decreased plasma oncotic pressure is the major cause of edema in the nephrotic syndrome, kwashiorkor, hydrops fetalis, and Ménétrier's disease. In the nephrotic syndrome, excessive glomerular permeability results in the loss of large amounts of protein (largely albumin) into the urine. Excessive protein loss is also the underlying problem in Ménétrier's disease, but, in this condition, protein is secreted into the gut in the form of mucus produced by hyperplastic gastric mucosal cells.

**(152 and 156)** Underproduction (rather than excessive loss) of plasma proteins is the underlying defect in both kwashiorkor and hydrops fetalis. In kwashiorkor, profound protein malnutrition produces severe protein deprivation in all tissues of the body, including the liver, severely limiting hepatic plasma protein production. In hydrops fetalis, the result of a hemolytic anemia produced by blood-group incompatibility between mother and child, hypoxic injury to the liver leads to markedly reduced synthesis of albumin and other major plasma proteins.

**(149)** Increased intravascular hydrostatic pressure is the major contributor to the edema associated with congestive heart failure, pregnancy, and constrictive pericarditis. In congestive heart failure, the most common cause of edema, the failing heart is unable to generate a normal cardiac output. Consequently, blood is not emptied adequately from the venous system of the lungs (left heart failure) or the systemic venous system (right heart failure), increasing venous hydrostatic pressure in the lungs or the periphery, respectively.

**(154 and 157)** In pregnancy and constrictive pericarditis, venous return to the heart is restricted by external compression, and hydrostatic pressure in the venous system proximal to the point of compression increases. Thus pregnancy-associated edema is primarily in the lower extremities, whereas the edema associated with constrictive pericarditis is characteristically systemic.

**(150)** In cirrhosis, hepatic scarring and obliteration of portal architecture greatly diminish portal flow through the liver and increase hydrostatic pressure in the portal system, producing ascites. In some cases of cirrhosis, decreased hepatic cell numbers and/or function also may lead to a decrease in albumin production and the resultant decrease in plasma oncotic pressure will contribute to the ascites/edema. Unless accompanied by severe malnutrition, however, decreased albumin production is seldom severe enough to be a major factor. The principal contribution to the edema/ascites in nearly all cases of cirrhosis is portal hypertension.

**(151)** Disruption of endothelial integrity with increased vascular permeability produces edema in thermal burns and bee stings. In thermal burns, direct tissue injury as well as mediators of vascular permeability generated in the accompanying inflammatory response lead to a massive outpouring of fluid into injured tissues. **(153)** Bee stings most commonly produce a mild inflammatory response and localized edema. In sensitized individuals, however, immunoglobulin E–mediated hypersensitivity responses lead to increased vascular permeability on a wider scale, producing either hives or anaphylaxis.

**(158)** Edema associated with metastatic carcinoma is most often the result of lymphatic blockage by tumor. Other mechanisms, such as venous compression by tumor, protein wasting, or hepatic replacement by metastatic tumor, are possible, but less common, causes.

**(155)** Excessive salt intake in normal individuals ordinarily does not cause edema. In those predisposed to sodium retention, however, edema may result from elevated osmotic pressure in interstitial fluid containing increased numbers of sodium ions. *(pp. 93–95)*

**160. (E); 161. (A); 162. (D); 163. (E); 164. (C); 165. (B); 166. (E); 167. (B); 168. (A)**

Morphological patterns of tissue necrosis depend on the balance between progressive enzymatic digestion of dead cells and coagulation of denatured proteins in the cytoplasm of dead cells. At least four distinctive morphologic patterns of necrosis can be recognized: coagulation necrosis, liquefaction necrosis, enzymatic fat necrosis, and caseous necrosis.

**(160)** Although many infectious diseases cause tissue necrosis of some type, a few notable exceptions exist. In cholera, for example, a severe secretory diarrhea is produced as a result of the pathophysiologic effects of an enterotoxin elaborated by *Vibrio cholerae* on small bowel absorptive cells. Although the toxin alters intracellular physiologic processes, it does not kill the cells. Thus, no cellular necrosis is produced in this disease.

**(161 and 168)** Coagulation necrosis is the most common pattern of necrosis and is characterized by preservation of the basic cellular shape, permitting recognition of the cell outlines and tissue architecture despite the loss of nuclei from the dead cells. It is the result of coagulation of denatured proteins in dead cells and delayed proteolysis by lysosomal enzymes. This type of necrosis commonly occurs in myocardial infarction with ischemic necrosis of myocytes. Coagulation necrosis also predominates in acute tubular necrosis resulting from sudden severe ischemia to the kidney or after chemical injury, such as mercuric chloride poisoning. In these injuries, entire renal tubules may undergo necrosis but the outlines of the tubular epithelial cells still can be recognized.

**(165 and 167)** Liquefaction necrosis is the result of enzymatic digestion of dead cells, resulting in obliteration of tissue architecture. This occurs when lysosomal enzymes within the dead and dying cells are activated (autolysis) or when the powerful hydrostatic enzymes of bacteria or leukocytes contribute to the digestion of dead cells (heterolysis). This pattern of necrosis characteristically occurs in wet gangrene of an extremity. In wet gangrene, the liquefactive action of bacteria (*Clostridia*) and attracted leukocytes both contribute to this pattern of necrosis. Liquefaction necrosis is also characteristic of ischemic destruction of brain tissue, but in this case the process is primarily autolytic in nature.

**(164)** Enzymatic fat necrosis is highly characteristic of acute pancreatitis. In this condition powerful lipases and proteases are released into the surrounding peripancreatic fat. They catalyze the decomposition of triglycerides that leak from the damaged adipose cells, producing free fatty acids. Indistinct outlines of necrotic adipose cells are seen in association with granular, basophilic deposits that represent calcium soaps formed by the reaction of calcium with the released free fatty acids.

**(162)** Pott's disease is the term by which tuberculous spondylitis is known. The granulomatous lesions of *Mycobacterium tuberculosis*, wherever they are found in the body, are characterized by a distinctive pattern of necrosis known as caseation. Caseous necrosis represents a combination of coagulative and liquefactive necrosis in which the outlines of the dead cells are neither totally destroyed nor well preserved. Grossly, caseous necrosis resembles clumped cheesy material, and, microscopically, distinctive amorphous granular debris is seen. This pattern of necrosis is highly characteristic of mycobacterial infection.

**(163)** Although tuberculoid granulomas are characteristic of the vigorous T cell–mediated immune response mounted by individuals infected with *Mycobacterium leprae* in tuberculoid leprosy, the granulomatous lesions do not characteristically undergo necrosis and instead remain as hard tubercles.

**(166)** Infection with the intestinal flagellate *Giardia lamblia* usually produces dramatic symptoms, including copious watery diarrhea, cramps, and even malabsorption (steatorrhea). Ironically, however, the organism often causes relatively few morphologic changes in the small bowel. Although the intestinal morphology may range from virtually normal to markedly abnormal with villous flattening, necrosis is virtually never seen. *(pp. 15–17; 326; 333–334; 339; 366; 534; 701–702; 900)*

**169. (B); 170. (D); 171. (A); 172. (C); 173. (C); 174. (D); 175. (B); 176. (A); 177. (E); 178. (E); 179. (E); 180. (D)**

Although immune responses are essential for survival in a world filled with microbes, they also can cause debilitating and even fatal diseases. Disorders resulting from tissue-damaging immune reactions can be separated into four major categories based on the immunologic mechanism that mediates the disease.

**(171 and 176)** Hay fever and penicillin-induced urticaria are both examples of type I (anaphylactic type) hypersensitivity responses. In type I disease (disease mediated by a type I hypersensitivity immune response), exposure to an antigen leads to the production of cytotropic immunoglobulin E antibodies that become affixed to mast cells and basophils. On re-exposure, antigen combines with the cell-bound antibody, triggering release of vasoactive amines (histamine and adenosine) from granules within the cell. These agents increase vascular permeability and produce edema within a few minutes following degranulation. Depending on the allergen and the portal of entry, localized reactions may take the form of cutaneous swellings (hives, or urticaria), nasal and conjunctival discharge, hay fever, bronchial asthma, or allergic gastroenteritis. Systemic reactions, often developing after an intravenous injection of the offending antigen, can produce a state of shock that is sometimes fatal. *(pp. 178–180)*

**(169 and 175)** Erythroblastosis fetalis (a hemolytic anemia in the newborn caused by blood group incompatibility between mother and child) and hemolytic anemia induced by the antihypertensive agent α-methyldopa (dopamine) are examples of type II diseases. Type II (cytotoxic type) hypersensitivity responses are caused by the formation of antibodies directed toward molecules present on the surface of cells or toward other tissue components. The antigen may be one intrinsic to the cell membrane or an adsorbed exogenous antigen. Antibody-coated cells are then susceptible to three separate modes of injury: (1) complement activation and direct complement-mediated membrane damage; (2) phagocytosis promoted by opsonization; or (3) antibody-dependent cell-mediated cytotoxicity (ADCC). In ADCC reactions, immunoglobulin G (IgG)–coated target cells are killed by nonsensitized cells bearing Fc receptors for IgG, such as monocytes, neutrophils, eosinophils, and natural killer (NK) cells. In erythroblastosis fetalis, the mother's immune system reacts to blood group antigens expressed by the fetal red blood cells. In the dopamine-induced hemolytic anemia, the drug initiates (in some unknown manner) the production of antibodies that are directed against intrinsic red blood cell antigens. The red cell antigens that are usually the target of the immunologic response in dopamine-induced hemolytic anemia are the Rh blood group antigens. *(pp. 182–184; 602)*

**(172 and 173)** Polyarteritis nodosa and acute poststreptococcal glomerulonephritis are examples of type III diseases (immune complex disorders). Type III hypersensitivity responses are caused by antigen-antibody complexes that cause tissue damage through their ability to activate a variety of serum mediators (principally complement). Such a reaction usually (but not always) requires at least two exposures to the antigen: a sensitizing exposure to induce circulating antibody followed by a second exposure sometime later. However, persistence of the antigen through the phase of the primary immune response when circulating antibody is present also can lead to immune complex formation. Polyarteritis nodosa is a necrotizing form of vasculitis thought to be produced by complement-fixing immune complexes that become localized to vessel walls, particularly those of small or medium-sized muscular arteries. Although the inciting antigen is not known in most cases, about 30% of patients with polyarteritis nodosa have hepatitis B antigen in their serum and circulating HBsAg-anti-HBs immune complexes. In acute poststreptococcal glomerulonephritis, immune responses to infection by nephritogenic strains of streptococci result in the formation of complement-fixing immune complexes that lodge in the glomerular basement membrane. This causes glomerular inflammation and injury and results in hematuria, proteinuria, and azotemia. *(pp. 184–186; 945–946)*

**(170, 174, and 180)** Hypersensitivity responses mediated by specifically sensitized T lymphocytes are known as type IV (cell-mediated) reactions. Poison ivy dermatitis, graft-versus-host disease, and chronic berylliosis are all examples of cell-mediated hypersensitivity. The eczematous dermatitis produced by poison ivy results from a delayed hypersensitivity response mounted against plant-derived antigens that have become affixed to epidermal cells. In graft-versus-host disease, the immunocompetent cells in the grafted tissue mount an immune response against the tissue antigens of the immunocompromised recipient. In chronic berylliosis, T cells immunized against beryllium initiate granuloma formation, the hallmark of chronic berylliosis. Through their production of lymphokines, the sensitized T cells are able to regulate macrophage activity and induce the formation of granulomas (clusters of epithelioid histiocytes). *(pp. 187–189; 194; 712; 1194–1195)*

**(177 through 179)** In cyclosporine-induced renal injury, chlorpromazine-induced cholestatic jaundice, and pulmonary asbestosis, the tissue injury is caused by the direct toxic effects of the causative agent. Immunologic responses are not known to play any direct role in these disorders. *(pp. 384; 388; 710)*

**181. (D); 182. (D); 183. (E); 184. (A); 185. (A); 186. (E); 187. (A); 188. (E); 189. (A); 190. (C); 191. (C); 192. (D)**

**(181, 182, and 192)** The three major cell types that comprise the immune system are T lymphocytes, B lymphocytes, and macrophages. In varying proportions, all of these cell types are found in the circulating blood (monocytes are the circulating form of macrophages) and in the peripheral lymphoid tissues, and all arise from stem cells in the bone marrow. In the cortex of lymph nodes, B cells are found primarily in the germinal centers, whereas T cells and macrophages are found predominantly in the paracortical zones. *(pp. 171–173; 629–630)*

**(184, 185, 187, and 189)** T lymphocytes are the major effector cells in cellular immune reactions such as delayed hypersensitivity responses and in the regulation (both initiation and termination) of all immune responses. Unlike B cells and macrophages/monocytes, the great majority of T lymphocytes do not display class II histocompatibility antigens (HLA-D) on their cell surface, nor do they have cell surface receptors for complement. *(pp. 172–173; 175–177)*

**(183)** B lymphocytes are the major effector cells in humoral immune responses. They express antigen-specific cell surface immunoglobulin (IgM) that constitutes the antigen-binding component of the B cell receptor. The cell surface immunoglobulin is identical in specificity to the immunoglobulin secreted by that cell when it differentiates into a plasma cell. *(p. 173)*

**(190 and 191)** Macrophages play several key roles in the immune response. They function as antigen-presenting cells and also act as powerful effector cells in cell-mediated immune responses (usually under the direction of cytokines produced by activated T cells). Along with mast cells and neutrophils, macrophages produce lipoxygenase derivatives of arachidonic acid, known as leukotrienes. Leukotrienes $C_4$, $D_4$, and $E_4$ are powerful mediators of anaphylaxis. In addition, macrophages respond chemotactically to another of these lipoxygenase derivatives, leukotriene $B_4$, a mediator of acute inflammation. *(pp. 65; 69; 173)*

**(186 and 188)** Although macrophages are capable of ingesting and lysing antibody-coated target cells, only natural killer (NK) cells are capable of lysing antibody-coated target cells by means of a nonphagocytic mechanism. This process, called antibody-dependent cellular cytotoxicity (ADCC), requires previous sensitization by the antigen and the production of cytophilic antibody. NK cells also are capable of lysing target cells, such as tumor cells or virus-infected cells, without previous sensitization. Although NK cells share some cell surface properties with T cells, B cells, and macrophages, they are thought to be distinct from any of these cell types. They are considered to be important as the first line of defense against tumors and viral infections. *(pp. 173–174)*

**193. (D); 194. (D); 195. (C); 196. (E); 197. (E); 198. (B); 199. (A); 200. (B); 201. (B); 202. (E)**

Pigment accumulation in cells is most often the result of a pathologic process. Normal examples of pigment accumulation are few and include melanin in melanocytes and in neighboring basal keratinocytes of the skin and iron stores in the form of hemosiderin in the bone marrow. Examples of pathologic accumulations of pigment in cells are much more numerous, however, and certain disorders characteristically produce accumulations of a specific pigment type.

**(193 and 194)** Lipofuscin, an insoluble brown pigment that is the product of cell membrane breakdown—often the result of lipid peroxidation by free radicals—is considered "wear-and-tear" or aging pigment. It is present in abundance in the heart and liver of elderly, malnourished individuals. In severe cases, when lipofuscin deposition is accompanied by organ shrinkage, the condition is known as "brown atrophy." Lipofuscin is not injurious to cells, nor does it interfere with cellular function.

**(195)** Ceroid pigment is lipofuscin that has been altered chemically, probably by auto-oxidation. It commonly is found in Kupffer's cells in the liver following hepatocellular injury. Lipofuscin is liberated from dying liver cells and taken up by sinusoidal phagocytes that convert it to ceroid pigment.

**(199)** In liver diseases that disrupt the flow of bile, such as large bile duct obstruction, profound cholestasis ensues, and bile "infarcts" (liver cell necrosis caused by spilled bile) may occur. In this setting, Kupffer's cells mop up the spilled bile and become laden with bilirubin, the major bile pigment.

**(198, 200, and 201)** Hemosiderin is an iron-containing pigment whose precise chemical composition is unknown. It commonly is seen within mononuclear phagocytes following a massive hemolytic crisis such as that which may occur in malaria or a hemolytic transfusion reaction. In conditions characterized by increased destruction of red blood cells, such as hereditary spherocytosis (see Chapter 7, Question 1), large deposits of hemosiderin are found in mononuclear phagocytes. Hemosiderin pigment also accumulates in any local or systemic excess of iron. Iron excess can result from any one of a number of conditions, including increased absorption of dietary iron, impaired utilization of iron, hemolytic anemias, or blood transfusions (an exogenous iron load).

**(196, 197, and 202)** Carbon is the pigment encountered in sinus histiocytes of the lungs and peribronchial lymph nodes of smokers. In tattooed skin, carbon is injected into the dermal tissues and taken up by dermal macrophages. The hyperpigmentation that occurs in Addison's disease, a condition caused by adrenal insufficiency, is seen microscopically as an accumulation of melanin in epidermal keratinocytes. Increased melanocytic production of melanin in Addison's disease is the result of increased adrenocorticotropic hormone released from the pituitary gland. One end of this molecule is homologous to melanocyte-stimulating hormone. *(pp. 28–29)*

**203. (A); 204. (E); 205. (B); 206. (B); 207. (A); 208. (C); 209. (D); 210. (C); 211. (C); 212. (C)**

The composition of the inflammatory cell infiltrate found in injured tissues is primarily determined by the type of underlying pathologic process (immunologic or inflammatory). However, there is much overlap in the cellular responses evoked by these two processes. Although lymphocytes, monocytes, and plasma cells characteristically predominate in most immunologically mediated reactions, the same cell types are also present in inflammatory responses of a chronic nature. Neutrophilic infiltrates usually are associated with acute inflammatory reactions, but they are also present in necrotizing immunologic responses mediated by complement-fixing antibody or immune complexes.

**(203 and 207)** Neutrophils are the predominant inflammatory cell type present in infarcted myocardium 12 to 72 hours after injury. In this setting, they represent an acute inflammatory response to the necrotic tissue. Neutrophilic infiltrates are also characteristic of the early phases of development of polyarteritis nodosa. In this immune-mediated vasculitis, neutrophils are attracted by chemotactic cleavage fragments of complement (activated by the circulating immune complexes that cause the disease). *(pp. 536; 490–491)*

**(204)** Although its name implies that it is an acute inflammatory reaction, acute viral hepatitis B is caused by a cellular immune response to virally infected hepatocytes. The effector cells in this disease are cytotoxic lymphocytes, and they are the predominant cell type seen in the affected liver. *(pp. 845–846; 852)*

**(205)** Sarcoidosis is a systemic disease of unknown etiology that produces lesions identical to those of a delayed hypersensitivity response, suggesting that the disease may be caused by a persistent, poorly degradable antigen. Noncaseating granulomas composed of epithelioid histiocytes (macrophages), often with numerous Langhans' or foreign body-type giant cells, occur in virtually any tissue or organ in this disease. *(pp. 712–713)*

**(206)** Primary pulmonary tuberculosis is characterized by the formation of granulomas (composed of monocytes/macrophages) subjacent to the pleura in the upper part of the lower lobe or lower part of the upper lobe. The pulmonary granulomas may be accompanied by granulomas in the draining hilar nodes (which become enlarged). This pattern of primary infection is known as a "Ghon complex." *(p. 700)*

**(209)** Although primary syphilis is an acute bacterial infection caused by the spirochete *Treponema pallidum*, the associated inflammatory response is characteristically composed principally of plasma cells. This rather unusual feature is an important clue in the histopathologic diagnosis of this infection. *(p. 369)*

**(208, 210, 211, and 212)** Eosinophilic inflammation is characteristic of both anaphylactic type hypersensitivity responses and parasitic infections. Löffler's syndrome and bronchial asthma are both examples of type I allergic reactions in the lung with prominent eosinophilic infiltrates. The nematode infection known as filariasis is caused by either *Wuchereria bancrofti* or *Brugia malayi*. Filariasis is just one of many examples of parasitic infections that induce florid eosinophilic inflammatory infiltrates. For unknown reasons (probably chemical chemotaxis), eosinophils are also the characteristic inflammatory cell type associated with reflux esophagitis. *(pp. 374; 692; 716; 761)*

**213. (A); 214. (E); 215. (B); 216. (B); 217. (D); 218. (F); 219. (F); 220. (D)**

Cytokines are soluble chemical mediators that serve to direct activities both of cells of the immune system and other cell types during induction and regulation of immune responses. Most of these factors are made by macrophages and activated T cells, but some also are produced by other cell types.

**(213 and 214)** Interleukin-1 (IL-1), for example, is produced by virtually all cells, including activated T cells. Tumor necrosis factor (TNF) is a product of macrophages, T cells, natural killer (NK) cells, and epithelial cells. IL-1 and TNF are both mediators of inflammation, have many of the same biologic effects, and act synergistically. Both IL-1 and TNF activate T cells, B cells, and endothelial cells. They induce acute phase reactions associated with infection or injury: fever, granulocytosis, ACTH and corticosteroid release, and shock. They also share with IL-2 and γ-interferon (γ-IFN) the ability to activate macrophages.

**(215 and 216)** Interleukin-2 (IL-2), in contrast, is made only by activated T cells. IL-2 stimulates the growth of activated T and B cells, but, unlike IL-1, TNF, or γ-IFN, IL-2 also promotes the growth of NK cells (see Questions 217, 219, and 220).

**(217 and 220)** Interferons were originally discovered for their antiviral activity. Sensitized T cells are induced to produce interferon-α, -β, and -γ during viral infections. These interferons inhibit intracellular viral replication and, therefore, constitute an important host defense mechanism in viral infection. γ-IFN also has the unique ability among the cytokines to induce class II histocompatibility antigens on the surfaces of macrophages and many other cells that do not normally express class II human leukocyte antigen molecules.

**(218 and 219)** No cytokine has the ability to directly kill bacteria, and neither IL-1, IL-2, TNF, nor $\gamma$-IFN stimulates the growth of mast cells. The cytokines that stimulate hematopoiesis include a family of growth factors known as colony-stimulating factors (CSFs) and stem cell factor (c-kit ligand), which acts on pluripotential cells. Individual CSFs are named for the myeloid cell type on which they have their primary effect (e.g., granulocyte CSF, macrophage CSF, granulocyte-macrophage CSF). *(pp. 41; 73; 174–175; 189)*

**221. (A); 222. (D); 223. (B); 224. (E); 225. (B); 226. (C); 227. (A)**

**(221)** CD8+ cytotoxic/suppressor T cells and natural killer (NK) cells are both capable of destroying tumor cells and virally infected cells. CD4+ helper T cells do not attack and destroy such cells directly. Indirectly, however, helper/inducer T cells abet cytotoxic immune responses by promoting the generation and/or activation of CD8+ T cells and NK cells. **(222)** None of these cell types is phagocytic.

**(223 through 225)** Both CD4+ helper/inducer T cells and CD8+ cytotoxic/suppressor T cells are small lymphocytes, and small lymphocytes do not contain granules in their cytoplasm. In contrast to T cells, NK cells are large lymphocytes that characteristically contain cytoplasmic granules. Thus, they sometimes are referred to as "large granular lymphocytes." Because NK cells lack both T-cell receptors and surface immunoglobulins (characteristic of mature T cells or B cells, respectively), they previously had been termed "null cells." However, it was recognized that NK cells have distinctive properties and capabilities unique among lymphocytes. They are able to react to and lyse cells (e.g., tumor cells or virally infected cells) *without* prior sensitization. Like macrophages, NK cells possess receptors for the Fc fragment of immunoglobulin G. One mechanism by which NK cells effect cellular killing is through binding of their Fc receptors to antibody-coated target cells, a phenomenon known as antibody-dependent cellular cytotoxicity (ADCC). A separate mechanism requires direct interaction with the target cell that is not dependent on antibodies.

**(226 and 227)** Class I and class II major histocompatibility complex (MHC) molecules each are involved in the initiation of responses of distinct subsets of T cells. CD8+ cytotoxic/suppressor T cells recognize antigens only in association with class I MHC molecules, whereas CD4+ helper/inducer T cells recognize antigens only in association with class II MHC molecules. For example, cytotoxic/suppressor T cells can recognize and lyse only virally infected cells that bear class I MHC antigens on their surface. Helper/inducer T cells can recognize antigen only when presented simultaneously with class II MHC molecules on the surface of macrophages or dendritic cells. Although NK cells can detect and destroy virus-infected cells, they are not dependent on the process of MHC-associated antigen presentation to achieve their cytotoxic effect. *(pp. 170–174; 183–184)*

**228. (D); 229. (E); 230. (C); 231. (B); 232. (D); 233. (B); 234. (A); 235. (A); 236. (E); 237. (C); 238. (D); 239. (B)**

Disease processes and tissue injuries of specific types usually are associated with a characteristic pattern of inflammation that helps the pathologist to identify and diagnose them.

**(228 and 232)** Both cat scratch disease (infectious lymphadenitis) and schistosomiasis characteristically produce granulomatous inflammation in the involved tissues. Granulomas of cat scratch disease (caused by the gram-negative bacillus *Rochalimaea henselae*) are distinctive because they typically coalesce to form large stellate structures with central necrosis. Schistosomiasis, a disease caused by either *Schistosoma mansoni*, *S. japonicum*, *S. mekongi*, or *S. haematobium* (depending on the endemic region), is the most common helminthic infection in the world. The organism and its ova (the principal antigenic stimulus) characteristically incite granuloma formation and fibrosis, often accompanied in early stages of infection by marked eosinophilia. Granulomatous inflammation in infectious diseases is the result of cell-mediated hypersensitivity in which activated, sensitized T cells release lymphokines and other effector molecules that attract macrophages. *(pp. 81; 371)*

**(229 and 236)** The immune system is the major host defense against viral infections. Inflammatory responses usually play only a minor or secondary role. Thus, the cellular infiltrates that are seen in acute viral pneumonia and acute viral hepatitis are composed predominantly of the mononuclear cells (lymphocytes, plasma cells, and monocytes), the effector cells of the immune system. These same cell types predominate in chronic inflammatory reactions as well. Therefore, even though they are acute in nature, viral pneumonia and viral hepatitis elicit cellular responses that are identical to those seen in chronic inflammatory conditions. *(pp. 52; 316; 320; 698; 850–851)*

**(230 and 237)** Acute appendicitis and acute ascending cholangitis are examples of suppurative (purulent) inflammation. Bacterial invasion, usually following luminal obstruction, plays a major role in the pathogenesis of both these processes. Masses of neutrophils are attracted to the site of infection and produce purulent exudate (pus). **(238)** In contrast to the suppurative cholangitis produced by the bile duct obstruction and ascending infection, nonsuppurative (characterized by mononuclear cells rather than granulocytes) inflammation, and granulomatous destruction of interlobular bile ducts characterize primary biliary cirrhosis. In this disease, bile duct injury is immunologically mediated, and mononuclear cell infiltrates with granuloma formation in and around the walls of the intrahepatic bile ducts are hallmarks of the early stage of the disease. Ultimately, the bile ducts are destroyed, and cirrhosis results. *(pp. 53; 83; 823; 867–869)*

**(231, 233, and 239)** Fibrinous inflammation is defined by exudation of large amounts of plasma proteins, including fibrinogen, and the formation of large masses of fibrin. It is typically the result of endothelial damage produced by the underlying pathologic disorder. Cellular infiltrates may be minimal in this type of inflammation, which occurs primarily as a result of alterations in vascular integrity and increased permeability. Examples of this type of inflammation include rheumatic pericarditis, uremic pericarditis, and adult hyaline membrane disease (adult respiratory distress syndrome with diffuse alveolar damage). Adult hyaline membrane disease is caused by direct injury to the alveolar walls from toxic or infectious insults. The initial injury in most cases is to capillary endothelium (less often, to capillary epithelium). The amount and type of accompanying cellular inflammation may vary somewhat, but the damage to the capillaries of the alveolar wall causes fibrinogen leakage. The "hyaline" membranes that form in the alveolar spaces are composed predominantly of fibrin. *(pp. 69; 83; 549; 567; 649–650; 677; 760)*

**(234 and 235)** Serous inflammation is characterized by an outpouring of acellular watery (having a low protein content) fluid caused by either leakage of serum from blood vessels (most commonly) or the secretion products of serous cells. Skin blisters resulting from mechanical friction or shallow thermal burns are common examples of serous inflammation. This type of inflammation is seen most often in mild injuries and often occurs early in the development of other types of acute inflammatory reactions before cellular infiltrates become prominent. *(p. 82)*

**240. (A); 241. (C); 242. (B); 243. (C); 244. (D); 245. (F); 246. (C)**

The generation of an acute inflammatory reaction in response to bacterial infection is dependent on both the delivery of leukocytes to the site of injury and the ability of leukocytes to ingest and destroy the invading microorganisms. These responses are mediated by chemical signaling and molecular interaction between leukocytes and the injured tissue.

**(240)** In order for circulating neutrophils to enter the injured tissue and have access to the offending organisms, they first must travel across blood vessel walls at the site of infection. Transmigration across vessels first requires that the neutrophils come in contact with the endothelium of the vessels (with normal blood flow, they are confined to a medial axial column within the vessel and do not touch the endothelium). Neutrophils "meet" the endothelium as a result of slowing of blood flow (hemostasis) in injured tissue (the consequence of increased vascular permeability), which is the earliest event in an acute inflammatory process. Hemostasis occurs with the release of endogenous vasoactive substances (such as histamine) that increase vascular permeability by inducing endothelial contraction. In addition, bacterial toxins may contribute to vascular leakage by causing direct injury to endothelial cells. Once in contact with endothelium, however, neutrophils must establish a firmly adherent bond with the endothelial surface before they can migrate across it. The process of neutrophil adhesion to endothelium is dependent on both the expression of adhesion molecules by endothelial cells and the expression of receptors for those molecules by neutrophils. Interleukin-1 (IL-1) induces endothelial cell expression of adhesion molecules for neutrophils. In specific, it induces *de novo* expression of E-selectin (ELAM-1) by endothelial cells and increases endothelial expression of intercellular adhesion molecule-1 (ICAM-1; see Question 241) and vascular cell adhesion molecule-1 (VCAM-1). ELAM-1, ICAM-1, and VCAM-1 are all leukocyte adhesion molecules, each of which is the ligand for a separate and distinctive receptor on the surface of neutrophils (and other leukocytes).

**(241 through 243)** Complement fragment C5a (produced when a pre-existing, circulating complement-fixing antibody binds to the bacterial target) stimulates neutrophil chemotaxis and other cellular responses that collectively are referred to as "leukocyte activation." One of the important events occurring as a result of activation is an increase in the binding avidity of LAF-1 on neutrophil surfaces for ICAM-1, a cell surface adhesion molecule of the immunoglobulin family that is expressed by endothelial cells and mediates leukocyte adhesion to and transmigration across blood vessels. LAF-1 (a $\beta_2$ integrin) is normally present on the surfaces of all leukocytes, but it does not bind to ICAM-1 under normal conditions. However, when neutrophils are activated by chemoattractants (such as C5a) or other stimuli, LFA-1 undergoes a conformational change that dramatically increases its avidity for ICAM-1. This conversion of LAF-1 to a high-affinity receptor for ICAM-1 leads to firm adhesion of neutrophils to endothelial cells, a step necessary for subsequent transmigration across the vessel wall into the tissue.

**(246)** Activation of neutrophils by chemoattractants (such as C5a) also leads to the production of arachidonic acid metabolites from phospholipids (catalyzed by phospholipase $A_2$). Neutrophil activation likewise induces both degranulation and activation of the oxygen burst that is essential for effective bactericidal activity. These two cellular events require protein phosphorylation, which is catalyzed by protein kinase C.

**(244)** Having arrived at the site of infection, neutrophils proceed to ingest (via phagocytosis) and kill (via generation of free radicals and other toxic metabolites) bacteria. Phagocytic uptake of the offending organisms is abetted by a process known as "opsonization," which renders the bacteria more appetizing to the neutrophils. Opsonization is accomplished in two ways: (1) bacteria become coated with naturally occurring circulating antibodies directed against them and the Fc regions of those antibodies bind to Fc receptors on neutrophil surfaces; and (2) the bound antibodies fix complement and generate the complement cleavage fragment C3b, which, in turn, binds to specific complement receptors on neutrophil surfaces (see Question 277).

**(245)** Once the target organism has been ingested, it is killed by the generation of toxic oxygen metabolites (hydrogen peroxide) within the neutrophil phagolysosomes. This is accomplished by rapid activation of NADPH oxidase, an enzyme that generates superoxide in the process of oxidizing reduced nicotinamide-adenine dinucleotide phosphate (NADPH). Superoxide is converted spontaneously to hydrogen peroxide by dismutation. Hydrogen peroxide itself is toxic to bacteria. However, in the presence of neutrophil myeloperoxidase (contained in the azurophilic granules), the interaction of hydrogen peroxide with halides (such as $Cl^-$) is catalyzed to produce halide free radicals ($HOCl^-$). These destroy bacterial by halogenation (covalent bonding of the halide to cellular constituents) or by oxidation of bacterial proteins and lipids. *(pp. 57–63)*

**247. (E); 248. (E); 249. (A); 250. (B); 251. (D); 252. (E); 253. (C)**

The diagnosis, either clinical or histologic, of many types of neoplasms can be aided greatly by the detection of an associated tumor cell product or other antigen. When dealing with an anaplastic tumor showing little or no evidence of differentiation, the identification of cell structural elements, surface antigens, or products that are restricted largely to specific classes of cells can be essential in classifying the malignancy. Often, effective treatment hinges on the precise identification of tumor type. Immunohistochemical staining of biopsy samples for tumor-specific or tumor-related antigens may aid the process of tumor identification significantly.

**(249)** Hepatocellular carcinomas (hepatomas) and yolk sac tumors of germ cell origin characteristically produce α-fetoprotein (AFP). Metastatic tumor is by far more common than primary malignancy in the liver, so the presence of AFP can help to identify positively the less common primary hepatoma. *(pp. 300–301)*

**(250)** Like many well-differentiated adenocarcinomas, colon cancers commonly produce abundant amounts of a glycoprotein normally found in embryonic tissues of the gut known as carcinoembryonic antigen (CEA). Blood levels of CEA often are elevated in patients with colonic carcinoma and fall below detectable levels after complete resection of the primary tumor. Monitoring of the blood levels of CEA following surgical resection has been used clinically to detect recurrences of the tumor. *(p. 300)*

**(251)** The production of large amounts of human chorionic gonadotropin (hCG) is characteristic of choriocarcinoma, a malignant tumor of placental or germ cell origin. Detection of hCG commonly is used in the initial diagnosis of this malignancy or in diagnosing recurrences. Although multinucleate, syncytiotrophoblastic-type cells capable of hCG expression may occur in such diverse tumors as seminoma or gastric carcinoma, these cells usually fail to generate the high serum levels of hCG so commonly found with choriocarcinoma. *(pp. 300; 1074)*

**(253)** In addition to hormones and oncofetal antigens, the identification of intermediate filaments can be helpful in determining the tissue of origin of a tumor. Desmin, for example, is a cytoskeletal intermediate filament found only in muscle cells. Thus, the detection of desmin in the cytoplasm of an anaplastic sarcoma can help to identify it as a neoplasm of myocyte origin (e.g., rhabdosarcoma, leiomyosarcoma), and tumors of other mesenchymal cell types then can be eliminated from the differential diagnosis. *(pp. 299; 1268)*

**(247, 248, and 252)** Lymphomas, neuroblastomas (primitive neural malignancies), and medullary carcinomas of the thyroid (malignancies of C cell origin) do not produce any of the substances listed as choices. They can be identified by other specific markers, however. Lymphomas are distinguished by their expression of lymphocyte-specific cell surface antigens recognized by monoclonal antibodies. Neuroblastomas commonly produce neuron-specific enolase, synaptophysin, or neurosecretory products (amines) that identify the tumor as neural in type and differentiate this neoplasm from the other "small round cell tumors" of childhood that it may resemble. Medullary carcinoma of the thyroid can be identified by its production of calcitonin and/or amyloid. *(pp. 458–459; 637; 1140–1141)*

**254. (B); 255. (E); 256. (A); 257. (A); 258. (B); 259. (E); 260. (E); 261. (E); 262. (D); 263. (E)**

**(256 and 257)** Although oncogenic viruses are known to be capable of inducing malignant tumor formation in a wide variety of animals, including primates, the evidence linking viruses to carcinogenesis in humans is limited. DNA viruses that have been related causally to human malignancy include certain types of human papillomavirus (HPV), hepatitis B virus (probably hepatitis C virus as well), and the Epstein-Barr virus (EBV). EBV has been implicated in the development of both the African type of Burkitt's lymphoma and undifferentiated nasopharyngeal carcinoma. *(pp. 287–289)*

**(254)** HPV is now known to be an important factor in the etiology of invasive uterine cervical carcinoma and the cervical intraepithelial neoplasia (precancerous cervical dysplasia) from which it develops. HPV DNA is present in these lesions in the vast majority of cases, and certain "high-risk" subtypes (HPV types 16, 18, 31, and 33) are more often present in malignant lesions than other subtypes. The exact role of HPV in oncogenesis is not yet clear, but it presently is believed that these viruses act as a promotors that act in concert with initiator cocarcinogens (e.g., other viruses, bacteria, or environmental agents) to produce cervical cancer. *(pp. 286–287; 1048)*

**(255)** Although breast cancer can be induced virally in the mouse by a retrovirus known as the mouse mammary tumor virus, there is no conclusive evidence that human breast cancer is induced virally.

**(258)** HPV also is linked to other types of squamous cell carcinomas such as those that arise in the cutaneous or mucosal warts produced by this virus. As in the uterine cervix, most of the lesions produced by HPV are benign. Anogenital mucosal warts (condylomata acuminata) rarely give rise to squamous cell carcinoma, but the less common HPV-induced lesion known as giant condyloma is locally invasive, like a squamous cell carcinoma. However, it does not metastasize. Bowenoid papulosis, a form of *in situ* squamous cell carcinoma of the external genitalia, and invasive squamous cell carcinoma of the penis both are known to be related to HPV as well. *(pp. 1008–1011)*

**(259)** Although a number of viruses are capable of inducing sarcomas in animals of various species (in hamsters sarcomas can be induced by various strains of adenovirus), human sarcomas are not known to be virally induced.

**(260)** At least two forms of human lymphoma/leukemia have been shown to be induced virally, however. The causative agent of adult T-cell lymphoma/leukemia is the retrovirus known as the human T-cell leukemia virus type I (HTLV-I). HTLV-I is the only retrovirus known to cause malignancy in humans. This virus is a close relative of human immunodeficiency virus (HIV) (see Question 55), the causal agent of acquired immunodeficiency syndrome, and, like HIV, can be transmitted sexually or parenterally. EBV is linked strongly to the pathogenesis of Burkitt's lymphoma, a B-cell malignancy that is the most common childhood tumor in Central Africa and New Guinea. Unlike HTLV-I, which alone is capable of malignant transformation of the affected cells, EBV probably requires additional factors (co-carcinogens or promotors) to produce malignancy. *(pp. 276–279; 281; 717–718)*

**(261 and 263)** In contrast to hepatocellular carcinoma (HCC), neither cholangiocarcinoma nor angiosarcoma of the liver is related causally to viral infection. However, both of these tumors are related to previous exposure to Thorotrast, a contrast agent formerly used in radiography of the biliary tract. Another chemical causally linked to the otherwise rare hepatic angiosarcoma is vinyl chloride. *(pp. 284; 879)*

**(262)** It is established firmly that hepatitis B virus (HBV) is causally related to HCC. However, the evidence suggests that the virus acts in concert with other factors to cause malignant transformation of hepatocytes. There is also strong evidence linking the naturally occurring chemical carcinogen aflatoxin with HCC induction, and it may be that these two carcinogenic agents act in concert in some cases. There is also evidence to suggest that the hepatitis C virus may be important in the development of HCC in some cases. *(pp. 289; 879)*

**264. (E); 265. (A); 266. (A); 267. (A); 268. (A); 269. (C); 270. (A); 271. (E); 272. (A); 273. (E)**

A paraneoplastic syndrome is a symptom complex occurring in a patient with a malignant tumor that can be ascribed neither to the effects of tumor spread nor to the production of indigenous tumor hormones (i.e., hormones appropriate to the tissue from which the tumor arose). Paraneoplastic syndromes occur in about 15% of patients with advanced malignancies. They can be difficult to control clinically and, depending on the type of syndrome, may even cause the death of the patient.

**(265, 266, 267, 268, 270, and 272)** Bronchogenic carcinoma is the most common form of malignancy underlying the major types of paraneoplastic syndromes. Hypercalcemia, caused by tumor production of parathyroid hormone, occurs most commonly with oat cell or squamous cell carcinomas of the lung. Similarly, hyponatremia, caused by tumor secretion of antidiuretic hormone, most often is caused by oat cell carcinoma. Hypertrophic osteoarthropathy with clubbing of the fingers is seen almost exclusively in patients with lung cancer. The less well understood cancer-associated dermatomyositis and myasthenia gravis syndromes both occur most commonly in lung cancer patients. Although the nephrotic syndrome, thought to be induced by immune complexes containing tumor antigens, may occur with gastric or colon carcinomas among other malignancies, it is caused most often by lung cancer.

**(269)** When polycythemia occurs as a paraneoplastic syndrome, it most often is caused by the elaboration of erythropoietin by renal cell carcinoma. This syndrome also occurs occasionally in association with cerebellar hemangioma and hepatocellular carcinoma, however.

**(264, 271, and 273)** None of the tumor types listed as choices constitutes the major form of cancer associated with acanthosis nigricans, anemia, or hypoglycemia. Gastric carcinoma is the tumor most often associated with the malignant form of acanthosis nigricans (lung cancer is second only to gastric cancer as the tumor most commonly associated with acanthosis nigricans). Although the causal mechanism is unknown, carcinoma of thymic origin is the most common type of tumor associated with the paraneoplastic syndrome of anemia. Hypoglycemia, usually caused by the production of insulin or an insulin-like substance by tumor cells, occurs most commonly and curiously with sarcomas, especially fibrosarcoma. *(pp. 295–297; 724–725)*

**274. (C); 275. (B); 276. (E); 277. (E); 278. (E); 279. (E); 280. (E); 281. (A); 282. (E)**

**(274, 275, and 281)** The surface markers given as choices are all primarily T-cell–associated antigens, and all are molecules related to specific cell functions. The CD3 molecule is part of the T-cell antigen–receptor (TCR) complex (both the $\alpha/\beta$ and $\gamma/\delta$ TCRs are bound noncovalently to CD3) and functions in T cell antigen recognition, but it does not bind antigen. The CD3 proteins are important in transduction of signals into the T cell once it has bound its antigen. The CD4 molecule (on helper/inducer T cells) binds to class II major histocompatibility complex (MHC) molecules during antigen presentation. Thus, CD4+ T cells can recognize only antigen in association with class II MHC molecules on the surface of the antigen-presenting cell. In contrast, the CD8 molecule (on suppressor/cytotoxic T cells) binds only to class I MHC molecules, and CD8+ T cells can recognize antigen only in association with class I MHC molecules. *(pp. 172; 175–176)*

**(276)** Interleukin-2 (IL-2), the cytokine made by activated T cells that stimulates the growth of activated T, B, and natural killer cells and directly activates monocytes and NK cells, binds to a high-affinity receptor (IL-2R) on the surface of target cells. Blockade of IL-2R by specific antireceptor antibodies prevents cellular activation by IL-2. IL-2R is a molecule that is unrelated to either CD3, CD4, or CD8. *(p. 175)*

**(277)** Several receptors for complement (complement receptors 1, 2, and 3 [CR1, CR2, and CR3]) are expressed by macrophages and neutrophils. These interact with C3b (the opsonic fragment of C3) and its stable form, C3bi. CR3, which binds C3bi, is a molecule identical to mac-1, the $\beta_2$-integrin that is involved in adhesion to endothelium. CR3 also binds the extracellular matrix components fibronectin and laminin.

**(278)** The receptor for the Fc fragment of immunoglobulin G (IgG) that is present on macrophages and neutrophils is a molecule called Fc$\gamma$R. The CD16 molecule, which is a low-affinity receptor for the Fc portion of IgG, is primarily an NK cell–associated molecule and is used to identify NK cells. *(pp. 61; 174)*

**(279 and 280)** The CD molecules are not part of histocompatibility complexes at all. CD4 and CD8 are *receptors* for human leukocyte antigen class II and HLA class I molecules, respectively. *(p. 172)*

**(282)** The monomeric immunoglobulin M (IgM) displayed on its surface serves as the antigen receptor of the B cell. On differentiation of a B cell into a plasma cell, the immunoglobulin secreted by that plasma cell has the same specificity as the surface IgM of the B cell from which it is derived. *(p. 173)*

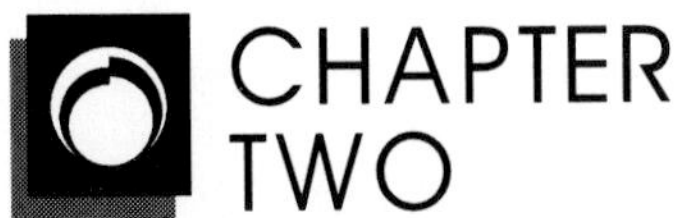

CHAPTER TWO

# Pediatric and Genetic Diseases

**DIRECTIONS:** For Questions 1 through 19, choose the ONE BEST answer to each question.

**1.** The leading cause of death in infancy (under 1 year of age) is:

A. Low birth weight
B. Hyaline membrane disease
C. Sudden infant death syndrome
D. Congenital anomalies
E. Injuries

**2.** Five minutes after birth, an infant appears pale and blue, has a heart rate of 90, and has slow, irregular respirations. His muscles are limp and he makes no response to a nasal catheter. His Apgar score is:

A. 0
B. 1
C. 2
D. 3
E. 4

**3.** Which one of the following statements about the prevention of Rh incompatibility (Rh-related erythroblastosis fetalis) is correct?

A. Anti-gammaglobulin antibody is adminstered to the affected infant of a sensitized mother after birth.
B. Anti-gammaglobulin antibody is administered in utero to the affected infant of a sensitized mother.
C. Anti-D immunoglobulin is given to a nonsensitized mother before delivery.
D. Anti-D immunoglobulin is given to a sensitized mother before birth.
E. Anti-D immunoglobulin is given to a sensitized mother throughout the last trimester of pregnancy.

**4.** The lesion pictured in Figure 2–1 arose on the face of a young child and grew rapidly to a large red-blue mass. This lesion:

A. Is known as a choristoma
B. Will most likely regress spontaneously
C. Is best treated by surgical excision
D. Is best treated by radiation therapy
E. Tends to metastasize to local lymph nodes

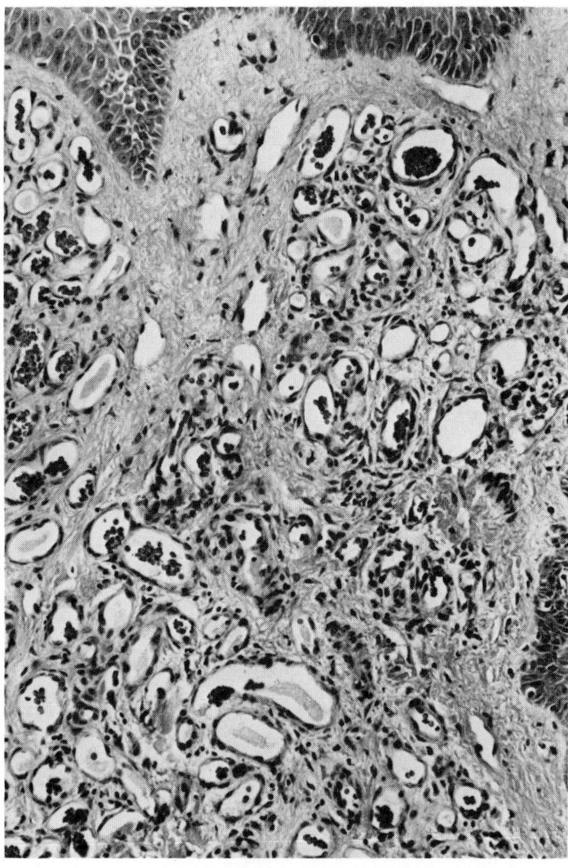

Figure 2–1

**5.** Conditions associated with impaired intrauterine fetal growth (intrauterine growth retardation) and low birth weight include all of the following EXCEPT:

A. First pregnancy
B. Chromosomal disorders of the fetus
C. Small placentas
D. Toxemia of pregnancy
E. Material alcohol abuse

**6.** Congenital malformations are associated with all of the following conditions EXCEPT:

A. Fetal chromosomal abnormalities
B. Maternal alcohol consumption
C. Maternal rubella infection during pregnancy
D. Maternal cytomegalovirus during pregnancy
E. Maternal cigarette smoking during pregnancy

**7.** In severe cases of erythroblastosis fetalis, all of the following findings are characteristic EXCEPT:

A. Anasarca
B. Yellow pigmentation of the brain
C. Extramedullary hematopoiesis
D. Enlarged placenta
E. Dark urine

**8.** All of the conditions listed below are associated with the disease process illustrated by the micrograph of the pancreas in Figure 2–2 EXCEPT:

A. Diabetes mellitus
B. Meconium ileus
C. Male infertility
D. *Pseudomonas* pneumonia
E. Vitamin K deficiency

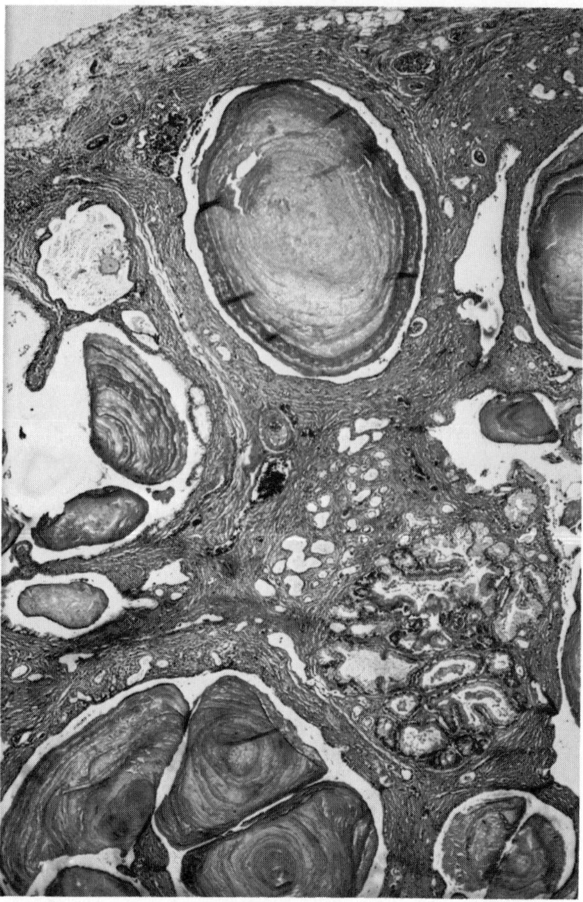

**Figure 2–2**

**9.** Malignancies that commonly occur in children under 4 years of age include all of the following EXCEPT:

A. Leukemia
B. Wilms' tumor
C. Retinoblastoma
D. Rhabdomyosarcoma
E. Osteosarcoma

**10.** Principal characteristics of the group of genetic disorders known as the mucopolysaccharidoses include all of the following EXCEPT:

A. Hepatomegaly
B. Muscular weakness
C. Skeletal deformities
D. Coronary artery disease
E. Cardiac valvular lesions

**11.** All of the following statements about congenital heart disease are true EXCEPT:

A. Most cases are associated with chromosomal abnormalities.
B. Males are more commonly affected.
C. The most common clinical presentation is cyanosis.
D. The involved heart is usually enlarged.
E. Most affected individuals survive into adulthood

**12.** All of the following are features of Down's syndrome EXCEPT:

A. Trisomy of chromosome 21
B. Normal parental karyotypes
C. Mental retardation
D. Higher frequency with increased maternal age
E. Average life expectancy of about 5 years

**13.** A 2,000-gm infant delivered at 39 weeks, gestational age:

A. Is considered preterm
B. Is an appropriate weight for gestational age
C. Is at high risk for hyaline membrane disease
D. Is unlikely to have experienced intrauterine growth retardation
E. Has a greater than 95% chance of survival

Questions 14 and 15 refer to Figure 2–3.

**14.** The condition shown in Figure 2–3 is most strongly associated with:

A. Diabetes in the mother
B. Male sex of the infant
C. Maternal alcohol consumption during pregnancy
D. Delivery by cesarean section
E. Preterm delivery

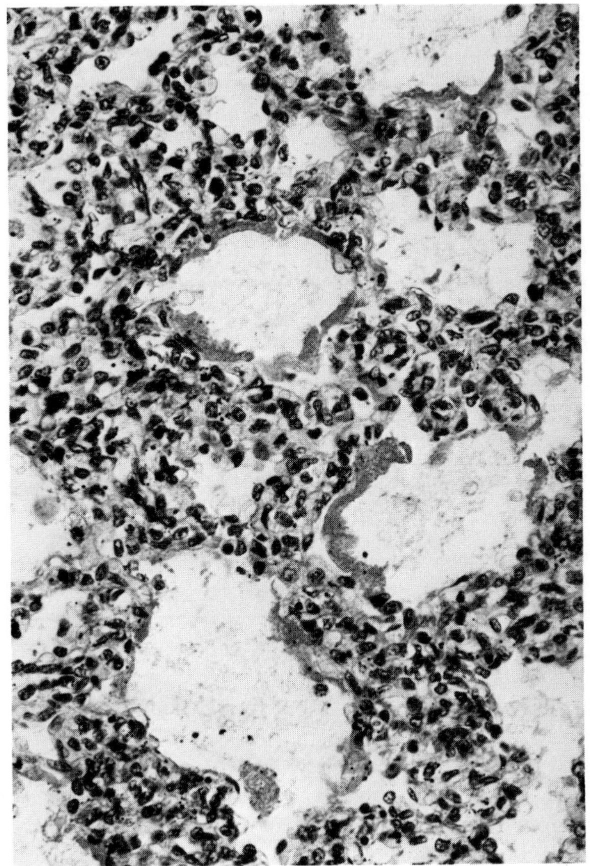

**Figure 2–3**

**15.** Infants recovering from this condition are at increased risk of:

A. Patent ductus arteriosus
B. Intraventricular cerebral hemorrhage
C. Necrotizing enterocolitis
D. All of the above
E. None of the above

**16.** All of the following statements about HOX genes are true EXCEPT:

A. They control morphogenetic embryonic patterning.
B. Their mutation results in congenital malformations.
C. Their homeobox has DNA-binding properties.
D. Their homeobox is highly variable among species.
E. Their expression is altered by retinoic acid.

**17.** All of the following disorders (lysosomal storage diseases) result from deficiency of a specific lysosomal acid hydrolase EXCEPT:

A. McArdle syndrome
B. Nieman-Pick disease
C. Tay-Sachs disease
D. Gaucher's disease
E. Pompe's disease

**18.** All of the following statements correctly describe the sudden infant death syndrome (SIDS) EXCEPT:

A. Infants with congenital malformations are affected most commonly.
B. Infant prematurity is an associated risk.
C. SIDS in a prior sibling of the infant is an associated risk.
D. Maternal narcotic abuse is an associated risk.
E. Autopsy reveals no anatomic cause of death.

**19.** Neurofibromatosis type 1 (von Recklinghausen's disease) is associated with all of the following EXCEPT:

A. Pigmented macular skin lesions
B. Scoliosis
C. Hemangioblastomas of the central nervous system
D. Bone cysts
E. Pigmented iris hamartomas

**DIRECTIONS:** For Questions 20 through 39, you are to decide whether EACH choice is TRUE or FALSE.

For each of the following statements about erythroblastosis fetalis (hemolytic disease of the newborn), choose whether it is TRUE or FALSE.

**20.** RH hemolytic disease is more common than ABO hemolytic disease.
**21.** ABO hemolytic disease is more severe than Rh hemolytic disease.
**22.** ABO hemolytic disease requires no prior sensitization of the mother.
**23.** ABO hemolytic disease occurs almost exclusively in infants of type O mothers.
**24.** ABO hemolytic disease cannot be prevented.

For each of the following statements about the ductus arteriosus, choose whether it is TRUE or FALSE

**25.** Closure normally occurs within the first 2 days of postnatal life.
**26.** Closure is delayed in premature infants.
**27.** Prostaglandins are essential to normal closure.
**28.** Patent ductus arteriosus presents with cyanosis during infancy.
**29.** Patent ductus arteriosus creates an early systolic blowing murmur.

For each of the following statements about coarctation of the aorta, describe whether it is TRUE or FALSE.

**30.** It occurs commonly in Turner's syndrome.
**31.** It usually occurs as a solitary congenital defect in an otherwise normal child.
**32.** Preductal coarctation causes right ventricular hypertrophy in utero.
**33.** Notching of the inner surfaces of the ribs on radiographs is associated with preductal coarctation.
**34.** The lesion often recurs after surgical resection.

For each of the following statements about tetralogy of Fallot, choose whether it is TRUE or FALSE.

**35.** The severity of clinical symptoms is related most directly to the degree of right ventricular outflow obstruction.
**36.** A patent ductus arteriosus is requisite to survival in most cases.
**37.** Most affected individuals are cyanotic from birth.
**38.** Polycythemia is a common complication.
**39.** Early corrective surgery is the treatment of choice

**DIRECTIONS:** For Questions 40 through 61, the set of lettered headings is followed by a list of numbered words or phrases. For each numbered word or phrase choose:
A—if the item is associated with (A) only
B—if the item is associated with (B) only
C—if the item is associated with *both* (A) and (B)
D—if the item is associated with *neither* (A) nor (B)

For each of the characteristics listed below, choose whether it describes phenylketonuria, alkaptonuria, both, or neither.

A. Phenylketonuria
B. Alkaptonuria
C. Both
D. Neither

**40.** A defect in tyrosine metabolism causes the disease.
**41.** Affected infants appear normal at birth.
**42.** Urine turns black on standing.
**43.** Untreated patients often develop mental retardation.
**44.** Dietary restriction is the treatment of choice.

For each of the characteristics listed below, choose whether it describes Marfan's syndrome, the Ehlers-Danlos syndromes, both, or neither.

A. Marfan's syndrome
B. Ehlers-Danlos syndromes
C. Both
D. Neither

**45.** Is caused by a single gene mutation
**46.** Is characterized by defective collagen synthesis
**47.** Is sometimes complicated by arterial rupture
**48.** Is characterized by long slender extremities
**49.** Typically produces joint inflexibility

For each of the following statements, choose whether it describes atrial septal defect, ventricular septal defect, both, or neither.

A. Atrial septal defect
B. Ventricular septal defect
C. Both
D. Neither

**50.** The lesion represents a common congenital cardiac defect.
**51.** The defect develops between the second and eighth weeks of embryogenesis.
**52.** The defect typically presents early in infancy.
**53.** A defect of small size predisposes to bacterial endocarditis.
**54.** The defect is a feature of tetralogy of Fallot.
**55.** Surgical correction of isolated defects in infancy is the treatment of choice.
**56.** The objective of surgical correction is prevention of pulmonary hypertension.

For each of the following characteristics, choose whether it describes tricuspid valve atresia, pulmonary valve atresia, both, or neither.

A. Tricuspid valve atresia
B. Pulmonary valve atresia
C. Both
D. Neither

**57.** Is commonly associated with a hypoplastic right ventricle
**58.** Is commonly associated with an atrial septal defect
**59.** Is frequently associated with a ventricular septal defect
**60.** Accounts for as much as 10% of congenital cyanotic heart disease
**61.** Surgical correction is usually possible

**DIRECTIONS:** Questions 62 through 70 are matching questions. For each numbered item, choose the most likely associated lettered item from those provided. Each numbered item has ONLY ONE answer. Within each group, each lettered item may be the answer to one, more than one, or none of the numbered items.

For each of the sexual disorders listed below, choose whether the most common associated karyotype is 45,X, 46,XY, 47,XXY, or none of these.

A. 45,X
B. 46,XY
C. 47,XXY
D. None of these

**62.** Klinefelter's syndrome
**63.** Turner's syndrome
**64.** True hermaphroditism
**65.** Testicular feminization syndrome

For each of the features listed below, choose whether it is characteristic of Fabry's disease, Lesch-Nyhan syndrome, von Hippel-Lindau disease, Wilson's disease, or none of these.

A. Fabry's disease
B. Lesch-Nyhan syndrome
C. Von Hippel-Lindau disease
D. Wilson's disease
E. None of these

**66.** Gout and self-mutilative behavior
**67.** Progressive renal failure and angiokeratomas
**68.** Xanthomas and accelerated atherosclerosis
**69.** Cirrhosis and cavitation of the brain
**70.** Retinal hemangioblastomas and renal cell carcinoma

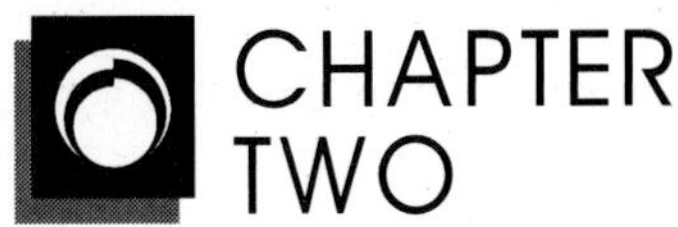

CHAPTER TWO

# Pediatric and Genetic Diseases

## ANSWERS

**1. (A)** In the United States, far more deaths occur in infancy (less than 1 year of age) than in any other period of childhood. Among neonates (less than 4 weeks of age), survival correlates with birth weight. Low birth rate is the leading cause of death in this age group. Low birth weight (less than 2500 gm) may result from either of two primary problems (although both may be present in any one case): (1) preterm birth (infant is immature) and (2) intrauterine growth retardation (infant is undergrown). With intrauterine growth retardation (IUGR), the infant's development *in utero* has been slowed by fetal or maternal factors or both and, at birth, the infant is small for the gestational age (even at term). This is a much more dire situation than preterm (premature) birth alone, in which the infant's birth weight is low but is appropriate for gestational age. Although both prematurity and IUGR cause low birth weights, IUGR is associated with significantly higher mortality rates for any given birth weight or gestational age.

Respiratory distress syndrome (hyaline membrane disease of the newborn) is most commonly the result of immature pulmonary development in infants of low birth weight and is second to IUGR/low birth weight as a cause of death in neonates. Congenital anomalies and sudden infant death syndrome also cause death in this age group, but not as commonly as perinatal conditions, including low birth weight, respiratory distress syndrome, and birth trauma. Death resulting from injury in infancy is related chiefly to birth trauma but is only one of several perinatal conditions contributing to mortality. In the older pediatric age groups, however, injuries assume major importance and are the leading cause of death among children from 1 to 14 years of age. *(pp. 432–433)*

**2. (C)** The Apgar score is a useful clinical method for rapid evaluation of the physiologic condition of a newborn infant. Five parameters are evaluated: heart rate, respiratory effort, muscle tone, response to nasal catheter, and color. The infant is evaluated at 1 and 5 minutes of life and each item is given a score of 0, 1, or 2. A score of 2 is normal, a score of 0 indicates absence of that function, and a score of 1 is an intermediate response. Thus, an infant with a heart rate of less than 100 (score 1), slow irregular respirations (score 1), and absence of muscle tone, pink color, or response to a nasal catheter (scores of 0) would have an overall Apgar score of 2. The Apgar score correlates well with the chances of survival during the first 28 days of life. Infants with Apgar scores of 0 or 1 at 5 minutes have a 50% risk of mortality during the first months of life. Prognosis improves with increasing Apgar scores, and mortality is almost zero when the score is 7 or greater. Although a good predictor of short-term survival, the Apgar score is not a reliable indicator of long-term neurologic morbidity. *(p. 436)*

**3. (C)** The principle of the therapeutic approach to Rh incompatibility is to prevent primary maternal immunization to the D antigen, an event that usually occurs during labor (or abortions). Thus, prior to delivery, anti-D immunoglobulin is administered to the nonsensitized, Rh-negative mother. The administered antibody coats the fetal red cells that leak into the maternal circulation. The antigenic determinants become masked and fail to stimulate the maternal immune system. This treatment must be given for the first and every subsequent pregnancy of the unsensitized mother. There is no theoretical or practical use for this treatment in the mother who has already become sensitized. The success of this therapeutic approach has now made fetomaternal ABO incompatibility (for which there is no similar treatment), rather than Rh incompatibility, the most common cause of erythroblastosis fetalis. *(p. 447)*

**4. (B)** The lesion pictured in the micrograph is a benign tumor of blood vessels known as a capillary hemangioma.

Hemangiomas are the most common tumors of infancy. This lesion is benign and tends to regress spontaneously, so it does not require surgical excision or radiation therapy and, of course, does not metastasize. A choristoma is the name applied to microscopically normal cells or tissues that are present in an abnormal location (e.g., a pancreatic rest in the duodenal submucosa). Although benign, a hemangioma is a true tumor and therefore would not be classifiable as a choristoma. *(pp. 456–457)*

**5. (A)** Low birth weight in small-for-gestational-age infants is frequently the result of impaired intrauterine growth (see Question 1). Impaired growth *in utero* may be caused by a variety of fetal, placental, or maternal factors. Fetal conditions that commonly reduce growth potential despite an adequate supply of nutrients from the mother include chromosomal disorders, congenital anomalies, and congenital infections. Small placentas and other placental conditions (infections, tumors, or vascular lesions) may produce placental insufficiency and retard intrauterine growth. In the vast majority of cases, however, impaired intrauterine growth is caused by maternal conditions that limit or interfere with fetal nourishment or oxygenation. In this category, maternal vascular diseases such as toxemia of pregnancy or chronic systemic hypertension are common underlying causes. Additional important maternal causes of impaired intrauterine growth include alcohol abuse, cigarette smoking, and narcotic abuse. First pregnancy, however, is not in itself associated with impaired intrauterine fetal growth. On the contrary, it is more likely that the small uterus of a first pregnancy may constrain a normally growing fetus and cause fetal deformation. *(pp. 432–434, 437)*

**6. (E).** Congenital malformations are intrinsic abnormalities occurring during fetal development that are seen at birth as structural defects. Major malformations resulting from defective embryogenesis are present in as many as 3% of newborn infants. Although the cause is unknown in at least 50% of cases, the remainder of the congenital malformations in humans are known to be related to either genetic or environmental factors. Fetal chromosomal abnormalities are among the most common genetic causes of congenital malformation. Environmental causes include infection, teratogenic drugs and chemicals, and irradiation. For example, maternal thalidomide use is an infamous cause of malformation. It recently has become recognized that alcohol, a readily available and widely used agent, is a teratogen. Affected infants manifest growth retardation, microcephaly, atrial septal defects, short palpebral fissures, maxillary hypoplasia, and other more minor anomalies. These changes have come to be known as the fetal alcohol syndrome. Rubella and cytomegalovirus are two of the most common infectious agents known to cause congenital malformations. Although heavy cigarette smoking throughout pregnancy is associated with infants that are small for gestational age, there is no definitive evidence that it leads to congenital malformations. *(pp. 434; 437–440)*

**7. (E)** In cases of severe erythroblastosis fetalis, (see Questions 20 through 24), hemolysis is extensive, and the oxygen-carrying capacity of the blood is severely impaired. Thus, the heart may suffer hypoxic damage, leading to circulatory failure. Circulatory failure, in turn, exacerbates the anemia-induced hypoxic damage to other organs. The liver, with its high metabolic rate, is especially prone to injury. Hepatic failure with a resultant decrease in albumin production (hypoproteinemia) accompanied by cardiac failure and increased venous capillary pressure results in generalized edema (anasarca), a situation known as hydrops fetalis.

Unconjugated hyperbilirubinemia, the hallmark of any hemolytic disease with jaundice, has severe consequences in the neonate that would not occur in an older child or an adult. In the neonate, unconjugated bilirubin, which is markedly lipophilic, passes readily through the immature blood-brain barrier, causing toxic damage to the brain and spinal cord. The brain becomes edematous and has a characteristic bright yellow pigmentation (kernicterus). Kernicterus is the most serious complication of erythroblastosis fetalis. The marked increase in erythropoietic activity in this hemolytic state characteristically induces extramedullary hematopoiesis in the spleen and liver and possibly other tissues as well. Enlarged, heavy, edematous placentas are also highly characteristic of severe erythroblastosis fetalis, with liver damage, hypoalbuminemia, and fetal edema.

Dark urine is a consequence of spillover into the urine of water-soluble conjugated bilirubin. This occurs in disorders in which bilirubin is conjugated but not excreted (e.g., cholestatic jaundice caused by large duct obstruction). In erythroblastosis fetalis, however, jaundice is caused by an excess production of unconjugated bilirubin and does not produce dark urine. *(pp. 447–448)*

**8. (A)** The pancreatic disease picture in Figure 2–2 is cystic fibrosis (CF), the most common lethal genetic disease that affects white populations. It is caused by mutation of the CF gene on chromosome 7 that encodes a chloride channel protein. The result is a primary defect in the regulation of epithelial sodium chloride transport. An increased concentration of sodium in sweat is one manifestation of this defect and constitutes the basis for a common clinical test for CF.

Although the pathologic changes in the pancreas pictured in the micrograph are characteristic of CF, they make it difficult to identify the tissue. Markedly dilated pancreatic ducts plugged with inspissated secretions dominate the pathologic picture. The obstruction leads to atrophy of the exocrine pancreas and its replacement by fibrous tissue. As is typical of any form of pancreatic ductal obstruction with secondary pancreatic atrophy, the endocrine pancreas largely is spared. Diabetes mellitus, therefore, is not commonly associated with CF or any other form of pancreatic ductal obstruction. The major physical defect in CF is the production in glandular structures of a highly viscous mucus that is difficult to mobilize and that tends to form plugs. Thus, primarily tissues that are organized around mucin-secreting tubal structures, such as the bronchial tree, the gastrointestinal mucosa, and the excretory ducts of the male genital system, are involved in this disease process. In newborns with this disease, small bowel obstruction (known as meconium ileus) may occur as a consequence of abnormal gastrointestinal mucous secretion and the absence of pancreatic amylases. Obstruction of wolffian duct derivatives (the epididymis and vas deferens) produces azoospermia and infertility in 95% of males with this disease. Pulmonary abnormalities are present in almost every case of CF. The bronchial tree becomes plugged with tenacious mucous secretions. Superimposed infections give rise to severe chronic bronchitis and marked bronchiectasis. *Pseudomonas aeruginosa* and *Staphylococcus aureus* are the two most common pathogens responsible for lung infections in this setting. Deficiency of vitamin K, a fat-soluble vitamin, often occurs as part of the malabsorption syndrome that results from the loss of pancreatic exocrine secretions. *(pp. 451–454)*

**9. (E)** Although benign tumors are far more common in infancy and childhood than malignant tumors, several malignancies exhibit sharp peaks in incidence in children under 5 years of age. Primary among these are leukemia (particularly acute lymphocytic leukemia), Wilms' tumor (nephroblastoma), retinoblastoma, and rhabdomyosarcoma, as well as neuroblastoma, hepatoblastoma, teratoma, and ependymoma. Osteosarcoma is virtually nonexistent in this age group and characteristically occurs in late childhood and adolescence, the period of most rapid bone growth. Knowledge of the characteristic age distribution in childhood neoplasms can be helpful in diagnosing malignant processes in early childhood. *(pp. 458–459)*

**10. (B)** The mucopolysaccharidoses are a group of genetic disorders resulting from deficiencies of specific lysosomal enzymes involved in the degradation of mucopolysaccharides (glycosaminoglycans). Mucopolysaccharides (i.e., dermatan sulfate, heparan sulfate, keratan sulfate, and chondroitin sulfate) typically accumulate in the mononuclear phagocyte system, causing hepatosplenomegaly. Accumulation in endothelial cells, intimal smooth muscle cells, and fibroblasts throughout the body is also common. The cardiovascular system usually is involved, especially the coronary arteries and valves. Skeletal and facial deformities also occur. Typically, the head is large and long, and the nose is broad and flat. Muscular weakness is not a characteristic symptom of the mucopolysaccharidoses. It is, however, one of the cardinal symptoms of glycogen storage diseases. *(pp. 144–147)*

**11. (A)** Only about 5% of cases of congenital heart disease (abnormalities of the heart or great vessels that are present from birth) are associated with chromosomal abnormalities (e.g., trisomies of chromosome 21, 18, 13, 22, or 9 or Turner's syndrome). Yet some genetic factors appear to play a role in the etiology of congenital heart disease (CHD), because about one third of affected individuals have one or more relatives with congenital heart disease. In addition, CHD appears more frequently in males, suggesting a sex-linked genetic influence. Although CHD covers a wide spectrum of anatomic anomalies, the physiologic end result of most of them is either a shunt (abnormal communication between heart chambers or major vessels or both) or an obstruction to blood flow. Shunts allow poorly oxygenated blood to enter the systemic circulation and produce some degree of cyanosis. The most common types of CHD are shunting defects. These include ventricular septal defect, patent ductus arteriosus, and tetralogy of Fallot, which together account for over half of all cases of CHD. Thus, cyanosis is the most common clinical presentation overall. Whether the defect produces a shunt or an obstruction, the altered hemodynamics usually result in cardiac dilation or hypertrophy or both. Nevertheless, with early diagnosis and surgical correction, most patients (more than 85%) with CHD survive into adulthood. *(pp. 571–573; 579)*

**12. (E)** Down's syndrome is the most common chromosomal disorder, affecting about 1 in 700 newborns in the United States, and is a major cause of mental retardation. About 95% of affected individuals have three complete copies of chromosome 21 and a chromosome count of 47. About 4% have 46 chromosomes, with an extra copy of genetic material from the long arm of chromosome 21 translocated to another acrocentric chromosome, (e.g., 14 or 22; translocation variant form of Down's syndrome). Parents of affected individuals have normal karyotypes, however. Full expression of Down's syndrome requires triplication of only a single region (band 21q22) of the long arm of chromosome 21, a band large enough to include several hundred genes. It is hoped that mapping of the genes in this "obligate Down's region" will provide new insight into the pathogenesis of this syndrome.

Major features of the Down's syndrome include severe mental retardation, distinctive facies (flat facial profile, oblique eyelids, and epicanthal folds), occurrence of congenital heart disease in about 40% of cases, and a 10- to 20-fold increased risk of developing acute leukemia in childhood. The incidence of the disease increases dramatically with maternal age (1 in 1550 live births for mothers under age 20; 1 in 25 births for mothers over age 45). With medical care, individuals with Down's syndrome have an average life expectancy of 30 years, and 25% live to age 50. *(pp. 154–156)*

**13. (E)** Only infants delivered before the 37th or 38th week of gestation are considered preterm. Infants born between the 38th and 42nd weeks of gestation are considered term infants. Their birth weight is considered appropriate for gestational age (AGA) if it falls between the 10th and the 90th percentiles of weights within that gestational age group. For a term infant at 39 weeks, an appropriate birth weight would range from approximately 2,300 to 3,600 gm, and a 2,000-gm infant would be considered small for gestational age (SGA). Intrauterine growth retardation (see Question 1) most commonly underlies SGA, so it is likely that the infant described here experienced IUGR.

Classifying infants on the basis of both their birth weight and their gestational age in this way is more accurately predictive of infant morbidity and mortality than classification by either parameter alone. For example, a 2,000-gm infant born at 34 weeks of gestation has an 8% mortality rate, and yet an infant of the same birth weight born at 39 weeks of gestation has only a 2% risk of mortality. Certain causes of infant morbidity are associated only with preterm delivery (irrespective of birth weight) and result from functional and structural immaturity of various organ systems. Hyaline membrane disease of the newborn, caused by functional immaturity of type II pneumocytes, is a prime example. A full-term infant would not be at increased risk for hyaline membrane disease. *(pp. 432–433; 444)*

**14. (E)** The micrograph of the lung illustrates the classic microscopic features of respiratory distress syndrome (RDS) of the newborn. This disorder is the result of structural and functional immaturity of the lungs, almost always occurring in infants delivered before term. Its incidence is inversely proportional to gestational age, and preterm delivery is the most important risk factor for RDS. The fundamental defect in RDS is deficient surfactant production by immature type II pneumocytes. As a consequence, the work of expanding the air spaces increases dramatically, and widespread atelectasis ensues. The resultant hypoxemia and acidosis not only further impair surfactant production but lead to pulmonary vasoconstriction and hypoperfusion. Capillary endothelial cells then suffer anoxic damage, and plasma proteins (particularly fibrinogen) leak into the alveolar spaces to form thick hyaline membranes, the characteristic pathologic feature of this disorder.

In addition to preterm delivery, other factors may pose a significant risk for RDS. For example, there are strong, but not invariable, associations of RDS with delivery by cesarean section and with maternal diabetes. In infants of diabetic mothers, the reactive hyperinsulinemia counteracts the normal inductive effects of corticosteroids on surfactant production in the fetal lung. Male sex is also a risk factor. RDS occurs twice as often in male infants as in female infants, as a result of the relatively early maturation of the female lung.

Maternal alcohol consumption, narcotic abuse, or heavy cigarette smoking during pregnancy are all associated with small-for-gestational-age infants, not necessarily with preterm delivery. Most infants who develop RDS are normal for gestational age, so it is clear that preterm delivery is more strongly associated with RDS than with being small for gestational age. *(pp. 434; 444–446)*

**15. (D)** In general, infants with RDS have an excellent chance of recovery if ventilatory therapy is successful in maintaining their life for the first 3 to 4 days. Unfortunately, however, recovery from RDS is associated with a variety of complications. Most significantly, the infant is at increased risk of patent ductus arteriosus, intraventricular cerebral hemorrhage, and necrotizing enterocolitis. Patent ductus arteriosus results from delayed closure of the ductus because of immaturity, hypoxia, and acidosis. Intraventricular hemorrhage is a consequence of anoxia and immaturity of the brain as well as the disproportionately large amount of cerebral blood flow through the periventricular circulation, where the vessel walls are fragile. The pathogenesis of necrotizing enterocolitis is less well understood but is thought to be related to intestinal ischemia resulting from hypoxia and secondary bacterial invasion. Interestingly, it may be the extrapulmonary consequences of hypoxia that pose the greatest risk to life in the recovery phase of neonatal RDS. *(p. 446)*

**16. (D)** HOX genes are one of a class of genes (morphogenesis genes) known to be important in embryonic patterning and control of normal morphogenesis during fetal development. These genes contain highly conserved regions thought to be important in transcriptional regulation. This region of the HOX genes (180 nucleotides) has been called the "homeobox" and has DNA-binding properties. The homeobox regions have been conserved highly among species (e.g., they are nearly identical in both insects and humans), attesting to their essential function. From animal studies, it is known that mutations of these genes or alterations in their expression result in congenital malformations, observations consistent with their critical role in embryonic patterning. Although the mechanisms by which HOX genes are controlled are not yet clear, it has been shown that retinoic acid is an upstream regulator of some HOX genes. In animals, exposure to retinoic acid causes reproducible changes in HOX gene expression and results in a wide range of congenital malformations. Retinoic acid is teratogenic in humans as well. Infants born to mothers being treated with retinoid acid for severe acne have central nervous system, cardiac, and craniofacial defects, a syndrome known as retinoic acid embryopathy. It is hoped that knowledge about the function and control of morphogenesis genes will greatly increase our understanding of human congenital malformations. *(p. 442)*

**17. (A)** Niemann-Pick disease, Tay-Sachs disease, Gaucher's disease, and Pompe's disease are lysosomal storage diseases (diseases that result from a deficiency in a single lysosomal acid hydrolase and characterized by accumulation or "storage" of the undegradable substrate within the "digesting" cell, causing cell dysfunction). In Neimann-Pick disease and Gaucher's disease, the deficient enzymes are sulfatidases and the accumulated substrates are sphingomyelin and glucocerebroside, respectively. In Tay-Sachs disease, the missing enzyme is hexaminidase and the undegraded substances are $GM_2$ gangliosides. In Pompe's disease, the lack of lysosomal glucosidase leads to accumulation of glycogen. The histopathologic and pathophysiologic characteristics of each disease are determined by which cell types normally degrade the metabolite in question and therefore are most affected by the enzyme deficit. In Neimann-Pick disease and Gaucher's disease, phagocytic cells (macrophages) throughout the body accumulate the metabolite. In Tay-Sachs disease, neurons in the central and autonomic nervous systems are the most profoundly affected. In Pompe's disease, glycogen accumulates in all organs, but the heart usually is involved most profoundly.

McArdle's syndrome does not involve lysosomal enzymes at all. It is a condition produced by a deficiency of phosphorylase in striated muscle, and in general its only effects are muscular weakness following periods of physical activity. *(pp. 138–143; 147)*

**18. (A)** The sudden infant death syndrome (SIDS) is an enigmatic disorder. Its very definition reflects the almost complete lack of understanding of this process: "the sudden death of an infant under 1 year of age that remains unexplained after a thorough case investigation, including performance of a complete autopsy, examination of the death scene, and review of the clinical history." There is no evidence that these deaths occur more frequently in infants with congenital malformations than in normal infants. Epidemiologic studies have shown that the risk of SIDS is increased if the mother is younger than 20 years of age, is unmarried, has abused narcotics or smoked cigarettes, or belongs to a low socioeconomic group, infant risk factors include prematurity, low birth weight, male sex, and prior siblings with SIDS. SIDS also occurs more commonly in infants who were products of multiple births or who were not the first sibling.

Most infants stricken by SIDS usually die at home during the night after a period of sleep, implicating apnea and abnormal temperature control as possible causative factors. It is postulated that a neurodevelopmental delay may be a common abnormality in the pathophysiology of SIDS, even though the underlying causes may be diverse. *(pp. 454–456)*

**19. (C)** Neurofibromatosis (von Recklinghausen's disease) is a genetic syndrome with three major features: (1) multiple tumors (neurofibromas) throughout the body; (2) pigmented skin lesions; and (3) pigmented iris hamartomas called Lisch nodules. Skeletal abnormalities such as scoliosis and bone cysts also commonly occur in this syndrome. The neurofibromatosis-1 gene (NF-1) has been mapped to chromosome 17q11.2. It belongs to the family of tumor suppressor genes that negatively regulate cell growth. It encodes a protein called neurofibromin, which down-regulates the function of the p21 *ras* oncoprotein. Although the defective gene is inherited as an autosomal dominant trait in 50% of cases, an equal number of cases are due to new mutations.

Hemangioblastomas of the central nervous system do not occur in von Recklinghausen's disease but are characteristic of another rare autosomal disorder known as von Hippel-Lindau's disease. *(pp. 148–149)*

**20. (False); 21. (False); 22. (True); 23. (True); 24. (False)**

**(20)** When the red blood cells of a fetus display antigenic determinants inherited from the father that differ from those of the mother, a maternal immune reaction against the fetal erythrocyte antigens may occur. The maternal antibodies cross the placenta and cause hemolysis in the infant (erythroblastosis fetalis). Although in theory many erythrocyte antigens could produce this phenomenon, in practice only ABO and Rh incompatibility are significant causes of hemolytic disease of the newborn. Although Rh incompatibility used to be the leading cause of erythroblastosis fetalis, routine prepuerperal therapy with anti-D immunoglobulin in Rh-negative women to prevent primary sensitization (see Question 3 and below) now has made fetomaternal ABO incompatibility the most common cause of erythroblastosis fetalis. **(21)** Happily, however, ABO incompatibility usually produces less severe hemolytic disease than Rh incompatibility. In fact, in most cases of ABO incompatibility, no hemolytic disease at all is produced. ABO incompatibility occurs in about 25% of pregnancies but produces laboratory evidence of hemolytic disease in only 10% of infants, and even then, only 0.5% of those infants manifest disease that is severe enough to require treatment. The mild nature of ABO incompatibility–related disease may be related to several factors: (1) most anti-ABO antibodies are of the IgM type and do not cross the placenta; (2) fetal red cells only weakly express ABO antigens; and (3) unlike Rh antigens, which are expressed only on erythrocytes, ABO antigens are expressed by many normal (epithelial and endothelial) cells that may bind (sop up) some of the transferred antibody.

**(22)** One of the major differences between ABO- and Rh-related erythroblastosis fetalis is the role played by prior maternal sensitization. In Rh hemolytic disease, an Rh-negative mother is exposed to the red cells of the Rh-positive infant during delivery, when the infant erythrocytes leak into the maternal circulation. The IgG antibodies formed in response to this exposure readily cross the placenta and cause disease in Rh-positive fetuses of subsequent pregnancies. In contrast, antibodies to A and B blood group antigens occur naturally in all individuals lacking one or both (type O blood) of these antigens. No previous sensitization is required.

**(23)** Naturally occurring antibodies to A and B antigens are mostly of the IgM type and do not cross the placenta. Type O individuals, however, often make IgG antibodies to these antigens as well. Thus, hemolytic disease occurs almost exclusively in infants of type O mothers.

**(24)** In contrast to Rh incompatibility-related disease, which can be prevented by therapeutic intervention to prevent sensitization, ABO incompatibility–related disease cannot be prevented. It can only be treated with supportive measures once it develops. *(pp. 446–449)*

**25. (True); 26. (True); 27. (False); 28. (False); 29. (False)**

**(25)** The ductus arteriosus is a vascular channel that connects the pulmonary artery with the aorta and serves to divert blood flow from the pulmonary vascular system during intrauterine life. Normally, during the first day or two of postnatal life, muscular contraction of the ductus arteriosus occurs. This produces functional closure of the conduit and shunting of blood ceases.

**(26)** In premature infants, however, this muscular contraction and functional closure are delayed, and the ductus arteriosus remains open. **(27)** This is due to alterations in the physiologic stimuli occurring after birth that normally cause the ductus to close, such as increasing arterial oxygen tensions and decreasing production of vasodilators, including prostaglandins. In short, vasodilatory prostaglandins delay (not induce) normal closure, and therapy with indomethacin to suppress prostaglandin E synthesis has proven an effective nonsurgical means of achieving closure of a patent ductus arteriosus (PDA).

**(28)** Most commonly (85 to 90% of cases), PDA occurs as an isolated defect and produces no functional defect at birth. During infancy, when the shunt is left to right, there is no cyanosis. It is only with the ultimate production of pulmonary hypertension and reversal of the right-to-left shunt that cyanosis develops. It is generally agreed that a PDA should be closed as early in life as feasible in order to prevent the development of pulmonary vascular disease.

**(29)** Although a PDA usually produces no functional difficulties at birth, it nevertheless may be recognized easily by ausculatory examination. It produces a harsh, continuous murmur that is described as "machinery-like." *(p. 575)*

**30. (True); 31. (False); 32. (True); 33. (False); 34. (False)**

**(30)** Coarctation (narrowing, constriction) of the aorta comprises about 5% of all congenital cardiovascular defects. Females with Turner's syndrome frequently have coarctation of the aorta. Overall, however, the defect is two to three times more common in males.

**(31)** Although coarctation of the aorta sometimes may occur as a solitary defect, in 75% of cases it occurs in association with other congenital cardiovascular defects, most commonly a bicuspid aortic valve.

**(32)** The position of the defect has a profound effect on the prognosis. Coarctations located proximal to the ductus arteriosus carry an ominous prognosis and require early surgical intervention. In such cases, the right side of the heart must supply the entire systemic circulation through the ductus arteriosus. Consequently, right ventricular hypertrophy occurs early, often *in utero*. Postpartum survival depends on the patency of the ductus arteriosus, but heart failure commonly supervenes, and many infants die in the neonatal period.

**(33)** When the coarctation is located distal to the ductus arteriosus (postductal coarctation), blood flow to the head and upper extremities is unimpaired, but blood flow to the lower half of the body depends on the development of collateral flow that bypasses the aortic obstruction. Blood frequently is diverted through the intercostal arteries, a common collateral bypass route. As they undergo enlargement, the intercostal arteries tend to produce erosion of the inner surface of the ribs that commonly appears radiographically as "notching."

**(34)** Surgical correction is the definitive treatment for coarctation and is curative in most cases. The defect does not tend to recur once it has been resected surgically, but persistent hypertension despite removal of the obstruction to flow is a complication in some patients. *(pp. 577–578)*

**35. (True); 36. (False); 37. (True); 38. (True); 39. (True)**

**(35)** Of the four features that comprise the tetralogy of Fallot—(1) ventricular septal defect (VSD), (2) an overriding aorta, (3) right ventricular outflow obstruction (subpulmonary stenosis), and (4) right ventricular hypertrophy—it is the degree of obstruction to the outflow from the right ventricle that determines the severity of the clinical symptoms.

**(36)** The subpulmonary stenosis, which usually consists of a narrowing of the infundibulum of the right ventricle (with or without pulmonary valvular stenosis), limits flow through the pulmonary arterial system. Patency of the ductus arteriosus does not alleviate this physiologic deficit and therefore does not affect survival.

**(37)** With limited pulmonary flow (and oxygenation of blood), most affected individuals are cyanotic from birth or soon after. Only in so-called pink tetralogy, with initially mild subpulmonary stenosis and shunting through the VSD (left-to-right shunt), is cyanosis avoided until increasing subpulmonary stenosis results in significant outflow obstruction and produces right-to-left shunting of blood.

**(38)** In profound cyanosis, the low oxygen tension is a stimulus to erythropoietin production, and thus polycythemia is a common part of the clinical picture.

**(39)** Corrective surgery should be performed as soon as possible in infants with tetralogy of Fallot, because the right ventricular outflow obstruction tends to increase with time. Complete surgical repair is possible for classical tetralogy but is more problematic when pulmonary atresia and dilated bronchial arteries are present. Untreated, most patients die before age 10 from cyanosis and congestive heart failure. *(pp. 575–576)*

**40. (C); 41. (C); 42. (B); 43. (A); 44. (A)**

**(40)** Phenylketonuria and alkaptonuria are both diseases caused by inborn errors of tyrosine metabolism. **(41)** The defect in classic PKU is a total lack of hepatic phenylalanine hydroxylase, which converts phenylalanine to tyrosine. In alkaptonuria, the metabolism of phenylalanine-tyrosine is blocked at the level of homogentisic acid as a result of the lack of homogentisic oxidase. In both diseases, the affected infant appears normal at birth.

**(42)** In alkaptonuria, homogentisic acid accumulates in the body and spills over into the urine. If the urine is allowed to stand, the homogentisic acid oxidizes and the urine turns black. The retained homogentisic acid in the body binds to connective tissues, tendons, and cartilage, producing a characteristic blue-black pigmentation (ochronosis) and arthritis that is often severe and painful.

**(43 and 44)** In PKU, the inability to metabolize phenylalanine has more profound consequences. Unless treated with dietary restriction that effectively prevents these complications, hyperphenylalaninemia leads to mental deterioration and retardation in most patients. It is important to recognize that uncommon variants of PKU exist that cannot be treated by dietary restriction and, therefore, have a poor prognosis. These variant forms result from deficiencies in enzymes other than phenylalanine hydroxylase and also may involve defective tyrosine and tryptophan metabolism. In contrast to PKU, there is no effective treatment for alcaptonuria. Dietary restriction of phenylalanine and tyrosine of the degree necessary to prevent disease is considered impractical and potentially deleterious in this disorder. *(pp. 147–148; 449–450)*

**45. (C); 46. (B); 47. (C); 48. (A); 49. (D)**

**(45)** Marfan's syndrome and Ehlers-Danlos syndromes (EDS) are hereditary disorders of connective tissue caused by mutations in single genes involved in structural protein synthesis. Marfan's syndrome is an uncommon autosomal dominant syndrome caused by mutation of the fibrillin gene on chromosome 15. Fibrillin is a glycoprotein essential to the formation of the microfibrillary scaffold of the elastin network in connective tissue. **(46)** The EDS include ten variants encompassing three different Mendelian patterns of inheritance, all related to mutation of genes involved in collagen synthesis. In both Marfan's syndrome and EDS, reduced tensile strength of connective tissue results from the structural protein defect.

**(47)** In both Marfan's syndrome and type IV EDS, vascular weakness is a prominent feature and arterial tearing is common. In Marfan's syndrome, tears in the aorta with formation of dissecting aortic aneurysms occur with a high frequency and constitute the major life-threatening complication. In type IV EDS, the result of an abnormality in type III collagen synthesis, blood vessels and intestine (both rich in type III collagen) are both prone to spontaneous rupture.

**(48)** The skeletal abnormalities of Marfan's syndrome are distinctive, however. Individuals with Marfan's syndrome characteristically have long, slender extremities with particular elongation of the fingers, and tall stature. **(49)** Although joint disorders are characteristic of both Marfan's syndrome and EDS, they are typified by joint ligament laxity and marked hypermobility of the joints rather than the inflexibility that occurs in most other joint diseases. *(pp. 132–134)*

**50. (C); 51. (C); 52. (B); 53. (B); 54. (B); 55. (D); 56. (D)**

**(50 and 52)** An atrial septal defect (ASD) is an abnormal opening in the atrial septum that allows free communication between the right and left atria. ASD constitutes the most frequent asymptomatic congenital cardiac anomaly of childhood. Although the physical signs are trivial and the oscultative findings subtle, most ASDs are diagnosed in childhood. Nevertheless, many escape diagnosis and come to clinical attention only in the adult. Ventricular septal defect (VSD) is the most common congenital cardiac anomaly overall. In contrast to ASD, it is usually symptomatic in childhood, even from birth, depending on the size of the defect. Only small defects may remain recognized in the infant. In some cases, small defects may even close spontaneously. **(51)** Both lesions occur during the same period of fetal development. Normally by the 8th week of gestational life, both the atrial and septal walls of the heart are completely formed. Thus, defects in the development of either septum are produced between the 2nd and 8th weeks of embryogenesis.

**(53)** Infective endocarditis is rare with ASD of any size. Small or moderate-sized VSDs, however, pose a well-defined risk of superimposed bacterial endocarditis at the site of the jet lesion (a complication rarely encountered in large lesions). **(54)** In contrast to ASD, VSD frequently is associated with other structural cardiac anomalies. It constitutes one of the four cardiac defects in the syndrome known as tetralogy of Fallot (see Questions 35–39), in which it is accompanied by an overriding aorta, right ventricular outflow obstruction, and right ventricular hypertrophy.

**(55 and 56)** In septal defects in the heart, whether atrial or ventricular, a left-to-right shunt is created that increases flow through the pulmonary system and may result in irreversible pulmonary hypertension, with cyanosis, respiratory difficulties, and, ultimately, cardiac failure. Overall, irreversible pulmonary hypertension occurs earlier and more frequently with VSD than ASD. Nevertheless, one of the primary goals of surgical correction of either of these defects is the prevention of this dire end-stage complication, which renders either condition inoperable. Surgical closure of an ASD generally is not indicated during infancy. Most are well tolerated during the first decade of life before pulmonary hypertension develops. Thus, the threat to life during infancy is less than that of the operative mortality associated with surgical closure. Surgical correction of isolated VSD (not associated with other structural defects) usually is not attempted in infancy, in hopes of spontaneous closure. If this does not occur, however, surgical correction before the onset of development of pulmonary hypertension is essential. *(pp. 573–575)*

**57. (C); 58. (C); 59. (A); 60. (B); 61. (C)**

**(57 and 58)** Tricuspid valve atresia and pulmonary valve atresia both are associated commonly with underdevelopment (hypoplasia) of the right ventricle and an atrial septal defect. **(59)** In addition, tricuspid valve atresia usually is associated with a ventricular septal defect. The ventricular septum usually is intact in pulmonary valve atresia. **(60)** Although neither is a common congenital cardiac defect, pulmonary valve stenosis or atresia accounts for 10% of congenital cardiac defects, whereas tricuspid atresia accounts for only about 1%. **(61)** Surgical correction is usually possible for both of these valvular atresias, but it is risky and complex as a result of the right ventricular hypoplasia. *(pp. 621; 625)*

**62. (C); 63. (A); 64. (D); 65. (B)**

**(62)** Cytogenetic disorders involving sex chromosomes occur more frequently than those involving autosomal aberrations. One of the most common is Klinefelter's syndrome, with an approximate incidence of 1 in every 850 live male births. The characteristic karyotype of Klinefelter's syndrome is 47,XXY, although numerous multiple-X chromosome variants and mosaics also occur. The major manifestation of Klinefelter's syndrome is hypogonadism, so the disorder rarely is diagnosed before puberty.

**(63)** Turner's syndrome results from complete or partial monosomy of the X chromosome and generally is associated with a 45,X karyotype. The major manifestation of Turner's syndrome is hypogonadism (with primary amenorrhea), but the disorder commonly is recognized from birth by the accompanying characteristic manifestations of webbing of the neck and peripheral lymphedema. Short stature and failure of development of secondary sex characteristics are evident in the adolescent and adult.

**(64)** True hermaphroditism is an extremely rare disorder that most often is associated with a 46,XX karyotype, although some mosaics have been described. The disorder is characterized by the presence of both ovarian and testicular tissue, either separated into separate organs or combined together in "ovotestes." The external genitalia are usually ambiguous.

**(65)** The syndrome of testicular feminization characteristically is associated with a 46,XY karyotype. This disorder is a form of male pseudohermaphroditism and is characterized by a female phenotype with good breast development but absence of uterus and fallopian tubes. Bilateral inguinal testes are usually present. *(pp. 133–136)*

**66. (B); 67. (A); 68 (E); 69. (D); 70. (C)**

**(66)** The Lesch-Nyhan syndrome is an X-linked disorder that is characterized by a deficiency of hypoxanthine guanine phosphoribosyltransferase (HGPRT), an enzyme involved in the "salvage" of free purine bases from the breakdown of nucleic acids. Without this enzyme, there is increased *de novo* synthesis of uric acid. Thus, uric acid is synthesized in excess, hyperuricemia results, and gout is produced. A variety of neurologic problems whose pathogenesis is less well understood also occur. Principal among them are self-mutilation, aggressive behavior, mental retardation, spastic cerebral palsy, and choreoathetosis.

**(67)** Fabry's disease, one of the lysosomal storage disorders (see Question 17), is an X-linked disorder of galacterocerebroside metabolism, resulting in the systemic accumulation of this compound. Although the cardiovascular system, the central nervous system, and the reticuloendothelial systems are all affected, the kidney is the most severely involved organ, and most patients die of progressive renal failure in middle life without chronic hemodialysis and/or renal transplantation. However, another aspect of Fabry's disease may dominate the clinical picture: red-blue elevated skin nodules known as angiokeratomas (dermal telangiectasias with lipid accumulation in the endothelial cells and hyperkeratotic thickening of the overlying epidermis).

**(68)** Xanthomas and accelerated atherosclerosis are the features of familial hypercholesterolemia, an autosomal dominant disorder that is possibly the most common disease with Mendelian inheritance. Familial hypercholesterolemia is caused by loss of feedback control mechanisms that regulate cholesterol synthesis. The result is widespread deposition of excess cholesterol in tissues such as the skin (xanthomas), coronary arteries, peripheral vessels, and other organs. Death from coronary artery disease and myocardial infarction at an early age is a common consequence.

**(69)** Wilson's disease is a rare inborn error of copper metabolism. Excess deposits of copper accumulate in the brain, liver, and cornea to produce the three characteristic pathologic consequences of this disorder: degenerative changes in the brain with focal cavitation, liver damage with cirrhosis, and the pathognomonic green-brown ring at the limbus of the cornea (Kayser-Fleischer ring). Characteristically, hepatic disease occurs long before the ocular or neurologic disease becomes clinically evident. The disease is important to recognize because it can be treated effectively with a low-copper diet and chelating agents.

**(70)** Von Hippel-Lindau (VHL) disease is a rare autosomal dominant disorder characterized by the occurrence of multiple benign and malignant neoplasms through the body. The most commonly occurring tumors in this disorder are retinal and cerebellar hemangioblastomas. Renal cell carcinomas, adrenal pheochromocytomas, angiomas of the liver and kidney, adenomas of the kidney and epididymis, and cysts in the pancreas, liver, and kidneys are also common. Renal cell carcinomas occur in about 25% of cases and, in this subgroup, are the major cause of death. It is now known that VHL is caused by mutation of a tumor suppressor gene (the VHL gene) on chromosome 3 that encodes a protein involved in signal transduction or cell adhesion. Mutations of this gene are believed to be important in the pathogenesis of sporadic and familial renal cell carcinoma as well. *(pp. 138; 135; 863–864; 986; 1255; 1354)*

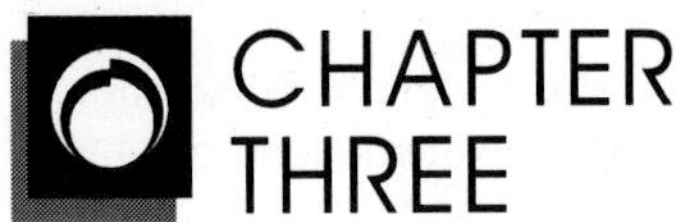

# Nutritional and Environmental Diseases

**DIRECTIONS:** For Questions 1 through 20, choose the ONE BEST answer to each question.

**1.** Deficient production of the vitamin K–dependent coagulation factors is *not* associated with:

A. Hepatic failure
B. Use of warfarin
C. Strict vegetarianism
D. Pancreatic insufficiency
E. Use of broad-spectrum antibiotics

**2.** All of the following statements correctly describe vitamin A–associated nutritional disorders EXCEPT:

A. Liver disease causes vitamin A deficiency.
B. Vitamin A deficiency causes blindness.
C. Vitamin A deficiency causes squamous metaplasia in glandular epithelia.
D. Vitamin A toxicity causes liver disease.
E. Vitamin A toxicity is associated with increased infections.

**3.** Hypovitaminosis A occurs in association with all of the following conditions EXCEPT:

A. Pseudomembranous colitis
B. Chronic pancreatitis
C. Whipple's disease
D. Abetalipoproteinemia
E. Celiac sprue

**4.** Deficiency of vitamin D is associated with all of the following conditions EXCEPT:

A. Strict vegetarianism
B. Celiac disease (sprue)
C. Cirrhosis
D. Hypoparathyroidism
E. Chronic renal failure

**5.** All of the following statements correctly describe vitamin E EXCEPT:

A. It is obtained from both animal and vegetable dietary sources.
B. Transport in the blood requires no specific protein carrier.
C. Deficiency causes neurologic damage.
D. Deficiency occurs with abetalipoproteinemia.
E. Toxicity reactions are unknown in humans.

**6.** All of the following statements about Vitamin $B_1$ (thiamine) are true EXCEPT:

A. It is a coenzyme involved in cleavage of ATP.
B. Deficiency produces polyneuropathy.
C. Deficiency produces cardiomyopathy.
D. Deficiency produces the Wernicke-Korsakoff syndrome.
E. Deficiency is common among chronic alcoholics.

**7.** The absorption of vitamin $B_{12}$ from food and its delivery to the cells of the body is dependent on all of the following factors EXCEPT:

A. Intrinsic factor
B. Cobalophilins
C. Pancreatic proteases
D. Bile salts
E. Transcobalamin II

**8.** At the cellular level, deficiency of vitamin $B_{12}$ results in all of the following consequences EXCEPT:

A. Increased intrinsic factor production
B. Folate deficiency
C. Synthesis of abnormal fatty acids
D. Reduced adenine synthesis
E. Reduced thymidine synthesis

**9.** Patients with scurvy develop defects of all of the following functions EXCEPT:

A. Metabolism of toxins by P-450 mixed-function oxidase
B. Iron absorption from the intestine
C. Cross-linking of collagen
D. Formation of hydroxyproline
E. Adhesion of platelets

**10.** Neurologic dysfunctions are known to result from deficiencies of all of the following nutrients EXCEPT:

A. Vitamin $B_1$ (thiamine)
B. Niacin
C. Vitamin $B_6$ (pyridoxine)
D. Vitamin $B_{12}$
E. Folate

**11.** All of the following statements about iron as a nutrient are true EXCEPT:

A. Daily requirements are greater for young women than young men.
B. Normally, most dietary iron is not absorbed.
C. Deficiency in adult males is often due to gastrointestinal blood loss.
D. Deficiency causes a drop in the total iron-binding capacity.
E. Deficiency causes abnormal mitochondrial function.

**12.** All of the following conditions increase in incidence with obesity EXCEPT:

A. Rheumatoid arthritis
B. Diabetes mellitus
C. Hyperlipidemia
D. Gallstones
E. Hypertension

**13.** All of the following statements correctly describe synthetic retinoids EXCEPT:

A. They effectively treat severe acne.
B. They effectively treat premalignant actinic keratosis.
C. They effectively treat acute promyelocytic leukemia.
D. They increase the incidence of urinary tract cancers.
E. They increase the incidence of fetal malformations when taken during pregnancy.

**14.** Which of the following statements correctly describes vitamin K deficiency?

A. Deficiency causes defects in both the intrinsic and extrinsic coagulation pathways.
B. Deficiency produces defects in platelet function.
C. Deficiency is associated with strict vegetarian diets.
D. Intestinal bacteria produce enough vitamin K to prevent deficiency under normal conditions.
E. Deficiency develops less frequently in breast-fed infants than in bottle-fed infants.

**15.** Vitamins that are ingested in an active form and do not require metabolic conversion for activity include all of the following EXCEPT:

A. Vitamin K
B. Vitamin E
C. Vitamin C
D. Vitamin D
E. Vitamin $B_{12}$

**16.** Use of oral contraceptives (as currently formulated) is associated with increased risk of:

A. Venous thrombosis
B. Ovarian cancer
C. Hepatocellular adenoma
D. Breast cancer
E. Endometrial cancer

**17.** All of the following conditions lead to vitamin $B_{12}$ deficiency EXCEPT:

A. Ulcerative colitis
B. Crohn's disease
C. Surgical resection of the stomach (gastrectomy)
D. Achlorhydria
E. Strict vegetarianism

**18.** Aspirin is associated with all of the following adverse drug reactions EXCEPT:

A. Gastric ulceration
B. Renal papillary necrosis
C. Massive hepatic necrosis
D. Tinnitus
E. Asthma

**19.** Which of the following nutrients is involved in free radical scavenging (antioxidant) reactions?

A. Biotin
B. Vitamin $B_6$
C. Vitamin $B_{12}$
D. Vitamin D
E. Vitamin E

**20.** Ionizing radiation causes cellular damage by all of the following mechanisms EXCEPT:

A. Elevation of temperature (generation of heat)
B. Formation of free radicals
C. Generation of autoimmunity
D. Breakage of chromosomes
E. Inhibition of mitosis

**DIRECTIONS:** For Questions 21 through 58, the set of lettered headings is followed by a list of numbered words or phrases. For each numbered word or phrase choose:

A—if the item is associated with (A) only
B—if the item is associated with (B) only
C—if the item is associated with *both* (A) and (B)
D—if the item is associated with *neither* (A) nor (B)

For each of the characteristics listed below, choose whether it describes kwashiorkor, marasmus, both, or neither.

A. Kwashiorkor
B. Marasmus
C. Both
D. Neither

**21.** Total caloric intake is adequate.
**22.** Affected infants are cachetic and ravenously hungry.
**23.** Edema is usually present.
**24.** Desquamative skin lesions are pathognomonic.
**25.** Fatty change usually is seen in the liver.
**26.** Intercurrent parasitic infection is common.
**27.** The pathologic changes caused by the disease are completely reversible with restoration of an adequate diet.

For each of the characteristics listed below, choose whether it describes rickets, osteomalacia, both, or neither.

A. Rickets
B. Osteomalacia
C. Both
D. Neither

**28.** Osteoid mineralization is retarded.
**29.** Endochondral ossification is retarded.
**30.** Osteitis fibrosa cystica frequently occurs concomitantly.
**31.** The disease has a hereditary autosomal recessive form.
**32.** The disease has a hereditary X-linked form.
**33.** Looser's zones seen on radiographs are pathognomonic.

For each of the characteristics listed below, choose whether it relates to calcium, phosphate, both, or neither.

A. Calcium
B. Phosphate
C. Both
D. Neither

**34.** Decreased serum levels induce synthesis of 1,25-$(OH)_2D_3$.
**35.** Intestinal absorption is increased by vitamin D.
**36.** Parathyroid hormone increases renal excretion.
**37.** Increased renal losses occur in the Fanconi syndrome.
**38.** Lamellar osteoid seams appear in bone in deficiency states.
**39.** Anticonvulsant drugs cause decreased intestinal absorption.
**40.** Calcitonin increases serum levels.

For each of the characteristics listed below, choose whether it describes disease caused by alcohol toxicity, thiamine deficiency, both, or neither.

A. Alcohol toxocity
B. Thiamine deficiency
C. Both
D. Neither

**41.** Produces a dilated cardiomyopathy
**42.** Causes cirrhosis
**43.** Is associated with a transketolase deficiency
**44.** Produces skeletal muscle weakness
**45.** Is associated with the Wernicke-Korsakoff syndrome

For each of the following conditions, choose whether it is associated with vitamin $B_{12}$ deficiency, folate deficiency, both, or neither.

A. Vitamin $B_{12}$ deficiency
B. Folate deficiency
C. Both
D. Neither

**46.** Occurs in pernicious anemia
**47.** Occurs commonly in alcoholism
**48.** Typically produces glossitis
**49.** Typically produces sideroblasts in the bone marrow
**50.** Results in hypersegmentation of neutrophils
**51.** Reduces fertility

For each of the physiologic processes listed below, choose whether it requires vitamin C, vitamin D, both, or neither.

A. Vitamin C
B. Vitamin D
C. Both
D. Neither

**52.** Osteoid production
**53.** Osteoid mineralization
**54.** Bone resorption
**55.** Bone remodeling
**56.** Cartilage resorption in endochondral bone growth
**57.** Tooth formation
**58.** Wound healing

**DIRECTIONS:** Questions 59 through 85 are matching questions. For each numbered item, choose the most likely associated lettered item from those provided. Each numbered item has ONLY ONE answer. Within each group, each lettered item may be the answer to one, more than one, or none of the numbered items.

For each of the environmental or occupational carcinogens listed below, choose whether it causes skin cancer, lung cancer, bladder cancer, stomach cancer, or none of these.

A. Skin cancer
B. Lung cancer
C. Bladder cancer
D. Stomach cancer
E. None of these

**59.** Aflatoxin B
**60.** $\beta$-Naphthylamine
**61.** Nitrites
**62.** Vinyl chloride
**63.** Uranium
**64.** Benzene
**65.** Asbestos

For each of the following characteristics, choose whether it is associated with riboflavin (vitamin $B_2$), niacin, pyridoxine (vitamin $B_6$), all of these, or none of these.

A. Riboflavin (vitamin $B_2$)
B. Niacin
C. Pyridoxine (vitamin $B_6$)
D. All of these
E. None of these

**66.** The molecule is a coenzyme in cellular oxidative metabolism.
**67.** The human body is capable of endogenous synthesis of the vitamin.
**68.** The molecule facilitates conduction of impulses in peripheral nerves.
**69.** No deficiency syndrome is known to occur.
**70.** A deficiency state causes a macrocytic anemia.
**71.** A deficiency state causes a dermatitis.
**72.** A deficiency state is associated with dementia.
**73.** Parenteral administration commonly produces toxic effects.

For each of the hematologic abnormalities listed below, choose whether it is associated with iron deficiency, vitamin $B_{12}$ deficiency, starvation, all of these, or none of these.

A. Iron deficiency
B. Vitamin $B_{12}$ deficiency
C. Starvation
D. All of these
E. None of these

**74.** Increased hemolysis
**75.** Increased osmotic fragility of erythrocytes
**76.** Hypochromic, microcytic anemia
**77.** Normochromic, macrocytic anemia
**78.** Hypochromic, normocytic anemia

For each of the adverse drug rections listed below, choose whether it is commonly associated with acetaminophen, tetracycline, penicillin, chloramphenicol, or none of these.

A. Acetaminophen
B. Tetracycline
C. Penicillin
D. Chloramphenicol
E. None of these

**79.** Massive hepatic necrosis
**80.** Fatty liver
**81.** Interstitial fibrosis of the lung
**82.** Aplastic anemia
**83.** Anaphylaxis
**84.** Hemolytic anemia
**85.** Drug-induced lupus

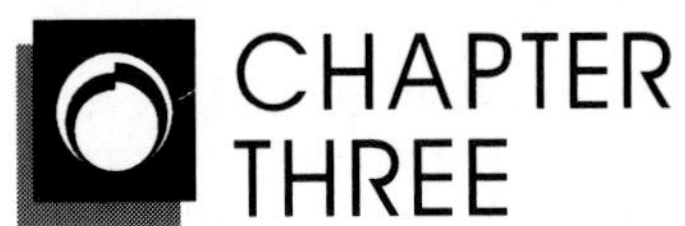

CHAPTER THREE

# Nutritional and Environmental Diseases

## ANSWERS

**1. (C)** Vitamin K is a fat-soluble vitamin that acts as a cofactor for a liver microsomal carboxylase that is important in the synthesis of four coagulation factors (factors II [prothrombin], VII, IX, and X). Thus, a coagulopathy secondary to decreased levels of the vitamin K–dependent coagulation factors may result from any type of diffuse liver disease, especially if it is severe enough to produce hepatic failure. The synthesis and secretion of all the vitamin K–dependent coagulation factors is reduced in hepatic failure.

Pancreatic exocrine insufficiency from any cause (e.g., cystic fibrosis, chronic pancreatitis, or surgical resection of the pancreas) decreases the secretion of all pancreatic enzymes. In turn, enzymatic hydrolysis of all ingested nutrients is compromised, but fat absorption especially is affected. Fat malabsorption results in deficiencies of essential fatty acids and of all the fat-soluble vitamins (vitamins A, D, E, and K).

Vitamin K deficiency also may be iatrogenic, because it can occur as a consequence of administration of certain drugs. Broad-spectrum antibiotics inhibit hepatic epoxide reductase, which is involved in recycling vitamin K (restoring the vitamin to its active form after it has participated in a carboxylase reaction) within the liver cell. Warfarin and dicumarol also are known to inhibit hepatic epoxide reductase and, for this reason, are used therapeutically as anticoagulants.

However, strict vegetarianism would not lead to vitamin K deficiency, because vitamin K is widely available in the diet from both plant (especially green vegetables) and animal sources. *(pp. 419–420; 796; 841; 904)*

**2. (E)** Vitamin A is known to be requisite to: (1) the processes of maturation and differentiation of epithelial cells, both glandular and squamous; and (2) the production of photosensitive pigments in the retina. Deficiencies of the vitamin lead to decreased production of rhodopsin in rods (impairing vision in dim light) and iodopsin in cones. Protracted deficiency leads to conjunctival and corneal desiccation and erosion, impeding transmission of light and predisposing to infection. Subsequent scarring or extrusion of the lens produces blindness. Vitamin A deficiency is the leading cause of blindness in many Asian and African countries, and, next to protein-calorie malnutrition, it is the most common nutritional disorder in the world.

Although hypovitaminosis A usually is caused by dietary deficiency, it also can occur with diseases that lead to decreased absorption or transport of the vitamin. Both the transportation of mobilized vitamin A stores in the blood and the uptake of vitamin A by peripheral tissues is dependent on retinol-binding protein (RBP), a protein that is synthesized by the liver. In chronic liver disease and cirrhosis, RBP production is decreased and circulating levels of vitamin A are consequently inadequate. Loss of RBP via the urine (e.g., in the nephrotic syndrome) has the same effect. Cirrhosis may also compromise hepatic retinyl ester stores (the principal reservoir of vitamin A in the body). Decreased uptake of Vitamin A occurs in any disease interfering with fat absorption (pancreatic, biliary tract, or small intestinal disease) (see Question 3), and a hypovitaminosis A results.

Vitamin A toxicity may be either acute or chronic. Acute toxicity produces symptoms suggestive of a brain tumor: headache, stupor, vomiting and papilledema. Chronic toxicity begins with anorexia, nausea, vomiting, cutaneous desquamation, and pruritus. Liver injury with hepatomegaly and fibrosis (sometimes severe enough to produce portal hypertension) occurs with more protracted disease.

In deficiency states, glandular epithelia (e.g., gastrointestinal, respiratory, and genitourinary mucosae) undergo squamous metaplasia. Squamous metaplasia in the bronchial tree destroys the natural host defense provided by ciliated epithelial surfaces and increases susceptibility to respiratory tract infection. Furthermore, the mortality rate from childhood infections is increased (four times greater than controls) in children with vitamin A deficiency. Vitamin A toxicity, in contrast, is not associated with increased infections. *(pp. 411–414)*

**3. (A)** Vitamin A is a fat-soluble vitamin. Therefore, a primary deficiency of the vitamin may occur in any disease causing impaired absorption of fat. In chronic pancreatitis, the resultant pancreatic insufficiency leads to defective intraluminal hydrolysis, solubility, and subsequent absorption of fat.

Whipple's disease is a rare systemic infection (mode of transmission unknown) that primarily affects the small bowel and causes a malabsorption syndrome. In this disease, the lamina propria of the small bowel mucosa is filled with macrophages containing the infecting organism (a gram-positive actinomycete named *Tropheryma whippelii*) in their cytoplasm.

In abetalipoproteinemia, an inherited defect in apolipoprotein A production by small intestinal absorptive cells results in an inability to synthesize the $\beta$ lipoproteins required for the export of triglycerides from the cell. Thus, fat can enter the absorptive cell, but it cannot exit. Fat accumulates within the mucosal cells, and severe hypolipidemia with hypovitaminosis A develops.

Celiac sprue is a hypersensitivity-mediated enteropathy caused by an immune reaction to gluten (wheat protein). Severe small bowel mucosal injury is produced, and malabsorption of many nutrients, including fats and fat-soluble vitamins, results.

Pseudomembranous colitis (caused by *Clostridium difficile*) is not usually associated with defects in nutrient absorption. The disease process is entirely limited to the mucosa of the colon, and nutrient absorption in the small bowel takes place normally. Therefore, absorption, transport, and storage of vitamin A are unaffected. *(pp. 795–800)*

**4. (D)** Vitamin D is a biochemical relative of cholesterol, and its principal dietary sources are animal products. Therefore, strict vegetarian diets can lead to vitamin D deficiency. This is especially true if endogenous sources of vitamin D are inadequate, as they are for most people living in the Northern hemisphere, where exposure to sunlight is limited. Dietary vitamin D is absorbed in the small intestine like other fats, so diseases that severely reduce the bowel's absorptive surface, such as celiac sprue (gluten enteropathy), compromise uptake of vitamin D.

The liver plays three key roles in vitamin D metabolism: (1) synthesis of serum transport proteins for vitamin D, (2) storage of vitamin D, and (3) 25-hydroxylation of vitamin $D_3$, the first step in the metabolic conversion of vitamin $D_3$ to its metabolically active form. Thus hepatic parenchymal diseases, such as cirrhosis, often are associated with a vitamin D deficiency state. The second step in the conversion of vitamin $D_3$ to its active form (1-hydroxylation) takes place in the kidney. Therefore, severe renal parenchymal disease with chronic renal failure also can lead to a functional vitamin D deficiency.

The parathyroid glands have no direct effect on vitamin D metabolism. Indirectly, however, the fall in serum calcium concentration caused by hypoparathyroidism would be expected to stimulate vitamin D metabolism. *(pp. 414–416; 1147)*

**5. (E)** "Vitamin E" actually encompasses a family of four different, but chemically related, tocopherols and tocotrienols. These are fat-soluble substances that are widely distributed in both plant and animal dietary sources. Following their absorption, the tocopherols are transported in chylomicrons in the blood. They require no specific serum transport proteins, nor do they require metabolic conversion for activity. Biologically, these compounds act as antitoxidants. They are especially important in the neutralization of free radicals, which are generated continuously (and are highly destructive) at the cellular level.

Deficiencies in vitamin E can result from diseases causing severe fat malabsorption, such as abetalipoproteinemia (see Question 3). Clinically, hypovitaminosis E is characterized primarily by neurologic damage (spinocerebellar degeneration) and skeletal muscle abnormalities, but deficiency of the vitamin is usually present for years before becoming clinically evident. Pathologically, axonal degeneration in the posterior columns and neuron loss from the dorsal root ganglia are the most common changes. Denervation atrophy and lipopigment accumulation occurs in skeletal muscle. In infants, vitamin E deficiency causes hemolytic anemia.

Vitamin E toxicity occurs with massive overdoses (e.g., megadose vitamin consumption) and produces a variety of gastrointestinal disturbances, platelet dysfunction, and coagulation defects. In infants, vitamin E therapy has been associated with necrotizing enterocolitis. *(pp. 418–419)*

**6. (A)** Vitamin $B_1$ (thiamine) is both a coenzyme involved in the synthesis (not cleavage) of ATP and a cofactor for transketolase in the pentose phosphate pathway. Thus, it is required for carbohydrate metabolism. It is also required for maintenance of nerve cell membranes and for normal nerve conduction. For this reason, the peripheral nerves and the brain are major targets of injury in thiamine deficiency. A thiamine deficiency syndrome characterized primarily by peripheral neuropathy is known as "dry beriberi." Involvement of the brain, with hemorrhagic necrosis in the mammilliary bodies and the adjacent ventricular system, causes clinical syndromes characterized by psychotic symptoms that begin abruptly (Wernicke's encephalopathy) or memory disturbances and confabulation (Korsakoff's syndrome). Frequently, the two occur together and are known as the Wernicke-Korsakoff syndrome. The heart is the third major target of thiamine deficiency. A deficiency syndrome characterized primarily by cardiomyopathy and heart failure is known as "wet beriberi."

Primary dietary deficiency of thiamine occurs in those populations whose diet consists largely of polished rice or milled grains, because the discarded husks contain most of the grains' thiamine. Increased losses of this water-soluble vitamin with diuretic therapy also cause deficiencies. Thiamine loss also may occur as a consequence of direct enzymatic degradation by thiaminases contained in raw foods such as fish, shellfish, or meat, and therefore, a diet consisting mainly of these foods may cause beriberi. However, chronic alcoholism is by far the most common cause of beriberi. Poor general nutrition with decreased thiamine intake, increased losses from vomiting and ethanol-induced diuresis, and an inherited transketolase abnormality that is common among chronic alcoholics all may contribute to thiamine deficiency. *(pp. 420–421; 1339)*

**7. (D)** Vitamin $B_{12}$ is an organometallic compound, known as cobalamin, that contains a cobalt atom in the center of a corrin ring (structurally similar to the porphyrin rings of hemoglobin, with their central iron atoms). Absorption of vitamin $B_{12}$ is a complex process requiring the interaction of a number of factors. When ingested, the vitamin is attached to animal protein (its only dietary source), from which it is released in the acid-peptic milieu of the stomach. It then complexes with secreted salivary proteins known as vitamin $B_{12}$–binding proteins or cobalophilins. These also are known as rapid (R)-binder proteins because of their electrophoretic mobility. R-binder proteins have a high affinity for cobalamin at a low pH and form R–vitamin $B_{12}$ complexes in the acid environment of the stomach. In the duodenum, R–vitamin $B_{12}$ complexes are broken down by pancreatic proteases, and the released cobalamin combines with intrinsic factor (IF), a glycoprotein synthesized by gastric parietal cells. The IF–vitamin $B_{12}$ complexes then are transported to the ileum, where they are bound by specific mucosal cell receptors, a process requiring calcium and a pH greater than 5.6. Once bound, the complex is taken up and transported across the ileal mucosal cell to the blood. Within the blood, vitamin $B_{12}$ is bound to its plasma transport protein, transcobalamin II, for delivery to the liver and other organs. None of the steps in this absorptive process is known to require the presence of bile salts. *(pp. 605–606)*

**8. (A)** Metabolic derivatives of vitamin $B_{12}$ are required for two important biochemical reactions: (1) conversion of homocysteine to methionine and (2) the conversion of methylmalonyl-coenzyme A to succinyl-coenzyme A. The first is essential to the synthesis of both purines and thymidine (essential precursors of DNA), and the second to fatty acid synthesis. Thus, in vitamin $B_{12}$ deficiency, the production of purines (adenine and guanine) and thymidine (a pyrimidine) is reduced (see below), and abnormal fatty acids are synthesized.

Normally, during the process of conversion of homocysteine to methionine, tetrahydrofolate ($FH_4$) is "liberated" from its methylated form by methyltransferase. This reaction is dependent on vitamin $B_{12}$, which serves as an essential cofactor for methyltransferase. With vitamin $B_{12}$ deficiency, transmethylation is decreased and folate is "trapped" in the form of methyltetrahydrofolate, creating a functional folate deficiency. The decreased availability of $FH_4$, in turn, decreases biosynthetic reactions in which $FH_4$ serves as an intermediate in the transfer of one-carbon structural units (formyl and methyl groups) from compound to compound. The transfer of one-carbon units is essential to the production of compounds such as methionine, purines, and dTMP (deoxythymidylate monophosphate—the form of thymidine that is the immediate precursor of DNA), so deficiencies of these compounds occur with either vitamin $B_{12}$ or folate deficiencies.

Although the availability of vitamin $B_{12}$ is dependent on the production of intrinsic factor (IF), vitamin $B_{12}$ is not known to exert any feedback control on the elaboration of IF by gastric parietal cells. Therefore, vitamin $B_{12}$ deficiency would not be expected to increase IF production. *(pp. 606–609)*

**9. (E)** Scurvy is the disease produced by vitamin C deficiency. Scurvy is an uncommon disorder because vitamin C is abundant in most foods, easily absorbed throughout the small bowel, and stored in substantial quantity in most tissues. Vitamin C is required for collagen cross-linking and the hydroxylation of proline (i.e., formation of hydroxyproline) as well as other biochemical events in collagen synthesis. Therefore, in vitamin C deficiency states, these essential functions are compromised and collagen production is impaired. The major clinical manifestations of scurvy reflect the consequences of abnormal collagen production and include: (1) weakened vascular walls with hemorrhage, (2) skeletal deformities in the growing child, and (3) defective wound repair. Vitamin C is also a component of the P-450 mixed-function oxidase system, which is critical in the metabolism of toxins by the liver and other organs in which this enzyme system is found. In addition, vitamin C enhances the absorption of inorganic (nonheme) iron from the intestine, participates in the synthesis of carnitine and neurotransmitters, and serves as a potent antioxidant that prevents free radical injury throughout the body. All of these processes are affected adversely by deficiency of vitamin C.

Although scurvy is associated with hemorrhagic diatheses (purpura, ecchymoses, subperiosteal hemorrhages and intracerebral hemorrhages), these are the result of vascular fragility caused by defective collagen in blood vessel walls and are not related to altered platelet function. Platelet functions are not known to be affected by vitamin C deficiency. *(pp. 13; 423–424)*

**10. (E)** Many nutritional deficiencies have profound effects on the nervous system that occasionally may dominate the clinical presentation. Vitamin $B_1$ (thiamine) is required both for maintenance of nerve cell membranes and for the normal conduction of impulses in peripheral nerves. Thus, the brain and the peripheral nerves are major targets of injury in thiamine deficiency. The thiamine deficiency syndrome dominated by peripheral neuropathy is known as "dry beriberi" (see Question 6). In contrast, brain dysfunction secondary to thiamine deficiency usually causes a clinical syndrome characterized by psychotic symptoms and memory disturbances, known as the Wernicke-Korsakoff syndrome.

Vitamin $B_6$ (pyridoxine) is known to participate (as a coenzyme) in numerous metabolic functions in the brain, including the synthesis of neurotransmitters. Consequently, pyridoxine deficiency states produce peripheral neuropathies and occasionally convulsions. Furthermore, pyridoxine-deficient mothers may produce mentally retarded infants.

Niacin deficiency typically is associated with degeneration of the ganglion cells of the brain and spinal cord tracts. Ganglion cell degeneration produces dementia that, along with diarrhea and dermatitis, forms the classic symptom triad ("the three D's") of pellagra.

Both vitamin $B_{12}$ and folate deficiencies produce megaloblastic anemia, but only vitamin $B_{12}$ deficiency is associated with neurologic abnormalities. Vitamin $B_{12}$ deficiency produces peripheral neuropathy and degeneration of the posterior and lateral spinal columns. The pathogenesis of these lesions is not completely understood but may be related to the derangement of cobalamin-dependent fatty acid biosynthesis and incorporation of abnormal fatty acids into the lipids of myelin. The neurologic manifestations of vitamin $B_{12}$ deficiency help to distinguish it from folate deficiency, which it resembles hematologically. *(pp. 412; 420–421)*

**11. (D)** The total iron content of the body is normally a closely regulated constant. In general, iron is recycled efficiently by the body, and daily losses of iron (in the form of intracellular ferritin) from sloughing of various epithelial cells (skin, gastrointestinal, and genitourinary) are fixed and quite small. Additional losses in the young adult female occur with menses and pregnancy. Therefore, women of reproductive age require approximately twice as much iron daily as their male counterparts. Normal losses are small, so iron balance is maintained by restricting intestinal absorption of dietary iron (most of which takes place in the duodenum). Enterocytes constitute a "mucosal barrier" to iron absorption by regulating uptake of iron from the gut lumen and transfer to the plasma. About 25% of ingested heme iron (from animal proteins such as hemoglobin and myoglobin) is absorbed, but only 1 to 2% of inorganic (nonheme) iron is absorbed. Overall, only about 5 to 10% of all ingested iron is absorbed.

In industrialized countries having abundant food supplies, iron deficiency in adult males often reflects occult bleeding from an infectious, inflammatory, or neoplastic process in the gastrointestinal tract. In nonindustrialized countries, however, iron deficiencies are usually the result of a lack of iron in the diet. Early manifestations of deficiency are: 1) the depletion of iron stores, indicated by a drop in serum ferritin; and 2) decreased iron transport, with low serum iron levels and INCREASED total iron-binding capacity. In other words, with decreased iron levels, the number of unused iron-binding sites on serum transferrin increases (transferrin is a glycoprotein made by the liver, which constitutes the serum transport system for iron). Iron deficiency causes qualitative and/or quantitative abnormalities of all normal iron-containing compounds, including mitochondrial enzymes involved in ATP synthesis, cytochromes, flavoproteins, myoglobin, and hemoglobin. Thus, the overall metabolic abnormalities of iron deficiency are as much a consequence of deficient enzymatic and mitochondrial function as of anemia. *(pp. 610–613)*

**12. (A)** In the United States, obesity is the single most common nutritional disorder. Obesity is known to predispose to a number of diseases that carry significant risks of morbidity and even mortality. Among the conditions that occur with increased frequency in obesity are hypertension, adult-onset diabetes mellitus, hyperlipidemia, and cholelithiasis (gallstones). Although degenerative osteoarthritis from increased stress on weight-bearing joints may be associated with obesity, there is no correlation between obesity and rheumatoid arthritis, a disease caused by immunologic injury. *(pp. 425–427; 1247; 1249)*

**13. (D)** Synthetic retinoids (vitamin A analogues) have antiproliferative and differentiation-promoting effects on both squamous and glandular epithelia and other cell types as well. They are highly effective, if not curative, in the treatment of many bothersome and disfiguring non-neoplastic skin diseases, such as severe acne, rosacea, and psoriasis. Several premalignant and malignant skin diseases, such as actinic keratosis, keratoacanthoma, and basal cell carcinoma, also can be treated effectively with synthetic retinoids. There is also evidence to suggest that retinoids (natural or synthetic) may be effective in preventing the development of and/or inducing the regression of metaplasias and premalignant dysplasia in other epithelial systems (besides the epidermis). Tumors of the urinary bladder, for example, have been reported to be susceptible to the anticancer effects of retinoids in both laboratory animals and humans. In addition, vitamin A derivatives have been used successfully to control acute promyelocytic leukemia by inducing differentiation of the immature leukemic cells. In sharp contrast to other forms of chemotherapy, retinoids themselves are not thought to be carcinogenic. They are not without their downside, however. For example, they are associated with an increased risk of fetal malformations (thus, their use is contraindicated in pregnancy). They also can cause acute toxic reactions and other complications. *(pp. 413–414; 1201)*

**14. (A)** Vitamin K is a cofactor for a hepatic carboxylase that converts the inactive proenzyme forms of clotting factors II (prothrombin), VII, XI, and X to their functionally active state. Vitamin K–dependent carboxylation of these factors is required for their calcium-dependent interaction with phospholipid surfaces involved in the generation of thrombin. Factor VII is activated in the extrinsic pathway, factor XI in the intrinsic pathway, and factors X and II in both (in the final common pathway). Thus, inactivity of these vitamin K–dependent clotting factors cause defects in both pathways. However, because vitamin K has no known role in platelet biology, vitamin K deficiency would not be expected to affect platelet function adversely.

Vitamin K is widely available in the diet and is especially plentiful in leafy green vegetables, as well as dairy products, liver, and bacon. Therefore, strict vegetarianism, although associated with deficiencies of most other fat-soluble vitamins, does not cause a vitamin K deficiency. Intestinal bacteria also contribute to the daily supply by synthesizing vitamin K but do not provide enough of this compound to meet the full vitamin K requirements without dietary supplementation. In infancy, when intestinal bacterial colonization is incomplete and hepatic reserves of vitamin K are small, the risk of developing vitamin K deficiency is increased by breast feeding because human breast milk contains less vitamin K than cow's milk. *(pp. 419–420)*

**15. (D)** Vitamins K and E (fat-soluble vitamins) as well as vitamins $B_{12}$ and C (water-soluble vitamins) all are obtained from dietary sources in their active form and require no metabolic conversion for biologic activity in humans. Vitamin K is obtained primarily from leafy green vegetables, dairy products, and other animal sources. Vitamin E also is obtained from leafy green vegetables, as well as cooking oils and whole grains. Although $\alpha$-tocopherol is the major dietary form of vitamin E, there are actually eight compounds (four tocopherols and four tocotrienols) that have vitamin E activity. All of these are absorbed directly from the diet and are utilizable in their absorbed form. Vitamin C (ascorbate) is an acid available in many foodstuffs, including fruits, vegetables, liver, fish, and milk. It too is absorbed directly in its biologically active form. Although the processes of uptake and transport of vitamin $B_{12}$ within the body require the participation of several different binding proteins (see Question 7), the vitamin itself requires no metabolic conversion for activity.

In contrast to these natively active compounds, vitamin D is absorbed from dietary sources (a variety of animal products) in a biologically inactive form known as cholecalciferol or vitamin $D_3$. Vitamin $D_3$ requires two separate metabolic conversions in order to acquire full biologic activity. In the liver, cholecalciferol is first hydroxylated at the 25-carbon position. In the kidney, a second hydroxylation occurs at the 1-carbon position, yielding the active form of vitamin D (1,25-$(OH)_2D_3$) (see Question 4). *(pp. 414–420; 423; 606–607)*

**16. (C)** Most of the serious adverse side effects that had been linked to the use of oral contraceptives (OCs) in the past were largely due to the steroid concentrations, the relative amounts of estrogenic versus progestogenic compounds in the formula, and the dosage schedules of the earlier regimens. As currently formulated, with greatly reduced doses of estrogenic and progestogenic steroids, many of the adverse effects of OCs have been reduced greatly and some have been virtually eliminated. Current data on the "minipill" OCs indicates that these new compounds do not increase the risk of breast cancer, nor do they increase the risk of venous thrombosis in the absence of other predisposing factors (e.g., cigarette smoking, diabetes mellitus, hypertension). The risk of developing either ovarian or endometrial cancer actually is decreased by the use of OCs, indicating that OCs have a protective effect in these diseases. In contrast, the occurrence of hepatocellular adenomas is increased among users of OCs. In fact, other than those that occur in users of OCs, these benign neoplasms are otherwise exceedingly rare. *(pp. 386–387)*

**17. (A)** Vitamin $B_{12}$ (cobalamin) is a metalloorganic compound obtained only from meats and dairy products. Fruits and vegetables are devoid of vitamin $B_{12}$, so strict vegetarian diets often produce deficiency states.

Achlorhydria is the consequence of any pathologic process that destroys gastric parietal cells (e.g., pernicious anemia). Parietal cells produce intrinsic factor as well as hydrochloric acid, so their destruction results in decreased vitamin $B_{12}$ absorption as well as achlorhydria. Surgical resection of the stomach (gastrectomy) has the same functional effect.

Crohn's disease causes small intestinal mucosal injury, resulting in an inadequate absorptive surface. Deficiencies of many nutrients may occur as a result. However, vitamin $B_{12}$ deficiency is especially common, because the ileum (the primary site of vitamin $B_{12}$ absorption) is the region of the small bowel that is affected most frequently in Crohn's disease. In contrast to Crohn's disease, which may affect either the small or large intestine, ulcerative colitis is a process limited to the large bowel. Thus, ulcerative colitis does not affect vitamin $B_{12}$ absorption and is not associated with vitamin $B_{12}$ deficiency. *(pp. 605–606; 804)*

**18. (C)** Aspirin is a readily available, inexpensive, and commonly used over-the-counter drug. Its use is so common that many patients overlook its importance as a potentially injurious substance and fail to report it when asked about their medical history of drug ingestion. Aspirin has toxic effects on a number of organ systems. Common side effects involving the central nervous system include tinnitus ("ringing" in the ears) and dizziness. Aspirin is also directly toxic to the gastric mucosa and commonly causes gastritis (either acute or chronic) that may be accompanied by gastric ulceration. Chronic ingestion of large amounts of aspirin (especially when combined with phenacetin in analgesic mixtures) may lead to a condition known as analgesic abuse nephropathy, which is characterized by chronic tubulointerstitial nephritis with papillary necrosis. Aspirin is one of several pharmacologic agents that are known to provoke asthma. In aspirin-induced asthma, in particular, susceptible individuals are extremely sensitive to small amounts of the drug and often develop urticaria as well as asthma on ingestion of aspirin. The pathogenesis of aspirin-induced asthma is believed to be related to the ability of aspirin to inhibit the cyclooxygenase pathway of arachidonic acid metabolism without affecting the lipoxygenase pathway, favoring the production of the bronchoconstrictor leukotrienes.

Massive hepatic necrosis is not an adverse drug reaction that is associated with aspirin. It is acetaminophen, another commonly used nonprescription analgesic, that is associated with this catastrophic reaction. Normally, during the metabolism of acetaminophen by the liver, the hepatocellular P-450 enzyme system converts the drug to toxic intermediates that are rendered innocuous by coupling with glutathione. With depletion of glutathione, the toxic metabolites bind instead to hepatocellular constituents and cause necrosis of the liver cells. The reaction is targeted to the centrilobular zone of the hepatic lobule where the greatest concentration of P-450 enzymes is located. *(pp. 384–385; 692; 857t; 973)*

**19. (E)** Free radicals are highly reactive chemical species with an unpaired electron in an outer orbit. Most are derived from oxygen and are generated in many different biologic and pathologic processes. Free radicals are highly injurious to cells. Normally, they are controlled by enzymes that break them down and antioxidant molecules that either block their initiation or inactivate ("scavenge") them. Several essential nutrients either are constituents of antioxidant compounds or are themselves antioxidants.

The major role of vitamin E is that of an antioxidant. It is the major lipid-soluble antioxidant in the body, and it plays an important role in terminating peroxide-generated autocatalytic chain reactions that result in loss of unsaturated fatty acids from phospholipids and extensive membrane damage. β-Carotene (a vitamin A precursor or "carotenoid" derived from plants) and selenium are the other major dietary elements that are involved in antioxidant, free radical–scavenging activity. Carotinoids have direct antioxidant activity, whereas the antioxidant role of selenium is more indirect. Selenium is a component of glutathione peroxidase, an enzyme that catalyzes the conversion of toxic oxygen species (hydroxyl radicals or peroxide) to water.

Biotin is a cofactor in carboxylation reactions. Vitamin $B_6$ (pyridoxine) is a coenzyme in many intermediary biochemical reactions, and vitamin $B_{12}$ is essential to folate metabolism and DNA synthesis. Vitamin D plays a major role in the maintenance of normal plasma levels of calcium and phosphorus. None of these essential nutrients is an antioxidant, however. *(pp. 412–413; 414; 418–419)*

**20. (C)** Ionizing radiation represents a physical transfer of energy (in the form of either electromagnetic waves or particulate radiation—neutrons and charged particles) from an active source to a biologic target that induces ionization of (i.e., ejection of electrons from) the atoms of the target. This powerful form of energy may cause cellular injury in a variety of ways. During the initial process of excitation and ionization of target atoms, heat is generated that may cause thermal injury to the tissue. The ionization process also causes injurious chemical changes in the target tissue. For example, the radiolysis of cellular water yields free radicals, which are highly interactive with and destructive to critical intracellular molecules, such as enzymes and DNA. Biologic damage is mediated either by free radical formation (an "indirect" effect) or by the direct impact of the ionizing energy on the cell. The injury produced depends on both the radiation (the dose and type) and the target tissue (its biologic susceptibility to radiation or "radiation sensitivity"). Injury may range from cell death to inhibition of cell division (mitosis) to chromosomal breakage or other genetic damage. The ability of ionizing radiation to produce genetic alterations forms the basis of its mutagenic, teratogenic, and carcinogenic effects on target tissues.

In general, the pathogenesis of radiation injury does not involve the participation of the immune system, and ionizing radiation does not generate autoimmune responses. Instead, ionizing radiation suppresses the immune system, as it would any rapidly proliferating cell system, by the injurious mechanisms outlined above. *(pp. 402–404)*

**21. (A); 22. (B); 23. (A); 24. (A); 25. (C); 26. (C); 27. (C)**

**(21)** Marasmus and kwashiorkor represent opposite ends of the spectrum of protein-energy malnutrition (PEM). Marasmus is caused by a marked deficiency in total caloric intake, whereas kwashiorkor is the result of severe protein deficiency despite sufficient caloric intake.

**(22)** Both of these diseases occur much more frequently in children than in adults. The diseases are readily distinguishable from one another by their clinical manifestations. The marasmic child appears obviously wasted, with loss of body fat and atrophy of muscle, but has a voracious appetite. **(23)** In contrast, the child with kwashiorkor appears bloated (edematous) and is often anorectic. **(24)** Also characteristic (even pathognomonic) of kwashiorkor, although not uniformly present, are skin lesions characterized by pigment changes and desquamation (resembling "flaky paint").

**(25)** Fatty change in the liver is a common finding in both kwashiorkor and marasmus. **(26)** Also common to both conditions is intercurrent parasitic infection with such organisms as *Ascaris*, *Trichuris*, *Strongyloides*, and amebae. Infectious processes exacerbate PEM by further increasing metabolic demand for calories and proteins, which are already in inadequate supply. **(27)** Typically, the pathologic changes in the body caused by PEM are fully reversible with restoration of an adequate diet in all but terminally ill patients. Affected children fed an adequate diet experience "catchup" growth and complete restoration of physical health. *(pp. 409–411)*

**28. (C); 29. (A); 30. (C); 31. (C); 32. (C); 33. (C)**

**(28)** Deficiency of vitamin D may cause skeletal disease either in children (rickets) or in adults (osteomalacia). Both rickets and osteomalacia are characterized by retarded or inadequate mineralization of newly formed osteoid in bone.

**(29)** A feature that readily distinguishes the two conditions is the defective endochondral ossification of epiphyseal cartilage that occurs in rickets but not in osteomalacia. It is somewhat artificial as a point of distinction, however, because it merely reflects ongoing bone growth in children whose epiphyses have not yet closed.

**(30)** In both disorders, the lack of vitamin D has profound effects on the regulation of serum calcium concentration. Hypovitaminosis D results in hypocalcemia, which stimulates the parathyroid glands to increase parathormone production. Parathormone, in turn, induces osteoclastic resorption of mineralized bones in order to mobilize calcium. The resorptive process causes scalloping and thinning of cancellous and cortical bone, along with fibrosis of the marrow (osteitis fibrosa cystica).

**(31, 32)** Two diseases having well-defined hereditary modes of transmission are known to produce rickets and osteomalacia. One is an autosomal recessive disease, known as vitamin D–dependent rickets type I, which is characterized by a defect in vitamin D metabolism. (Hereditary contributions to type II vitamin D–dependent rickets, characterized by end-organ resistance to vitamin D, are presently undefined). A second is an X-linked dominant disease known as hypophosphatemic rickets or vitamin D–resistant rickets. In this disorder, renal phosphate wasting leads to marked hypophosphatemia, but affected individuals are usually normocalcemic. With the decreasing incidence of dietary deficiencies of vitamin D in developed nations, these metabolic diseases have emerged as relatively important causes of rickets and osteomalacia.

**(33)** Looser's zones or Milkman's fractures are early pathognomonic lesions of either rickets or osteomalacia. On radiographs, they appear as radiolucent lines lying at right angles or oblique to the cortical outlines of bones. They are often bilaterally symmetrical and commonly affect the scapulae, lower ribs, femoral necks, and proximal ulnas. They are thought to arise either from inadequately healed stress fractures or from bony erosion caused by penetrating nutrient arteries. For obvious reasons, these sites are vulnerable to fracture. *(pp. 414–418; 1226)*

**34. (C); 35. (C); 36. (B); 37. (B); 38. (A); 39. (C); 40. (D)**

**(34)** Although the role of phosphate in vitamin D metabolism is poorly understood, it is known to parallel calcium in some of its effects. Like hypocalcemia, hypophosphatemia stimulates synthesis of 1,25-$(OH)_2D_3$. Conversely, elevated serum levels of either phosphate or calcium increase production of 24,25-$(OH)_2D_3$, the less metabolically active form of the vitamin. **(35)** In turn, vitamin D plays an important role in the homeostasis of both calcium and phosphate. Vitamin D increases the intestinal absorption of both elements, although it apparently does so through independent mechanisms for each.

**(36)** Parathyroid hormone (PTH) affects the renal handling of phosphate but not of calcium. Increased secretion of PTH secondary to hypocalcemia not only mobilizes calcium and phosphate from bone but causes renal wasting of the mobilized phosphate. With inadequate supplies of phosphate available for calcium hydroxyapatite formation, bony mineralization is defective. This series of events is characteristic of hypovitaminosis D, in which the decreased intestinal uptake of calcium caused by the vitamin deficiency stimulates PTH output by the parathyroid glands.

**(37)** Increased phosphate losses also occur in several forms of renal tubular disorders, including the Fanconi syndrome and renal tubular acidosis. The resultant hypophosphatemia stimulates synthesis of 1,25-$(OH)_2D_3$, and intestinal absorption of phosphate increases (see Question 35). If losses exceed uptake, however, defects in bony mineralization ensue and widened osteoid seams are characteristically produced in affected bones.

**(38)** In hypophosphatemic states, osteoid seams composed only of woven osteoid are seen in the bone. Excessive woven osteoid results from defective mineralization of newly laid down osteoid matrix. In hypocalcemic states, both lamellar osteoid and woven osteoid are characteristically present. Lamellar osteoid is produced by mobilization of the mineral phase of lamellar bone in response to the PTH generated in a hypocalcemic state.

**(39)** The intricate mechanisms that control calcium and phosphate homeostasis can be compromised in a variety of ways by drugs. Virtually all anticonvulsant medications, for example, increase hepatic degradation of vitamin D. Thus, intestinal absorption of both calcium and phosphate are affected (both are decreased). In addition, anticonvulsants act directly on intestinal absorptive cells to inhibit calcium transport.

**(40)** Calcitonin affects calcium homeostasis only. It *lowers* serum calcium levels in response to hypercalcemia but has no effect on the regulation of phosphate. *(pp. 414–419; 1144–1146; 1215)*

**41. (C); 42. (A); 43. (C); 44. (C); 45. (C)**

**(41)** Both alcoholism and beriberi cause dilated cardiomyopathies. Alcoholic cardiomyopathy is thought to result from the direct toxic effects of alcohol and its metabolites on cardiac muscle. Beriberi heart disease is probably the result of metabolic derangements in the myofibers induced by thiamine deficiency. The two disorders have many similar manifestations and can be difficult to differentiate from one another.

**(42)** Hepatic cirrhosis is a common consequence of alcohol toxicity. In contrast, beriberi does not produce liver injury of any kind.

**(43)** Chronic alcoholics frequently are affected by beriberi. In the alcoholic, beriberi appears to be the result of a combination of factors: poor general nutrition and an apparent increased incidence of hereditary transketolase abnormalities compared to the general population. Thiamine is a cofactor for transketolase, an enzyme involved in the pentose phosphate pathway of carbohydrate metabolism. Thus, a transketolase abnormality would predispose to clinical manifestations of beriberi.

**(44)** Both disorders may also be associated with skeletal muscle weakness, although the pathogenesis may differ in the t vo conditions. In alcoholism, muscle weakness may result either from the direct toxic effect of ethanol on skeletal muscle fibers (rhabdomyolysis) or from an alcohol-induced polyneuropathy. In beriberi, however, weakness is primarily the result of the peripheral neuropathy caused by myelin degeneration, a characteristic feature of many thiamine deficiency states.

**(45)** Wernicke-Korsakoff's encephalopathy is associated with both thiamine deficiency and alcoholism. Frequently, both disorders are present concomitantly. Clinically, Wernicke's encephalopathy is characterized by mental confusion, nystagmus, extraocular palsies, and ataxia. Korsakoff's syndrome refers to a profound deficit in both recent and remote memory. Although thiamine administration for Wernicke-Korsakoff's encephalopathy is frequently therapeutic in alcoholics with beriberi, only about 20% of affected individuals recover completely with vitamin administration. Most have a residual Korsakoff's syndrome after treatment. This suggests that Korsakoff's syndrome is primarily the result of the direct neurotoxicity of alcohol but may be compounded by thiamine deficiency. *(pp. 390; 420–422; 564)*

**46. (A); 47. (C); 48. (C); 49. (D); 50. (C); 51. (A)**

**(46)** Pernicious anemia refers specifically to the megaloblastic anemia resulting from autoimmune gastritis. It produces gastric atrophy, decreased intrinsic factor production, and impaired vitamin $B_{12}$ absorption.

**(47)** Alcoholism may cause deficiencies of both vitamin $B_{12}$ and folate for several reasons. The general nutritional intake, including that of vitamin $B_{12}$ and folate, is inadequate in many alcoholic patients. Alcohol-associated gastritis and pancreatitis also may lead to defective vitamin $B_{12}$ absorption, which requires both gastric intrinsic factor and pancreatic proteases.

**(48)** Glossitis is a feature of both vitamin $B_{12}$ and folate deficiencies. Because these vitamins are critical to the biochemical events in cell division, rapidly dividing cells in the bone marrow and gastrointestinal tract (including oral mucosal cells) characteristically are affected adversely.

**(49)** The primary manifestation of both vitamin $B_{12}$ and folate deficiencies is megaloblastic anemia with prominent megaloblasts (not sideroblasts) in the bone marrow. Sideroblastic anemias constitute a separate group of disorders characterized by hypochromic, microcytic erythrocytes and red cell precursors (sideroblasts) containing granules of nonheme iron in their cytoplasm. Sideroblastic anemias have a number of causes, but the common defect is impaired iron utilization. In megaloblastic anemias, the defect is related to DNA synthesis (see Question 8).

**(50)** In megaloblastic anemia resulting from either folate or vitamin $B_{12}$ deficiency, the myeloid and megakaryocytic as well as the erythroid series are affected. Neutrophils are enlarged and, characteristically, have hypersegmented nuclei (see Chapter 7, Question 2).

**(51)** Two defects occur in vitamin $B_{12}$ deficiency that are not seen in folate deficiency: greatly reduced fertility (both sexes are affected) and peripheral neuropathy. *(pp. 586t; 603–610)*

**52. (A); 53. (B); 54. (B); 55. (C); 56. (C); 57. (C); 58. (A)**

**(52)** Vitamin C is essential to the synthesis of all collagen (see Question 9) and is therefore requisite to the production of osteoid, a specialized type of collagen. **(53)** The process of mineralization of osteoid, however, is regulated by vitamin D through its effects on calcium and phosphorus metabolism. **(54)** Bone resorption is also dependent on vitamin D, because only previously mineralized bone can be resorbed by osteoclasts. **(55)** Bone remodeling is the combined result of both bone formation and resorption. Therefore, both vitamin C and vitamin D are required for this process.

**(56)** In endochondral bone formation, cartilage at the expanding edge of the epiphysis is replaced by osteoid (requiring vitamin C), which then is mineralized. In this process, the cartilage first must undergo provisional mineralization before it can be resorbed and replaced by osteoid. Like mineralization of osteoid, mineralization of cartilage is a vitamin D–dependent process. **(57)** Tooth enamel formation is also a complex process requiring both collagen matrix synthesis and subsequent mineralization. Therefore, tooth formation, like normal bone formation, is dependent on both vitamins.

**(58)** Only vitamin C is essential for wound healing, because this is a process based almost completely on collagen and new vessel formation (hence vascular wall and basement membrane collagen production). *(pp. 414–416; 423–424; 1213–1216)*

**59. (E); 60. (C); 61. (D); 62. (E); 63. (B); 64. (E); 65. (B)**

A number of chemicals are known to be important in the initiation and/or promotion of human cancers. By definition, carcinogenic chemicals are capable of causing genetic damage and inducing neoplastic transformation of cells. These chemicals initiate carcinogenesis by causing permanent and irreversible genetic damage (mutations) in the target cell population. Initiated cells then must be induced to proliferate in order to generate a tumor, and they often undergo additional genetic alterations in the process. Chemicals that promote proliferation of initiated cells (called "promoters") are not themselves tumorogenic (i.e., they do not affect DNA directly and their effects are not permanent). Some chemicals, known as "complete" or "perfect" carcinogens, are capable of both initiation and promotion of carcinogenesis.

Chemicals that initiate neoplastic transformation include a wide variety of compounds that may be either synthetic or naturally occurring. Some may be capable of acting directly on the cell ("direct-acting" compounds), whereas others require metabolic conversion from a "procarcinogen" to an "ultimate carcinogen" before they can interact with cellular DNA. **(59)** Aflatoxin B is a well-known example of a naturally occurring, indirect-acting chemical carcinogen. It is a product of some strains of *Aspergillus flavus*, a fungus that commonly contaminates improperly stored grains and peanuts. Aflatoxin B causes hepatocellular carcinoma (hepatoma), and the incidence of hepatoma correlates directly with the dietary level of the carcinogen.

**(60)** β-Naphthylamine (2-naphthylamine), an azo dye used in the rubber and aniline dye industries, has been responsible for a 50-fold increase in bladder cancer in heavily exposed industrial workers in the past. This procarcinogen requires hydroxylation for metabolic activation. The hydroxylated carcinogen is inactivated when coupled to glucuronic acid, but, in the presence of urinary glucuronidases, the active compound is split off and is free to interact with the bladder mucosa.

**(61)** Nitrites (derived from nitrates—salts of nitric acid) are common contaminants of water and are used as food preservatives. In the acid environment of the stomach, nitrites combine with protein breakdown products to form nitrosamines and nitrosamides, which are carcinogenic and have been causally linked to stomach cancer.

**(62)** Vinyl chloride is the monomer from which the polymer polyvinyl chloride is made. Industrial exposure to this procarcinogen has been found to increase the incidence of an otherwise extremely rare malignant tumor, angiosarcoma of the liver.

**(63 and 65)** Uranium and asbestos both have been shown to increase the incidence of lung cancer (bronchogenic carcinomas) in industrially exposed individuals. Uranium is weakly radioactive, but lung cancer among nonsmoking uranium miners is four times more common than among the general population. Although asbestos is notorious as a cause of malignant mesothelioma, an otherwise much rarer tumor than lung cancer, bronchogenic carcinoma is actually the most frequently occurring cancer among persons exposed to asbestos.

**(64)** Benzene, a chemical widely used in the rubber, cement, dye and distillation industries, is one of several chemicals that increase the risk of leukemias and non-Hodgkin's lymphomas. In particular, benzene has been causally linked to myelogenous leukemia. *(pp. 283–284; 392–393; 658; 709–710; 721; 780; 879; 1001)*

**66. (D); 67. (B); 68. (E); 69. (E); 70. (E); 71. (D); 72. (B); 73. (B)**

**(66)** Riboflavin (vitamin $B_2$), niacin, and pyridoxine (vitamin $B_6$) are all B vitamins that function as coenzymes in a variety of important reactions in cellular oxidative metabolism. **(67)** Niacin is unique among the B vitamins, because it can be synthesized endogenously from tryptophan. Thus, the dietary requirements for niacin vary inversely with the tryptophan content of the diet, and a niacin deficiency state (pellagra) usually reflects a deficiency of both niacin and tryptophan. **(68)** Thiamine (vitamin $B_1$) facilitates conduction of impulses in peripheral nerves. No similar function exists for riboflavin, niacin, or pyridoxine.

**(69)** Deficiency states for all three of these vitamins—riboflavin, niacin, or pyridoxine—are well known and clearly defined by clinical criteria. Among the water-soluble vitamins, only biotin and pantothenic acid have no clearly defined deficiency state in humans. **(70)** Experimental deficiency states of any one of the three vitamins may produce an anemia. Clinically, however, anemia rarely occurs in association with deficiencies of these nutrients. Moreover, when anemia does occur, it is usually normocytic. (Macrocytic anemias are associated with deficiencies of two other B group vitamins; cyanocobalamin [vitamin $B_{12}$] and folate.) **(71)** Dermatitis is a characteristic clinical feature of the deficiency states of all three vitamins. **(72)** Dementia, however, is associated only with niacin deficiency. It is usually accompanied by a desquamative dermatitis and diarrhea and may be followed by death (the "four D's" of pellagra). **(73)** Because they are water soluble and can be eliminated rapidly in the urine, B group vitamins do not produce persistent toxic disorders. However, parenteral administration of niacin commonly produces transient toxic effects such as abdominal pain and peripheral vasodilation. Toxic reactions are not associated with either riboflavin or pyridoxine. *(p. 412t)*

**74. (E); 75. (E); 76. (A); 77. (B); 78. (C)**

**(74)** Iron deficiency, vitamin $B_{12}$ deficiency, and starvation all produce anemia. The anemia in all three cases is based primarily on red cell production and maturation defects rather than increased erythrocyte destruction. Neither increased hemolysis **(75)** nor osmotic fragility is associated with these anemias. Osmotic fragility reflects a defect (usually hereditary) in the red cell membrane, and membrane defects are not associated with the anemias of nutritional deficiency.

**(76)** Iron deficiency leads to insufficient production of hemoglobin. Red cells are pale and decreased in size, constituting a hypochromic, microcytic anemia.

**(77)** Vitamin $B_{12}$ deficiency produces a defect in DNA synthesis. Red cell precursors grow in size as their cytoplasm develops, but they cannot divide. Hemoglobin production is not affected, however. Megaloblasts produce abnormally large erythrocytes, and the resultant anemia is characterized as normochromic, macrocytic.

**(78)** For reasons less well understood, the characteristic anemia of starvation is hypochromic and normocytic. In general, normal red cell morphology is not typical of any of these deficiency states, although a normochromic, normocytic anemia sometimes may occur in starvation. *(pp. 608; 612–513)*

**79. (A); 80. (B); 81. (E); 82. (D); 83. (C); 84. (C); 85. (E)**

An adverse drug reaction (ADR) is defined as "any response to a drug that is noxious and unintended and occurs at doses used in humans for prophylaxis, diagnosis, or therapy, excluding failure to accomplish the intended purpose." ADRs are common hazards for the treating physician and the patient alike. With the use of any drug, the potential risks always must be weighed against the potential benefits. ADRs usually fall into one of two categories: (1) an exaggerated pharmacologic effect of the compound that is predictable and dose dependent, and (2) an idiosyncratic response that is neither predictable nor dose dependent. Many idiosyncratic ADRs are related to individual immunologic responses to the drug or to completely unexpected cytotoxicity. Physicians must be aware of the well-recognized ADRs related to specific, commonly used pharmacologic agents.

**(79)** Massive hepatic necrosis is a known consequence of acetaminophen toxicity. The drug is broken down to toxic metabolites in the liver, but metabolites usually are detoxified by coupling to glutathione. When the glutathione coupling system is overwhelmed, the metabolites cause direct toxic injury to the liver cells and result in widespread hepatocellular necrosis.

**(80)** Fatty change in the liver is a common (and usually innocuous) consequence of tetracycline use. In contrast to most other agents (such as alcohol) that produce fatty liver, tetracycline characteristically produces microvesicular rather than macrovesicular fatty change.

**(81)** Interstitial fibrosis of the lung is a potential consequence of exposure to certain specific chemotherapeutic (busulfan; bleomycin), antibiotic (nitrofurantoin), antiarrhythmic (amidiodarone), and other therapeutic (gold; penicillamine) agents.

**(82)** Aplastic anemia is a dire and well-known consequence of usage of certain chemotherapeutic and immunosuppressive agents as well as the antibiotic chloramphenicol.

**(83)** Anaphylaxis produced by a type I hypersensitivity immune reaction is a relatively common problem associated with the antibiotic penicillin. Penicillin allergy is one of the most common drug allergies in the general population. Thus, it is important to question patients about previous hypersensitivity responses to penicillin that might presage systemic anaphylaxis on re-exposure before administering this antibiotic.

**(84)** Penicillin also may act as a hapten, combining with the red blood cell (RBC) membrane to induce an antibody response to the RBC-drug complex. This results in binding of the antibody-coated RBCs to monocytes and macrophages and partial phagocytosis of the erythrocyte membrane, with spheroidal transformation of the RBC. The resultant spherocytes are sequestered avidly and destroyed in the spleen, producing a hemolytic anemia.

**(85)** A systemic lupus erythematosus syndrome (drug-induced lupus) is an ADR linked with hydralazine, procainamide, and isoniazid, but it is not commonly associated with acetaminophen, tetracycline, penicillin, or chloramphenicol. *(pp. 182; 384–385; 602; 704; 856–857)*

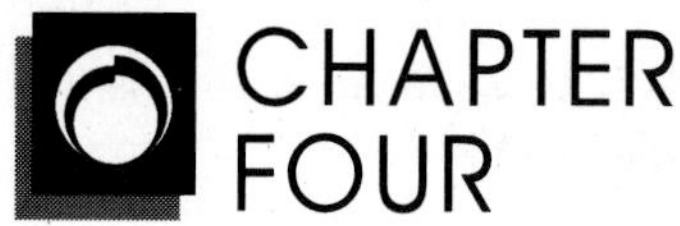

CHAPTER FOUR

# Infectious Diseases

**DIRECTIONS:** For Questions 1 through 15, choose the ONE BEST answer to each question.

**1.** Which of the following is the most common cause of diarrhea in infants?

A. *Yersinia enterocolitica*
B. Rotavirus
C. *Giardia lamblia*
D. Enteropathogenic *Escherichia coli*
E. *Campylobacter jejuni*

**2.** Sexually transmitted chlamydia produce all of the following problems EXCEPT:

A. Pelvic inflammatory disease
B. Acute epididymitis
C. Reiter's syndrome
D. Condylomata lata
E. Lymphogranuloma venereum

**3.** Ulcerated lesions on the penis occur in the acute form of all the following sexually transmitted infectious diseases EXCEPT:

A. Herpes simplex virus type 2 infection
B. Syphilis
C. Chancroid
D. Granuloma inguinale
E. Gonorrhea

**4.** All of the following statements correctly describe Lyme disease EXCEPT:

A. It is caused by a rickettsia.
B. It is transmitted by a tick.
C. It causes erythema chronicum migrans.
D. It causes meningitis.
E. It causes chronic arthritis.

**5.** Trichomoniasis causes lesions referred to as:

A. Raspberry tongue
B. Strawberry mucosa
C. Strawberry gallbladder
D. Anchovy paste abscesses
E. Chocolate cysts

**6.** All of the following statements correctly describe the mumps virus EXCEPT:

A. It is an RNA virus.
B. It is spread by respiratory droplets.
C. It produces diagnostic cell inclusions.
D. It replicates in T lymphocytes.
E. It produces pancreatitis.

**7.** All of the following organisms cause atypical pneumonia (diffuse alveolar damage) EXCEPT:

A. *Chlamydia pneumoniae*
B. *Pneumocystis carinii*
C. *Mycoplasma pneumoniae*
D. Influenza virus
E. *Haemophilus influenzae*

**8.** Body lice are the principal vectors of transmission of the causative organism in:

A. Bubonic plague
B. Babesiosis
C. Scrub typhus
D. Q fever
E. Epidemic typhus

**9.** Organisms that propagate outside of cells (extracellularly) during human infection include all of the following EXCEPT:

A. *Chlamydia trachomatis*
B. *Mycoplasma pneumoniae*
C. *Streptococcus pneumoniae*
D. *Trypanosoma gambiense*
E. *Wuchereria bancrofti* (filaria)

**10.** Intercellular adhesion molecule-1 (ICAM-1) is the cellular receptor for:

A. Rhinovirus
B. Rabies virus
C. Influenza virus
D. Epstein-Barr virus
E. Human immunodeficiency virus

**11.** All of the following statements correctly describe *Neisseria gonorrhoeae* EXCEPT:

A. Its binding to target cells is mediated by pili on the bacterial surface.
B. Its entry into cells is mediated by adhesins.
C. It makes enzymes that lyse immunoglobulin A.
D. Its virulence is determined by capsular polysaccharides.
E. It produces exotoxins that mediate cell injury.

**12.** All of the following diseases are mediated by bacterial exotoxins EXCEPT:

A. Tetanus
B. Diphtheria
C. Legionnaires' disease
D. Botulism
E. Antibiotic-associated pseudomembranous colitis

**13.** Organisms that typically induce granuloma formation include all of the following EXCEPT:

A. *Histoplasma capsulatum*
B. *Cryptococcus neoformans*
C. *Mycobacterium leprae*
D. *Giardia lamblia*
E. *Schistosoma mansoni*

**14.** All of the following statements correctly describe the organisms shown in Figure 4–1 EXCEPT:

A. Trophozoites are the only infectious form of the life cycle.
B. Trophozoites lack mitochondria.
C. Infection by trophozoites is often asymptomatic.
D. Trophozoite invasion of the colonic mucosa produces dysentery.
E. Flask-shaped ulcers in the colon are characteristic.

**15.** Which of the following diseases is acquired by ingestion of raw or undercooked animal flesh (meat or fish)?

A. Schistosomiasis
B. Liver fluke infection
C. Filariasis
D. Tapeworm infection
E. Hookworm infection

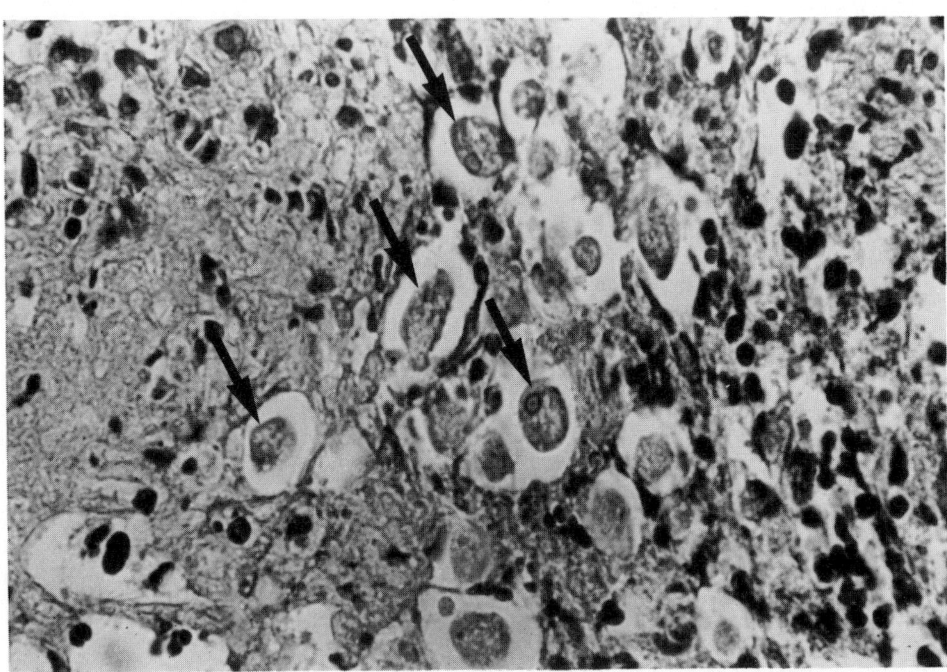

**Figure 4–1**

**DIRECTIONS:** For Questions 16 through 20, you are to decide whether EACH choice is TRUE or FALSE.

For each of the following statements about infectious mononucleosis, choose whether it is TRUE or FALSE.

**16.** The causative agent is the Epstein-Barr virus.
**17.** The abnormal circulating mononuclear cells are infected T lymphocytes.
**18.** Microscopic changes produced in the lymph nodes resemble Hodgkin's disease.
**19.** Heterophil antibodies are virtually diagnostic.
**20.** Burkitt's lymphoma is a complication of latent infection.

**DIRECTIONS:** For Questions 21 through 38, the set of lettered headings is followed by a list of numbered words or phrases. For each numbered word or phrase choose:

A—if the item is accociated with (A) only
B—if the item is associated with (B) only
C—if the item is associated with *both* (A) and (B)
D—if the item is associated with *neither* (A) nor (B)

For each of the diseases listed below, choose whether it is caused by streptococci, staphylococci, both, or neither.

A. Streptococci
B. Staphylococci
C. Both
D. Neither

**21.** Impetigo
**22.** Erysipelas
**23.** Erythema nodosum
**24.** Carbuncles
**25.** Toxin-induced food poisoning
**26.** Toxic shock syndrome
**27.** Acute glomerulonephritis
**28.** Scarlet fever

For each of the statements listed below, choose whether it describes lepromatous leprosy, tuberculoid leprosy, both, or neither.

A. Lepromatous leprosy
B. Tuberculoid leprosy
C. Both
D. Neither

**29.** The causative organism has never been cultivated *in vitro*.
**30.** Lesions typically contain large numbers of organisms.
**31.** Nerve involvement is typical.
**32.** Hypergammaglobulinemia often occurs.
**33.** Life-threatening vasculitis is an associated complication.

For each of the features listed below, choose whether it is characteristic of cryptosporidiosis, toxoplasmosis, both, or neither.

A. Cryptosporidiosis
B. Toxoplasmosis
C. Both
D. Neither

**34.** The causative agent is a protozoan.
**35.** Infection does not occur in normal (immunocompetent) individuals.
**36.** Person-to-person spread is the major mode of transmission.
**37.** Gastrointestinal tract disease is the major manifestation of infection.
**38.** Abscesses characteristically are produced.

**DIRECTIONS:** Questions 39 through 113 are matching questions. For each numbered item, choose the most likely associated lettered item from those provided. Each numbered item has ONLY ONE answer. Within each group, each lettered item may be the answer to one, more than one, or none of the numbered items.

For each of the following statements about respiratory viruses, choose whether it describes adenovirus, influenza virus, coxsackievirus, rhinovirus, or none of these.

A. Adenovirus
B. Influenza virus
C. Coxsackievirus
D. Rhinovirus
E. None of these

**39.** It is the major cause of the common cold.
**40.** It is associated with the Guillain-Barré syndrome.
**41.** It causes diarrhea.
**42.** It causes herpangina.
**43.** It is the most common cause of croup (lethal bronchiolitis) in infants.
**44.** It causes epidemic hemorrhagic keratoconjunctivitis.
**45.** It produces characteristic inclusion bodies in infected cells.

For each of the features of childhood infectious disease, choose whether it is characteristic of measles (rubeola), German measles (rubella), chickenpox (varicella zoster), all of these, or none of these.

A. Measles (rubeola)
B. German measles (rubella)
C. Chickenpox (varicella zoster)
D. All of these
E. None of these

**46.** The causative organism is an RNA virus.
**47.** It is highly contagious by droplet aspiration.
**48.** Koplik's spots are clinically diagnostic.
**49.** Multinucleate ("Warthin-Finkeldey") giant cells are pathognomonic.
**50.** Maternal infection is *not* associated with congenital malformations.
**51.** Skin lesions are characteristically pustular.
**52.** "Giant cell" pneumonia sometimes is produced.
**53.** A latent phase of infection is a common consequence.
**54.** Recovery confers lifelong immunity.

For each of the infectious disorders listed below, choose whether it is caused by viral, chlamydial, bacterial, or protozoal infection or none of these.

A. Viral infection
B. Chlamydial infection
C. Bacterial infection
D. Protozoal infection
E. None of these

**55.** Condyloma acuminatum
**56.** "Cold sores"
**57.** Rocky mountain spotted fever
**58.** Gas gangrene
**59.** Smallpox
**60.** Oral thrush
**61.** Whooping cough
**62.** Typhoid fever
**63.** Cat-scratch disease
**64.** Athlete's foot
**65.** Trachoma
**66.** Sleeping sickness
**67.** Poliomyelitis
**68.** Rabies

For each of the bacterial organisms listed below, decide whether it causes pathogenicity in humans by one of the mechanisms listed below or whether it acts by none of these mechanisms.

A. Formation of a phagocyte-resistant capsule
B. Production of leukocyte-killing substances
C. Avoidance of immune mechanisms by programmed antigenic variation
D. Interference with normal phagosome function
E. None of these

**69.** Pneumococcus (*Streptococcus pneumoniae*)
**70.** *Borrelia recurrentis*
**71.** *Mycobacterium tuberculosis*
**72.** *Clostridium perfringens*
**73.** *Neisseria gonorrhoeae*
**74.** *Vibrio cholerae*
**75.** *Clostridium botulinum*

For each of the characteristics listed below, choose whether it describes *Escherichia coli*, *Proteus mirabilis*, *Pseudomonas aeruginosa*, all of these, or none of these.

A. *Escherichia coli*
B. *Proteus mirabilis*
C. *Pseudomonas aeruginosa*
D. All of these
E. None of these

**76.** It is a source of endotoxin.
**77.** It grows best in anaerobic conditions.
**78.** It is *not* a cause of infectious enterocolitis.
**79.** It causes urinary tract infection.
**80.** It causes gram-negative pneumonia.
**81.** It is *not* associated with suppurative infections of the abdominal cavity.
**82.** It is associated with epidemics in burn units.

For each of the features listed below, choose whether it is characteristic of primary syphilis, secondary syphilis, tertiary syphilis, all of these stages, or none of these stages.

A. Primary syphilis
B. Secondary syphilis
C. Tertiary syphilis
D. All of these
E. None of these

**83.** A generalized skin eruption typically occurs.
**84.** The syphilitic gumma is the histologic hallmark.
**85.** Obliterative endarteritis is the histologic hallmark.
**86.** Treponemes are extremely difficult to demonstrate in lesions.
**87.** Tabes dorsalis develops.
**88.** Charcot's joints develop.
**89.** Hutchinson's teeth develop.

For each of the characteristics listed below, choose whether it describes *Candida albicans*, *Mucor*, *Aspergillus fumigatus*, *Cryptococcus neoformans*, or none of these.

A. *Candida albicans*
B. *Mucor*
C. *Aspergillus fumigatus*
D. *Cryptococcus neoformans*
E. None of these

**90.** It is the most common deep fungal infection in humans.
**91.** It typically forms pseudohyphae.
**92.** It rarely, if ever, infects immunologically normal individuals.
**93.** India ink preps aid in identification.
**94.** The most common clinical manifestation of infection is meningitis.
**95.** It causes hypersensitivity pneumonitis without lung infection.
**96.** It causes oral infection in infants who are bottle-fed.

For each of the features listed below, choose whether it is characteristic of blastomycosis, coccidioidomycosis, histoplasmosis, all of these, or none of these.

A. Blastomycosis
B. Coccidioidomycosis
C. Histoplasmosis
D. All of these
E. None of these

**97.** It is most prevalent in the southwest of the United States.
**98.** It is acquired from inhalation of contaminated soil.
**99.** The causative fungus grows in tissue as a yeast form.
**100.** It commonly produces asymptomatic primary disease.
**101.** It commonly produces skin involvement in disseminated disease.
**102.** It causes granulomatous lung disease.
**103.** It occasionally causes sclerosing mediastinitis.

For each of the features listed below, choose whether it is characteristic of malaria, babesiosis, Chagas' disease, all of these, or none of these.

A. Malaria
B. Babesiosis
C. Chagas' disease
D. All of these
E. None of these

**104.** Mosquitoes transmit the disease.
**105.** Pigment is typically found in phagocytes.
**106.** Sickle cell hemoglobin limits parasitemia.
**107.** Myocarditis is common in adult infection.
**108.** Progressive brain dysfunction occurs in the late stage of the disease.

For each of the characteristics listed below, choose whether it describes infection by *Ascaris lumbricoides*, hookworm, *Strongyloides*, pinworm, or none of these.

A. *Ascaris lumbricoides*
B. Hookworm
C. *Strongyloides*
D. Pinworm
E. None of these

**109.** It occasionally causes appendicitis in children.
**110.** It typically invades striated muscle.
**111.** It is diagnosed by duodenal aspiration.
**112.** It causes mechanical obstruction of the gastrointestinal tract.
**113.** It causes disease by sucking blood.

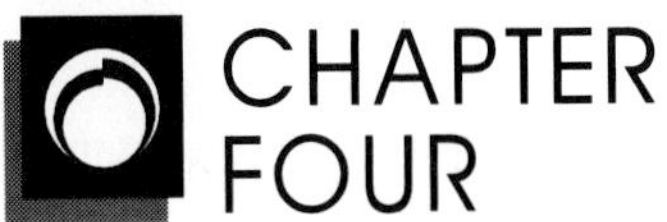

# Infectious Diseases

## ANSWERS

**1. (B)** Acute self-limited infectious diarrhea is a major cause of morbidity in children and can be devastating in the infant. In the pediatric age group, infectious diarrhea most often is caused by enteroviruses, primarily rotaviruses. Fortunately, rotavirus infection usually produces disease that is mild and self-limited. Although less common, bacterial or parasitic forms of childhood enteritis are often more debilitating than viral enteritides. For example, *Yersinia enterocolitica*, enteropathogenic *Escherichia coli*, and *Campylobacter jejuni* are all major causes of bacterial enteritis in the pediatric age group and are highly invasive and virulent enteric pathogens that cause severe ulcerating enterocolitis. *Giardia lamblia* rarely causes childhood diarrhea. *(pp. 328–329; 791)*

**2. (D)** *Chlamydia trachomatis* is an obligate intracellular pathogen that infects columnar epithelial cells and is a common cause of sexually transmitted urethritis and cervicitis. In the female, chlamydial infection is a major cause of pelvic inflammatory disease. In the male, it causes nongonorrheal urethritis and may extend to produce acute epididymitis. In some men, genital infection is accompanied by conjunctivitis and polyarthritis, a triad known as Reiter's syndrome. Lymphogranuloma venereum, caused by a specific strain of *Chlamydia trachomatis*, results in granulomatous inflammation of the inguinal, pelvic, and rectal lymph nodes. Lymphogranuloma venereum should not be confused with granuloma inguinale, a sexually transmitted disease caused by the bacterium *Calymmatobacterium donovani*. Condylomata lata are not produced by chlamydia; they are the characteristic papular lesions found on the penis or vulva in secondary syphilis, a disease caused by *Treponema pallidum*. *(pp. 341–342; 1004)*

**3. (E)** Ulcerated lesions characteristically occur on the penis in a number of sexually transmitted infections, including herpes simplex type 2 (HSV-2, or genital herpes) infection, syphilis, chancroid, and granuloma inguinale. Obviously, then, among patients with an ulcerated penile lesion, bacteriologic, serologic, or immunohistochemical testing may be required to make a diagnosis. However, gonorrhea does not produce a penile ulcer. In the male, gonococcal infection produces a mucopurulent discharge and meatal inflammation but no ulceration. Infection may extend retrograde to the posterior urethra, epididymus, prostate, and seminal vesicles. Urethral strictures and sterility are consequences of chronic infection in untreated cases. *(pp. 340–341; 343–344)*

**4. (A)** Lyme disease, named for the Connecticut town where an epidemic took place in 1976, is caused by the spirochete *Borrelia burgdorferi*. The organism is transmitted to humans from rodents by deer ticks. Lyme disease should not be confused with Rocky Mountain spotted fever, another tick-borne disease indigenous to the United States that produces fever and a rash but is caused by a rickettsia. Like syphilis, another major spirochetal disease, Lyme disease evolves in stages. Initially (stage 1), *Borrelia* spirochetes multiply in the dermis at the site of the tick bite and cause an expanding area of redness with a pale center. This skin lesion, called erythema chronicum migrans, may be accompanied by fever and lymphadenopathy but regresses within a few weeks. The organisms then disseminate throughout the body (stage 2), causing secondary annular skin lesions and inflammation in the lymph nodes, joints, meninges, and heart. At this stage, untreated patients develop antibodies to spirochete flagellar and outer membrane proteins that may be useful in the serodiagnosis of the disease. In the late disseminated stage (stage 3), chronic destructive arthritis is usually the major manifestation, but encephalitis also may persist and sometimes may be debilitating. *(pp. 359; 361–362)*

**5. (B)** Trichomoniasis is a common sexually transmitted parasitic infection caused by the flagellate *Trichomonas vaginalis*. The trophozoite adheres to the mucosal surfaces of the male and female genital tracts but does not invade the underlying tissues. Infection occurs most commonly in the female vagina and in the male urethra. The affected mucosa is typically erythematous, edematous, and spotted with small blisters or granules, and its appearance is referred to as "strawberry mucosa."

Raspberry tongue refers to the bright red color and edematous papillae of the tongue in the early stage of scarlet fever. Strawberry gallbladder refers to the gross appearance of the gallbladder mucosa in cholesterolosis. In this condition, the gallbladder mucosa is diffusely erythematous and studded with small yellow "seeds," which are actually collections of cholesterol-laden macrophages in the lamina propria. Anchovy paste abscesses occur in amebiasis with liver involvement. Amebic liver abscesses contain debris from digested red blood cells and liver cells that appears grossly as a brown-colored, pasty material resembling "anchovy paste." Chocolate cysts are foci of endometriosis which, with repeated bleeding during menstrual cycles, develop cystic change and become filled with brown, hemosiderin-laden fluid (see Chapter 11, Question 57). As should be obvious from this discussion, pathologists are exceedingly fond of food similes. *(pp. 334; 338; 346)*

**6. (C)** Mumps is an acute contagious disease caused by a single-stranded RNA paramyxovirus that causes acute inflammation of the parotid glands and, less often, the testes, pancreas, and central nervous system. It most commonly occurs in children but may affect adults. The virus is spread by respiratory droplets and multiplies in the upper respiratory epithelial cells, salivary glands, and T cells in local draining lymph nodes. A transient viremia disseminates the virus to other glands and to the central nervous system (via the choroid plexus). Mumps virus principally involves the parotid glands, usually bilaterally, producing the characteristic swelling by which it is recognized. Mumps pancreatitis tends to be mild and self-limited. Orchitis is common only in the adult patient, but it is unilateral in 70% of cases and thus rarely causes sterility. Mumps encephalitis may cause focal demyelinization. Unlike its close relative, the measles virus, mumps virus does not produce intracellular inclusions by which it can be identified microscopically. *(pp. 346–347; 1014)*

**7. (E)** Given that bronchopneumonia, a process usually caused by bacteria and characterized by purulent exudative inflammation, is considered the "typical" pattern of pulmonary infection, pneumonia characterized by a pattern of diffuse alveolar damage with hyaline membranes is considered "atypical." Organisms that characteristically produce atypical pneumonia include respiratory viruses (e.g., influenza virus types A and B, respiratory syncytial virus, adenovirus), *Mycoplasma pneumoniae* (the most common cause of atypical pneumonia), *Chlamydia pneumoniae*, *C. psittaci* (psittacosis), and *Pneumocystis carinii*. Although bronchopneumonia is always infectious in origin, the pattern of diffuse alveolar damage that characterizes atypical pneumonia can be produced by toxic injury, shock, and other noninfectious causes.

*Haemophilus influenzae* (not to be confused with influenza virus) is a gram-negative bacillus that causes life-threatening respiratory infections and meningitis in young children. It causes a severe (but "typical") bronchopneumonia with a high mortality rate. *(pp. 323; 698–699)*

**8. (E)** Body lice are the principal vectors of transmission of the rickettsial organisms causing epidemic typhus (typhus fever), a disease associated with wars and other dire human conditions that compromise normal hygiene. The causative agent, *Rickettsia prowazekii*, is a small, bacteria-like obligate intracellular parasite that infects endothelial cells and multiplies intracellularly. Ultimately, the burden of organisms becomes so great that the infected cells burst. The result is a widespread vasculitis with fever and a centrifugal rash. In severe cases, gangrenous necrosis may occur in the skin of the extremities and hemorrhages may be found in the brain, heart, lungs, and kidneys.

Scrub typhus and Q fever are also rickettsial diseases causing vasculitis, but they are transmitted by chiggers and droplet inhalation (no arthropod vector), respectively. Bubonic plague, caused by *Yersinia pestis*, is transmitted to humans by fleas from infected rodents. Babesiosis, a parasitic infection of red blood cells causing fever and hemolytic anemia, is caused by the malaria-like protozoan *Babesia microti*. This organism is transmitted by the same deer ticks that carry Lyme disease (see Question 4). *(pp. 358–360; 363)*

**9. (A)** With the notable exception of viruses, chlamydia, and rickettsia, all other classes of human endoparasites (organisms that can enter the human host) have members that propagate extracellularly. Mycoplasma are the smallest free-living pathogens and do not depend on a host cell for propagation, as exemplified by *Mycoplasma pneumoniae*. *Streptococcus pneumoniae*, the cause of pneumonococcal pneumonia, is an example of a bacterium that propagates extracellularly. *Trypanosoma gambiense*, the cause of sleeping sickness, and *Wuchereria bancrofti*, the cause of filariasis, are examples of extracellularly propagating protozoans and helminths, respectively.

All chlamydia (including *Chlamydia trachomatis*) are obligate intracellular parasites that are dependent on host metabolic capabilities for propagation. *(p. 307)*

**10. (A)** All viral infection is dependent on entry of the virus into the host cell, a process mediated by specific receptors for the virus on the surface of the target host cell. The tropism of viruses for specific cell types, excluding other cell types altogether, is largely determined by these host cell receptors. Rhinoviruses are the cause of more than 50% of all common colds. They bind to their target cells via the intracellular adhesion molecule ICAM-1, the same cell surface molecule that mediates antigen-specific T- cell responses as well as leukocyte emigration into inflammatory sites. Thus, any epithelial or endothelial cell expressing ICAM-1 may become infected with rhinovirus, but the disease is usually limited to the upper respiratory tract because viral replication is temperature sensitive. Rhinovirus replication proceeds optimally at temperatures slightly lower (33 to 35° C) than core body temperature (37.5° C).

Rabies virus binds to the acetylcholine receptor on neurons. Influenza virus binds to the sialic acid–containing proteins and lipids on the host cells in the upper airways. Epstein-Barr virus binds to the complement receptor on macrophages (CD2). Human immunodeficiency virus binds to the protein involved with antigen presentation (CD4) on the surface of helper T cells. *(pp. 315; 322)*

**11. (E)** *Neisseria gonorrhoeae* is the causative agent of the common sexually transmitted disease gonorrhea, otherwise known as "clap." It commonly causes pelvic inflammatory disease in the female and urethritis (or more extensive genitourinary tract involvement) in the male. Gonococcal bacteremia may result in an arthritis-dermatitis syndrome. *Neisseria gonorrhoeae* is a facultative intracellular pathogen that binds to and invades host epithelial cells. Binding is mediated by adhesin-bearing pili on the bacterial surface and internalization is mediated by a second set of adhesins (called the opacity outer membrane proteins). Capsular polysaccharides contribute to the virulence of the organism by inhibiting phagocytosis in the absence of anti-gonococcal antibodies. In addition, pathogenic *Neisseria* make proteases that are capable of lysing immunoglobulin A. Although *Neisseria* release endotoxins, which induce host secretion of tumor necrosis factor $\alpha$, causing shock and mediating cellular injury, no exotoxins are produced by these organisms. *(p. 343)*

**12. (C)** Exotoxins are bacterial products that are protein in nature, are released from the bacterium during exponential growth, and are toxic for target cells. Although exotoxins occur in many forms, most have both a binding domain and an enzymatic domain. It is the enzymatic domain that produces the toxic effect once the molecule is inside the cell. Despite this enzymatic action, exotoxins usually are categorized separately from other bacterial enzymes that are not unique to any single bacterial species (e.g., coagulases, hyaluronidases, leukocydins, hemolysins) and that play less specific (or undefined) pathogenic roles during *in vivo* infection. Unlike other enzymes, exotoxins are typically responsible for most of the biologic effects of infection by their organism of origin. Classic examples of exotoxin-mediated diseases include infections by clostridial organisms (prodigious exotoxin producers) and diphtheria.

*Clostridium tetani* are anaerobic, gram-positive organisms that proliferate in the devitalized tissue of penetrating wounds. They elaborate a powerful neurotoxin (tetanospasmin) that causes convulsive contractions of skeletal muscles, the characteristic feature of tetanus (also known as "lockjaw"). Another clostridial organism, *Clostrium difficile*, produces a severe toxin-mediated colitis characterized by mucosal inflammation and necrosis with the formation of pseudomembranes (coagula of fibrin, dead epithelial cells, and inflammatory cells). Overgrowth of *C. difficile*, a normal gut denizen, is most commonly the result of antibiotic administration, which alters the ecology of the intestinal flora. Thus, the disease is largely iatrogenic in origin. Yet another clostridial agent, *Clostridium botulinum*, produces a powerful neurotoxin that blocks synaptic release of acetylcholine and causes severe paralysis of respiratory and skeletal muscles (a disorder known as botulism). By far the most common mode of acquisition of botulism is ingestion of contaminated foods containing the preformed botulinum neurotoxin. *Corynebacterium diphtheriae* is a gram-positive bacillus that is transmitted by droplet inhalation. It causes upper respiratory tract infection with pseudomembrane formation, and toxemia with systemic manifestations including myocarditis, polyneuritis, and parenchymal injury in the kidneys, liver, and adrenals. Diphtheria toxin produces cell injury and death by completely inhibiting protein synthesis. The toxin is so powerful that a single molecule can kill a cell. Happily, vaccination has made diphtheria a rare childhood illness, but disease can result from infection of neglected skin wounds in adults.

*Legionella pneumophila* are gram-negative bacilli (usually revealed by silver staining) that cause a mild, self-limited fever (Potomac fever) in otherwise healthy persons. However, in smokers, immunosuppressed individuals, or those with chronic lung disease, they produce a severe pneumonia (legionnaires' disease). These organisms are unique among bacteria because they have the ability to proliferate within macrophages and eventually burst the cell. However, their pathogenicity is not related to exotoxin production. *(pp. 318–319; 338–339; 353)*

**13. (D)** A granulomatous response to infection commonly is associated with mycobacteria, spirochetes, fungi, and parasites. Less commonly, bacterial organisms also may be associated with granulomatous responses in the host. Principal among these are *Brucella suis* (brucellosis), *Pseudomonas mallei* (glanders), *Francisella tularensis* (tularemia), and *Yersinia pestis* (plague). *Histoplasma capsulatum* and *Cryptococcus neoformans* are both yeasts that typically elicit granulomas in the lung and other affected organs in disseminated disease. *Mycobacterium leprae*, like other mycobacteria (most notably, *M. tuberculosis*), characteristically produces chronic granulomatous inflammation. In leprosy, the skin and peripheral nerves are the primary sites of involvement, and disabling deformities of the extremities result. Schistosomiasis is the most globally important helminthic infection in humans and is a classic example of a parasitic granulomatous disease. In infection by *Schistosoma mansoni*, thousands of eggs are produced by the adult female worms, which take up residence in the portal venous system. The ova elicit brisk granulomatous responses wherever they lodge in the liver and gastrointestinal tract. Infection with *Giardia lamblia* is an exception to the parasite-granuloma rule. *Giardia lamblia* is an extremely common pathogenic intestinal protozoan. It causes injury by binding to the surfaces of small intestinal absorptive cells (via sugar groups on their cell membranes) and damaging their brush border. With the loss of brush border enzymes from damaged absorptive cells, nutrient malabsorption and diarrhea ensue. However, *Giardia* are lumen dwellers and do not invade the intestinal mucosa or elicit granulomas. *(pp. 320; 327; 334; 355; 366)*

**14. (A)** The organisms shown in Figure 4–1 are trophozoites of *Entamoeba histolytica*. Amebic infection is limited primarily to the lumen of the colon, but systemic spread of the organism with metastatic abscess formation may occur following infiltration of organisms into the colonic wall. The disease is acquired by ingestion of *E. histolytica* cysts (in contaminated food or water), which, unlike trophozoites, have a chitinous wall and are resistant to gastric acid. In the colonic lumen, cysts release trophozoites. In most cases, this does not result in disease because the trophozoites do not invade the colonic mucosa. Instead, an asymptomatic carrier state is produced. Asympotomatic infected individuals then shed organisms that can infect others (the principal mechanism of disease transmission). However, in 10% of infected individuals, trophozoite invasion of the colonic wall occurs, and a severe ulcerating colitis with dysentery results. Amebic colitis most often affects the cecum and ascending colon but occasionally involves the sigmoid, rectum, or appendix. The organisms typically produce ulcerations that have a flask-shaped contour (a narrow neck and a broad base) when viewed in transverse tissue sections. Because they lack mitochondria and Krebs cycle enzymes, amebic trophozoites are obligate fermenters of glucose to alcohol. This metabolic limitation is the basis of their susceptibility to treatment with metronidazole, a drug that targets ferredoxin-dependent pyruvate oxidoreductase. This enzyme is critical to the fermentation process in amebae but is absent in human cells. *(pp. 333–334)*

**15. (D)** Parasitic worms have complex life cycles that usually involve sexual reproduction in the definitive host, asexual multiplication in an intermediate host, and diverse mechanisms of entry into the host organisms. Humans may be either the definitive or the intermediate host, depending on the worm. Tapeworm (a flatworm) infection is usually contracted by ingestion of undercooked meat or fish containing encysted larvae. Human infection by either hookworms (roundworms or nematodes) or schistosomes (flukes or trematodes) is acquired by transcutaneous penetration of the infective forms of the worm, which have the ability to penetrate intact skin. Liver fluke infection is acquired by eating contaminated watercress containing the metacercarial form of the parasite. Filariasis, a group of roundworm infections, is transmitted to humans by insect bites. *(pp. 310–311; 315; 371–373)*

**16. (True); 17. (False); 18. (True); 19. (True); 20. (True)**

**(16)** Infectious mononucleosis is a benign, self-limited lymphoproliferative disease caused by the Epstein-Barr virus (EBV), a member of the herpes family. It is transmitted by close human contact, often via saliva. The disease is characterized by fever, generalized lymphadenopathy, splenomegaly, sore throat, and the appearance of atypical activated lymphocytes in the peripheral blood.

**(17)** EBV binds to the CD21 protein (the complement receptor) present on epithelial cells and B cells. After penetrating epithelial cells of the oropharynx, nasopharynx, and salivary glands, EBV infects B lymphocytes in the underlying lymphoid tissues. Within the infected B cells, the virus associates with the host cell genome (the source of latent infection). Infected B cells then undergo polyclonal activation and proliferation and display viral-directed antigens on their surface that are recognized by T cells. Activated, virus-specific cytotoxic T cells as well as suppressor T cells (not EBV specific) are generated and appear in the peripheral blood as atypical "mononuclear cells" (mononucleosis cells). Thus, the atypical circulating mononuclear cells represent a lymphocytic immune response to virally infected cells, but they themselves are not virally infected.

**(18)** The diagnosis of infectious mononucleosis can be difficult, because the disease may mimic other disorders both clinically and pathologically. Affected lymph nodes have markedly expanded paracortical (T cell) zones that occasionally contain large binucleate cells resembling Reed-Sternberg cells. Thus, a histologic appearance resembling Hodgkin's disease is produced. The microscopic changes produced in the liver resemble those of viral hepatitis, with mononuclear inflammation of the portal tracts and focal hepatocellular necrosis. **(19)** A helpful diagnostic feature is the presence of heterophil antibodies, immunoglobulins secreted by infected B cells that agglutinate sheep erythrocytes. These are present in about 90% of cases and can be detected easily with a commercially available spot kit (Monospot test). The test is both sensitive and specific (rarely, false-positive tests occur in patients with lymphoma or hepatitis). Together with tests for specific EBV antigens (capsid or nuclear proteins), the Monospot test and the atypical lymphocytosis establish the diagnosis conclusively.

**(20)** The ability of EBV to associate with the host genome and produce latent infection (i.e., no viral replication takes place and the cell is not killed) in B cells and epithelial cells has several potential long-term consequences. Latent EBV infection immortalizes B cells (they acquire the ability to propagate indefinitely *in vitro*). It also is related causally to malignant transformation of affected cells. In specific, it is associated with the development of the African form of Burkitt's lymphoma, nasopharyngeal carcinoma, some cases of Hodgkin's disease, and, in the immunosuppressed AIDS patient, true monoclonal B cell lymphoma. *(pp. 287; 347–349)*

**21. (C); 22. (A); 23. (A); 24. (B); 25. (B); 26. (B); 27. (A); 28. (A)**

**(21)** Streptococci and staphylococci are two of the most common and versatile human bacterial pathogens. Impetigo, a common superficial infection of the skin characterized by erosive lesions covered by honey- colored crust, can be caused by either group A streptococci (90% of cases) or staphylococci (10% of cases). *(pp. 336; 338; 1207)*

**(22)** Erysipelas is a disorder characterized by a rapidly spreading edematous and erythematous cutaneous infection, usually on the face. It is caused by group A $\beta$-hemolytic streptococcal infection. *(p. 338)*

**(23)** Erythema nodosum, the most common type of panniculitis, commonly is associated with $\gamma$-hemolytic streptococcal infection. Erythema nodosum may occur in association with other infectious diseases, such as tuberculosis, leprosy, coccidioidomycosis, or histoplasmosis, but it is not associated with staphylococcal infection. *(p. 1196)*

**(24)** Carbuncles are deep-seated suppurative lesions of the skin and subcutaneous tissues that spread laterally beneath the deep subcutaneous fascia and then erupt onto the skin surface, forming multiple adjacent skin sinuses. They typically appear on the upper back and posterior neck and are caused by staphylococcal infection. *(p. 337)*

**(25 and 26)** Food poisoning and the toxic shock syndrome are two examples of diseases caused by staphylococcal toxin production. Staphylococcal food poisoning results from the ingestion of a preformed enterotoxin without invasive staphylococcal enterocolitis. The toxic shock syndrome is caused by unique toxins produced by staphylococci that propagate in blood-soaked vaginal tampons during menstruation. In both situations, the systemic effects of the toxin are mediated by massive stimulation of T-cell cytokine release. T-cell stimulation occurs following binding of the toxin to both the major histocompatibility and the T-cell receptor $\gamma$ chain on the surface of macrophages. In contrast to staphylococci, streptococci do not normally elaborate exotoxins; they commonly produce disease either via the direct effects of suppurative spreading infection or indirectly via complications of a host immune response induced by the organism (e.g., glomerulonephritis, see below). *(p. 335)*

**(27)** Acute proliferative glomerulonephritis is a fairly common consequence of streptococcal infection of the pharynx or skin. More than 90% of cases are associated (in order of frequency) with types 12, 4, and 1 (identified by typing of the M protein of the cell wall). Glomerular disease occurs abruptly about 1 to 2 weeks after recovery from the acute streptococcal infection. It is caused by circulating streptococcal-antistreptococcal immune complexes that lodge in the glomerular basement membrane, activate complement, and cause leukocytic infiltration with glomerular injury. Full recovery with conservative therapy can be expected in children, but, in adults, chronic disease develops in about 40% of cases. *(pp. 337; 945–946)*

**(28)** Scarlet fever is an acute illness caused by streptococcal infection and mediated by a phage-encoded pyrogenic exotoxin that produces both fever and rash. It is characterized by pharyngitis, tonsillitis, and an erythematous rash over the trunk, face, and inner aspects of the extremities. The disease is rare before age 3 or after age 15. Although the disease is self-limited, it requires prompt treatment to prevent poststreptococcal complications such as glomerulonephritis. *(p. 338)*

**29. (C); 30. (A); 31. (C); 32. (A); 33. (A)**

**(29)** Leprosy is an indolent but debilitating disease caused by chronic infection by *Mycobacterium leprae*, an acid-fast obligate intracellular organism. The disease is acquired from infected individuals by droplet inhalation. Infection primarily involves the skin and peripheral nerves, typically taking one of two forms, lepromatous leprosy or tuberculoid leprosy, depending on the host response to the organism. *Mycobacterium leprae* has never been cultured successfully *in vitro* from patients with either form of the disease, but it can be propagated in the armadillo, which has a core body temperature similar to that of human skin (32 to 34° C).

**(30)** In lepromatous leprosy, large numbers of mycobacteria are typically demonstrable in the lesions (loose aggregates of macrophages that do not form granulomas) because infected individuals are immunologically anergic to the invading organisms (possibly as a result of the generation of suppressor T cells). In tuberculoid leprosy, a brisk cellular immune response to the organisms occurs and the resultant granulomas contain few demonstrable organisms. Because of the relative deficiency of immunologic control over the infecting organisms in the lepromatous form of the disease, it is more contagious than the tuberculoid form.

**(31)**Regardless of the type of host response and subsequent form of disease, peripheral nerve injury always occurs. In tuberculoid leprosy, granulomas form in the nerve sheaths, and in lepromatous leprosy, nerve damage is produced by widespread invasion of the mycobacteria into Schwann cells and macrophages in the endoneurium and perineurium.

**(32)** Although patients with lepromatous leprosy fail to produce an adequate cellular immune response, they often have a polyclonal hypergammaglobulinemia thought to be due to both massive lepra antigen exposure and suppressor T-cell production of interleukin-4, which induces antibody production by B cells. **(33)** The antibodies are ineffective in curbing the disease but lead to the formation of antigen-antibody complexes that produce serious complications such as life-threatening vasculitis or glomerulonephritis. *(pp. 365–367)*

**34. (C); 35. (D); 36. (D); 37. (A); 38. (D)**

**(34)** Crytosporidiosis and toxoplasmosis are parasitic diseases caused by the protozoans *Cryptosporidium parvum* and *Toxoplasma gondii*, respectively. **(35)** Both of these organisms are capable of infecting immunocompetent individuals. *Cryptosporidium parvum* causes a transient watery diarrhea in normal children, and *T. gondii* causes mild lymphadenopathy in infected adults. However, both organisms produce profound disease in immunosuppressed individuals and are two of the most common opportunistic infections in patients with AIDS.

**(36)** Cryptosporidiosis is acquired by drinking contaminated water. *Cryptosporidium parvum* is not killed by chlorine, so filtration through sand is required to remove these organisms from municipal water supplies. *Toxoplasma gondii* infection is acquired either by ingesting oocytes derived from the feces of domestic cats (sexual reproduction of the organism occurs in the cat intestine) or by ingesting *Toxoplasma* cysts, which are filled with bradyzoites, from incompletely cooked lamb or pork. Person-to-person spread does not occur at all with *C. parvum* and occurs with *T. gondii* only during maternal-fetal transplacental parasitemia if acute maternal infection occurs during the first trimester of pregnancy. This is an important and highly consequential circumstance causing destructive infection of the developing brain, heart, and lungs of the fetus, but it is obviously not the major mode of spread.

**(37)** Gastrointestinal tract disease is the only manifestation of infection by *C. parvum*. Sporozoites of *C. parvum* adhere to (via lectins on the parasite cell surface) and invade small and large intestinal epithelial cells. The disruption of the small intestinal microvilli causes malabsorption and a secretory diarrhea. *Toxoplasma gondii*, after entering the body via the gastrointestinal tract, spreads systemically and penetrates into any type of host cell. Its ability to infect any cell type is a unique feature that occurs because the organism binds the extracellular matrix protein laminin on its cell surface, which, in turn, binds to laminin receptors on the surface of the host cells.

**(38)** Neither organism produces abscesses in the tissues they infect. The inflammatory response to *C. parvum* is usually minimal because it does not spread beyond the infected epithelial cells, and the response to *T. gondii* is not pyogenic. *(pp. 357–358)*

**39. (D); 40. (C); 41. (A); 42. (C); 43. (E); 44. (A); 45. (A)**

**(39)** Viral diseases of the respiratory tract are the most common and least preventable of all human infectious diseases. Among the myriad species and serotypes responsible, adenovirus, influenza virus, coxsackievirus, and rhinovirus are among the most important. Rhinovirus is the major cause of the common cold (see Question 10). Although it is the cause of the single most frequent infectious disease, it seldom produces serious sequelae.

**(40 and 42)** Coxsackieviruses produce many patterns of disease besides upper respiratory tract infection. For example, coxsackie B virus can cause the Guillain-Barré syndrome and myocarditis. Coxsackie A strains may cause herpangina, a blistering inflammation of the pharynx.

**(41)** Adenoviruses cause both upper and lower respiratory tract infections as well as conjunctivitis. In contrast to the other respiratory viruses, however, they are also enteric pathogens and may cause acute, self-limited infectious diarrhea, most commonly in infants and children.

**(43)** Also of particular importance among viral respiratory pathogens affecting infants and children are the parainfluenza and respiratory syncytial viruses, which produce croup (lethal bronchiolitis) or pneumonia. Adenovirus also may cause croup but does so infrequently.

**(44)** Adenoviruses produce a number of febrile respiratory syndromes of varying severity but also are associated commonly with eye infections, particularly acute conjunctivitis. Adenovirus-induced keratoconjunctivitis, a more severe condition, may occur in sharp outbreaks related to inadequately chlorinated swimming pools.

**(45)** Among the major respiratory viruses, only adenovirus produces characteristic inclusion bodies that are diagnostic by light microscopy. Other viral agents that produce characteristic inclusion bodies and may involve the respiratory tract include the varicella zoster and rubeola (measles) viruses and cytomegalovirus in the immunosuppressed patient. *(pp. 308; 329; 346–347; 745)*

**46. (A); 47. (D); 48. (A); 49. (A); 50. (A); 51. (E); 52. (A); 53. (C); 54. (D)**

**(46)** Measles (rubeola), German measles (rubella), and chickenpox (varicella zoster) are three common viral infections of childhood with varying acute and chronic consequences. Measles (like mumps) is caused by a single-stranded RNA paramyxovirus. German measles is caused by a single-stranded DNA virus of the togavirus family. Chickenpox is caused by varicella zoster, a double-stranded DNA herpesvirus. **(47)** All of these diseases are highly contagious by droplet aspiration and hence spread rapidly among unimmunized children and nonimmune adults.

**(48)** Measles infection produces several unique clinical and pathologic features. The earliest diagnostic sign is the appearance of small blistering, ulcerating lesions (small areas of epithelial necrosis, neutrophilic inflammation, and neovascularization), known as Koplik's spots, on the cheek mucosa near the opening of Stensen's ducts. Their appearance may precede the skin rash. **(49)** A pathognomonic histologic feature of measles is the presence of Warthin-Finkeldey cells in involved lymphoid organs. These multinucleated giant cells characteristically contain eosinophilic nuclear and intracytoplasmic inclusion bodies. **(52)** A unique (and sometimes life-threatening) complication of measles infection is an interstitial pneumonia characterized by an abundance of giant cells, a feature for which it is named ("giant cell" pneumonia).

**(50)** In contrast to measles or chickenpox, German measles is a relatively mild childhood infection with few, if any, serious sequelae. Its major importance is its ability to produce congenital malformations in the offspring of affected mothers. Maternal varicella infection during the first trimester of pregnancy also has been associated with congenital malformations. In contrast, maternal measles infection is not known to cause fetal anomalies.

**(51)** Although skin lesions occur in all three of these systemic viral diseases, none are pustular in character. Measles and German measles both produce a maculopapular rash, and chickenpox characteristically causes macular lesions that rapidly progress to a vesicular stage without forming pustules.

**(53 and 54)** Although recovery from all three of these childhood infections confers lifelong immunity to reinfection, only varicella zoster causes latent disease. Following the production of chickenpox, the virus may remain latent for years in the sensory dorsal root ganglia. With advancing age or immunosuppression, the virus may become reactivated and cause a painful localized vesicular eruption in the distribution of the corresponding dermatomes, known as "shingles." Most frequently, this occurs in the distribution of the trigeminal nerve. *(pp. 308; 346; 349–350)*.

**55. (A); 56. (A); 57. (C); 58. (C); 59. (A); 60. (E); 61. (C); 62. (C); 63. (C); 64. (E); 65. (E); 66. (D); 67. (A); 68. (A)**

**(55)** Condylomata acuminata are genital warts caused by human papillomavirus (HPV). Among the various genetically distinctive types of HPV, types 6 and 11 have been associated most clearly with condyloma production. Most of these lesions remain benign throughout their course. *(p. 1008)*

**(56)** "Cold sores" are cutaneous or mucosal vesicles (usually on the face, lips, and/or nostrils) caused by herpes simplex type 1 (HSV-1), a double-stranded DNA virus. Herpes simplex type 2 (genital herpes) also causes these lesions but much less commonly than HSV-1. On primary infection transmitted by local contact (e.g., kissing), the virus replicates within epithelial cells. Infected cells develop intranuclear (Cowdry type A) inclusion bodies and undergo lysis, producing an inflamed vesicle. The virus then may enter a latent phase, inhabiting sensory ganglia that it reaches by traveling along sensory nerve pathways. Reactivation (by mechanisms still largely unknown) of latent disease causes recurrence of skin lesions. *(pp. 340–341)*

**(57)** Rocky mountain spotted fever is an acute febrile illness with rash caused by the bacterium *Rickettsia rickettsii*. The disease is most common in the southeastern and southwestern United States. The organism is transmitted to humans by dog and rodent ticks, invades vascular endothelial and smooth muscle cells, and causes a widespread vasculitis that is manifested as a hemorrhagic rash over the entire body. *(pp. 359–360)*

**(58)** Gas gangrene is a cellulitis that occurs as a complication of wound infection caused by anaerobic bacteria, chiefly *Clostridium perfringens* and *C. septicum*. These organisms proliferate in the devitalized tissue of wounds and produce numerous powerful exotoxins. The $\alpha$ toxin of *C. perfringens* (one of 12 exotoxins produced by this organism) destroys red blood cells, platelets, and muscle cells, causing myonecrosis. *(pp. 338–339)*

**(59)** Smallpox is a highly contagious febrile illness characterized by a vesicular/pustular skin eruption (pocks). It is caused by variola virus, a double-stranded DNA virus that only infects humans. Variola virus is a close relative of vaccinia virus, the cause of cowpox, and immunization with vaccinia confers immunity to smallpox. In 1798, Edward Jenner first published his historic discovery that inoculation of pustular material from cowpox lesions protected against smallpox. Since then, the worldwide practice of inoculation of vaccinia ("vaccination") has eradicated this once epidemic disease. *(p. 308)*

**(60)** Oral thrush is an infection of the oral cavity by *Candida albicans* (a fungus). It is one of the most common forms of candidiasis and occurs most commonly in bottle-fed newborns and immunosuppressed or antibiotic-treated adults. *(p. 354)*

**(61)** Whooping cough is an acute, highly contagious respiratory disease of childhood caused by *Bordetella pertussis*, a gram-negative coccobacillus. It is characterized clinically by paroxysms of violent coughing followed by loud inspiratory "whoops." *Bordetella pertussis* attach to the brush border of the bronchial epithelium, where they replicate without invading and also infect pulmonary macrophages. They produce exotoxins that cause both systemic symptoms (lymphocytosis, malaise, weight loss) and local injury to the ciliated respiratory epithelial cells. Recovery and immunity depend on secretory immunoglobulin A antibodies that prevent bacterial adhesion to the respiratory mucosa. Diphtheria-pertussis-tetanus vaccine, which contains heat-killed organisms, has reduced the prevalence of whooping cough greatly in the United States. *(p. 350)*

**(62)** Typhoid fever is a life-threatening febrile systemic illness caused by *Salmonella typhi*, a flagellated gram-negative bacterium. Humans are the only host of *S. typhi*, which is shed in stool, urine, and secretions by acutely ill patients and by chronic carriers with no overt disease. The organism invades the gastrointestinal tract, infecting intestinal epithelial cells and macrophages. In the small and large intestine, it causes mucosal lymphoid hyperplasia and mucosal necrosis. Acute disease causes fever and chills progressing to rash and abdominal pain and finally to intestinal bleeding and shock. *(pp. 331–332)*

**(63)** Cat-scratch disease is a self-limited, localized lymphadenopathy caused by *Rochalimaea henseii*, a streptobacillus of the genus *Rothia* that colonizes the teeth of cats. Coalescent granulomas with central abscess formation ("stellate granulomas") in affected lymph nodes, similar to those seen in lymphogranuloma venereum, are characteristic. *(pp. 309; 342)*

**(64)**"Athlete's foot" is a very common, superficial fungal infection of the plantar skin caused by a dermatophytic fungus known as *Tinea pedis*. About 30 to 40% of the population are affected at some time during their lives. The dermatophytic fungi (there are several types) infect only the nonviable keratinaceous structures of skin (stratum corneum, hair, and nails) and do not invade vital tissues (in contrast to fungi that cause "deep" infection, such as *Candida albicans*). They are troublesome but not dangerous. *(pp. 1207–1208)*

**(65)** Trachoma is a chronic suppurative eye disease caused by *Chlamydia trachomatis*. It is characterized clinically by follicular keratoconjunctivitis. It is one of the leading global causes of blindness. Infection is usually acquired during childhood through human contact or arthropod transmission. It is most common in dry, sandy regions of the world and among those living in poor socioeconomic conditions. *(p. 365)*

**(66)** "Sleeping sickness" is the common name for African trypanosomiasis, caused by the protozoans *Trypanosoma rhodesiense* and *T. gambiense*. The disease begins with parasitemia following a bite by an infected tsetse fly and an acute febrile illness with purpura and disseminated intravascular coagulation. Chronic bouts of fever with lymphadenopathy and splenomegaly follow. The final stage of the disease is characterized by a demyelinating panencephalitis that produces increasing lethargy and leads to death in coma. *(pp. 369–370)*

**(67)** Poliomyelitis (polio) is a systemic disease of varying severity that predominantly affects the central nervous system and can produce permanent paralysis. It is caused by poliovirus, a single-stranded RNA enterovirus belonging to the family Picornaviridae. Once a devastating scourge, poliomyelitis has been virtually eradicated in industrialized countries by immunization programs using either the Salk formalin-fixed (killed) vaccine or the Sabine attenuated (live) oral vaccine. *(p. 349)*

**(68)** Rabies is an acute encephalitis caused by a single-stranded RNA virus of the Rhabdovirus family. The organism is transmitted by the bite of a rabid animal and, from the wound site, travels along the peripheral nerves to the central nervous system (CNS). Fever, malaise, headache and paresthesias around the wound site are diagnostic. With progression of the infection, extraordinary CNS excitability is produced, with violent motor (convulsions) and sensory (pain) effects. Meningismus and flaccid paralysis are followed by alternating mania and stupor, coma, and death from respiratory paralysis. *(p. 1320)*

**69. (A); 70. (C); 71. (D); 72. (B); 73. (C); 74. (E); 75. (E)**

**(69)** Bacterial agents have evolved numerous clever ways of combating human biologic defense mechanisms. Some organisms, like the pneumococcus, are particularly resistant to engulfment by neutrophils by virtue of the carbohydrate capsule on their surface, which allows them to shed antigens that would trigger phagocytosis.

**(70 and 73)** Other bacteria, such as *Borrelia recurrentis*, the agent of relapsing fever, and *Neisseria gonorrhoeae*, the cause of gonorrhea, elude immunologic defense mechanisms by continuously changing their antigenic surface determinants. This genetically programmed variation in surface antigens allows each successive generation of organisms to survive while the preceding generations are immunologically exterminated.

**(71)** Granuloma-forming facultative intracellular bacteria such as *Mycobacterium tuberculosis* have evolved mechanisms to escape destruction following ingestion by phagocytes. The cell wall of *M. tuberculosis* contains sulfatides (surface glycoproteins containing sulfur) that interfere with the fusion of phagocytic vacuoles and lysosomes, thus forestalling the enzymatic reactions that would lead to their digestion. In addition, complement activated on the surface of the mycobacteria may facilitate uptake into macrophages via their complement receptor CR3 (MAC-1 integrin) without triggering the respiratory burst necessary to kill the organisms.

**(72)** *Clostridium perfringens* is a prime example of an organism that digests the cells of its host's defense system before it can be digested. It produces a plethora of bacterial enzymes, including alpha toxin (a lecithinase), which disrupts the plasma membranes of platelets, erythrocytes, and other host cells. Theta toxin binds cholesterol and causes membrane destabilization that leads to the lysis of neutrophils (explaining why so few inflammatory cells are present in the lesions of gas gangrene).

**(74 and 75)** In contrast, *Vibrio cholerae* and *Clostridium botulinum* are organisms that do not need to invade the tissues of their host to produce disease. These bacteria produce powerful, selective exotoxins that drastically alter the physiologic functions of their target tissues (the intestinal epithelium and the cholinergic nerves, respectively), producing cellular injury without direct tissue invasion by the organism. *(pp. 319; 338–339; 361)*

**76. (D); 77. (E); 78. (B); 79. (D); 80. (D); 81. (C); 82. (C)**

**(76)** All gram-negative organisms have cell walls that contain lipopolysaccharide-protein complexes known as "endotoxins." The release of endotoxins from disintegrating bacteria is responsible for the dramatic systemic effects of gram-negative sepsis, such as high fever, increased capillary permeability with shock, and disseminated intravascular coagulation.

**(77)** All of the gram-negative bacilli grow best in the presence of oxygen and, except for *Enterobacter* species, are only facultatively anaerobic.

**(78, 79, and 80)** *Escherichia coli*, *Proteus* species, and *Pseudomonas* species are all well-known causes of both urinary tract infection and gram-negative bronchopneumonia. *Escherichia coli* is the most common cause of primary uncomplicated urinary tract infection. It and *Pseudomonas aeruginosa* are intestinal pathogens as well, and both have been implicated as primary causes of necrotizing enterocolitis in infants. *Escherichia coli* is an especially versatile enteric pathogen; different strains cause disease either by direct mucosal invasion or by elaboration of toxins that cause enterocyte secretory dysfunction. None of the *Proteus* species are known to be enterotoxic.

**(81)** *Escherichia coli* and *Proteus* species are members of the family Enterobacteriaceae and are part of the indigenous intestinal flora. Enteric organisms, such as *E. coli*, *Proteus* species, and *Enterobacter* commonly are associated with various suppurative infections within the abdominal cavity, such as acute cholecystitis, diverticulitis, and cholangitis. *Pseudomonas aeruginosa*, in contrast, does not usually colonize the intestine and is not commonly associated with suppurative intra-abdominal processes.

**(82)** Unlike *E. coli*, *P. aeruginosa* is of low virulence for normal individuals and usually causes only nosocomial and opportunistic infections. It is virtually ubiquitous in hospitals and commonly is associated with epidemic infections in burn units, nurseries, and critical care units. It is, in fact, the most common cause of skin infections and generalized sepsis in burn patients. *(pp. 352–353; 792–794; 891)*

**83. (B); 84. (C); 85. (D); 86. (C); 87. (C); 88. (C); 89. (E)**

**(83)** Syphilis is a sexually transmitted disease caused by *Treponema pallidum*. The untreated disease has three stages, each with its own unique features. Primary syphilis is manifested only by the painless chancre that occurs on the external genitalia at the site of treponemal invasion. Secondary syphilis appears following a latent period of 2 weeks to 6 months after the primary stage. It is characterized by a generalized skin eruption that disappears spontaneously in about 4 to 12 weeks.

**(84)** The teritary stage of syphilis, which appears years or decades later, has the most devastating consequences. During this final stage of disease, localized destructive lesions known as syphilitic gummas appear in virtually any tissue.

**(85)** Whatever the stage of the disease, the histologic hallmark of the syphilitic lesion is an obliterative endarteritis with plasma cell infiltrates. Swelling and proliferation of endothelial cells in affected arterioles and small arteries produce a characteristic concentric "onionskin" appearance and luminal narrowing.

**(86)** Treponemes are characteristically extremely difficult to demonstrate in the gummas of tertiary syphilis, in contrast to the ease with which they are demonstrated in the lesions of primary and secondary syphilis.

**(87)** Central nervous system involvement is also characteristic of teritary syphilis. Two classic complications of such involvement (neurosyphilis) are tabes dorsalis, a locomotor ataxia resulting from degeneration of the posterior columns of the spinal cord, and **(88)** "Charcot's joint," a rapidly destructive arthritis of the knee joint resulting from spinal cord sensory loss.

**(89)** In contrast to the characteristics of sexually transmitted *Treponema pallidum* in the adult, Hutchinson's teeth are associated only with congenital syphilis infection contracted *in utero* from the mother. *(pp. 343–348; 1317–1318)*

**90. (A); 91. (A); 92. (B); 93. (D); 94. (D); 95. (C); 96. (A)**

**(90)** Among the fungal species that infect human beings, *Candida albicans* (an endogenous yeast), *Mucor* (a "bread mold"), *Aspergillus fumigatus* (a ubiquitous filamentous fungus), and *Cryptococcus neoformans* (a soil-dwelling encapsulated yeast) are the most important. *Candida albicans* is the single most common form of deep human fungal disease. **(91)** The organism can be recognized by its formation of pseudohyphae, which represent concatenations of individual elongated yeast forms and look like strings of sausages. *Candida* also form true septated hyphae as well.

**(92)** Although most fungal infection tends to occur in immunosuppressed or chronically debilitated patients, many fungal species are capable of causing disease in otherwise healthy individuals. Mucormycosis seldom, if ever, occurs in healthy individuals and is most often encountered in patients with diabetes, acidosis, advanced malignancy, or some form of immunodeficiency. Examples of fungal infections occurring in immunocompetent individuals are (1) vaginal candidiasis in women taking oral contraceptives; (2) colonizing aspergillosis (aspergilloma) occurring at the site of a previous lung abscess or infarct; and (3) cryptococcosis arising in a healthy individual exposed to contaminated bird excreta.

**(93)** *Cryptococcus neoformans* is a round budding yeast about the size of an erythrocyte that has a heavy gelatinous capsule and can be identified by a simple laboratory test known as an India ink prep. The carbon particles of the ink serve as a contrast medium that offsets the gelatinous capsule and permits ready identification of the organism. **(94)** In contrast to the other fungi, *Cryptococcus neoformans* has a special affinity for the central nervous system (CNS). Reasons for this include: (1) absence of anticryptococcal factors (normally found in serum) from the cerebrospinal fluid; (2) production of phenol oxidase by the organism, protecting it against the epinephrine oxidative system; and (3) dearth of complement in cerebrospinal fluid. Complement binding to the fungal cell surface and activation of the alternative pathway facilitate phagocytosis and killing by inflammatory cells outside of the CNS. Thus, the organism frequently produces meningitis as a result of seeding from a primary focus in the lung, where the infection may be mild or asymptomatic. Meningitis is the most common form of cryptococcal infection to come to clinical attention.

**(95)** Aspergillus is distinctive among the fungi in its ability to produce disease in the absence of true infection. In some sensitized individuals, inhalation of aspergillus spores leads to a florid hypersensitivity pneumonitis. This immunologically mediated lung disease, known as allergic bronchopulmonary aspergillosis, can produce marked pulmonary pathology in the absence of actual colonization or infiltration of the lung by organisms.

**(96)** Oral thrush is the name by which candidiasis of the oral cavity is commonly known (see Question 60). Although it may occur in adults receiving broad-spectrum antibiotic therapy, it is encountered most commonly in neonates, especially those who are bottle-fed. In infants, the disease is usually self-limited and disappears when the normal microflora of the mouth develop. *(pp. 354–357; 716)*

**97. (B); 98. (D); 99. (D); 100. (D); 101. (A); 102. (D); 103. (C)**

**(97)** In the United States there are three major mycotic infections that occur in the normal host and establish systemic infection. They are caused by *Blastomyces dermatitidis*, *Coccidioides immitis*, and *Histoplasma capsulatum*. In contrast to blastomycosis and histoplasmosis, which occur most frequently in the midwestern United States, particularly in the Mississippi-Ohio River basins, coccidioidomycosis is most prevalent in the western and southwestern United States, especially in the San Joaquin Valley of California.

**(98)** The fungal agents in each of these diseases are dimorphic. That is, they grow in nature as mycelium (mold)-bearing infectious spores, which are aerosolized from contaminated soil and inhaled, but **(99)** they produce yeast-like forms in the host.

**(100)** The diseases have many clinical as well as microbiologic features in common. Each of these infections may produce acute disease, chronic progressive disease, or no symptoms at all. In fact, asymptomatic disease is the most common outcome of infection in all three of these disorders.

**(101)** In the systemic form of blastomycosis, the skin commonly is involved and may be the only site of active infection. Skin lesions typically consist of fleshy fungating ulcers that may be confused with cutaneous malignancies. Although coccidioidomycosis and histoplasmosis may cause cutaneous infection with dissemination, this does not occur commonly.

**(102)** All of these fungal infections produce granulomatous inflammation, and all may be counted among the causes of granulomatous long disease. **(103)** However, only histoplasmosis is known to produce the condition known as sclerosing mediastinitis. This results from extension of the histoplasma infection from the mediastinal lymph nodes into the surrounding tissues, causing progressive scarring and contraction of mediastinal structures. This condition may appear as a mediastinal mass and can be confused with a malignancy, such as lymphoma. *(pp. 391–396)*

**104. (A); 105. (A); 106. (A); 107. (C); 108. (E)**

**(104)** Malaria, babesiosis, and Chagas' disease are protozoal diseases caused by *Plasmodia* species, *Babesia* species, and *Trypanosoma cruzi*, respectively. Although all of these diseases are transmitted to humans by insects, only malaria is transmitted by mosquitoes. Babesiosis is transmitted by a tick, and Chagas' disease is transmitted by "kissing bugs" (reduviid bugs).

**(105)** The protozoal agents of both malaria and babesiosis characteristically invade red blood cells and may be difficult to differentiate from one another. A distinguishing feature of malaria, however, is the characteristic gray or black hemozoin pigment found in parasitized red blood cells or cells of the monocyte-phagocyte system. The pigment represents products of heme digestion that are released into the bloodstream on destruction of the infected erythrocytes. In babesiosis, hemozoin pigment is not found in erythrocytes in the peripheral blood (on blood smears) or in the cells of the monocyte-phagocyte system (on spleen or liver tissue specimens).

**(106)** Sickle cell hemoglobin has a protective effect in infection by plasmodia, both because it forces the parasites to leave the cell when sickling begins and because erythrocytes have a shortened life span in sickle cell disease.

**(107)** In contrast to malaria and babesiosis, Chagas' disease is produced by an organism that does not multiply within the bloodstream. The trypanosomes of Chagas' disease invade tissues to proliferate, and the subsequent tissue injury induces inflammation. The heart is the organ most frequently involved by parasitic invasion. Thus, both acute myocarditis and chronic heart disease with progressive cardiac failure occur in of Chagas' disease.

**(108)** Progressive brain dysfunction is not a feature of any of these three diseases. It does occur, however, in another parasitic protozoal infection (caused by *Trypanosoma rhodesiense*) known as African trypanosomiasis or "sleeping sickness" (see Question 66). *(pp. 363–364; 369–371)*

**109. (D); 110. (E); 111. (C); 112. (A); 113. (B)**

Worms are the largest of the human parasites and produce a number of distinctive diseases. Among the most common helminthic diseases are ascariasis, hookworm infection, strongyloidiasis, and pinworm infection (enterobiasis).

**(109)** The pinworm, *Enterobius vermicularis*, causes the childhood "night itch" syndrome in children when the female worms migrate to the anal skin for egg laying during the night. These organisms also may cause appendicitis in children by producing appendiceal obstruction. In such cases, a ball of worms is found in the lumen of the surgically resected appendix.

**(110)** The worm that typically invades striated muscle is *Trichinella spiralis*. Trichinosis is acquired by ingesting viable cysts present in meat that has been cooked inadequately.

**(111)** *Strongyloides stercoralis* is a roundworm that causes human disease principally by inhabiting the gut lumen, damaging the mucosa, and giving rise to a malabsorption syndrome. Its eggs mature high in the intestine, so duodenal aspiration or biopsy may be particularly helpful in diagnosing this form of helminthic infection.

**(112)** *Ascaris lumbricoides* is another intestinal roundworm that tends to be a luminal dweller. In contrast to the malabsorption syndrome of strongyloidiasis, intestinal obstruction by worms tends to be more characteristic of ascariasis.

**(113)** Like strongyloidiasis, hookworm infection is acquired by larval penetration of the skin, migration to the lung via the blood, and finally intestinal luminal habitation after being coughed up and swallowed by the host. Once in the small intestine, hookworms attach to the mucosal villi and continuously suck blood from the underlying capillaries, causing chronic blood loss. *(pp. 310–311; 312–313; 364; 823)*

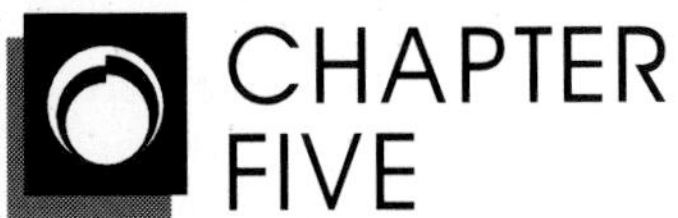

CHAPTER FIVE

# The Cardiovascular System

**DIRECTIONS:** For Questions 1 through 27, choose the ONE BEST answer to each question.

**1.** Myocardial hypertrophy is assessed most accurately by:

A. Left ventricular wall thickness
B. Histologic appearance of left ventricular myocardium
C. Weight of the heart
D. Measurement of the heart size by chest radiograph
E. None of these

**2.** Which of the following situations is the most common outcome of an acute myocardial infarction?

A. Sudden cardiac death
B. Recovery without complications
C. Left ventricular congestive failure
D. Cardiogenic shock
E. Cardiac arrhythmias

**3.** Systemic hypertension is associated with all of the following disorders EXCEPT:

A. Cerebrovascular infarction (stroke)
B. Aortic aneurysm rupture
C. Senile cardiac amyloidosis
D. Malignant nephrosclerosis
E. Berry aneurysm rupture

**4.** Which of the following is the LEAST important independent risk factor for the cardiac disorder shown in Figure 5–1?

A. Cigarette smoking
B. Hyperlipidemia
C. Systemic hypertension
D. Obesity
E. Diabetes mellitus

**5.** *Immediate* consequences of a first ischemic cardiac event include all of the following EXCEPT:

A. No symptoms
B. Angina pectoris
C. Transmural infarction
D. Sudden death without infarction
E. Cardiac rupture

**6.** The most common cause of sudden cardiac death is:

A. Aortic valve stenosis
B. Cocaine use
C. Ischemic heart disease
D. Hypertensive heart disease
E. Conduction system abnormalities

**7.** Following recovery from a myocardial infarction, all of the following therapeutic approaches are beneficial for the postinfarction patient EXCEPT:

A. Treatment with tissue-type plasminogen activator
B. Treatment with $\beta$ adrenergic blocking agents
C. Treatment with calcium channel blocking agents
D. Aspirin administration
E. Coronary artery bypass surgery

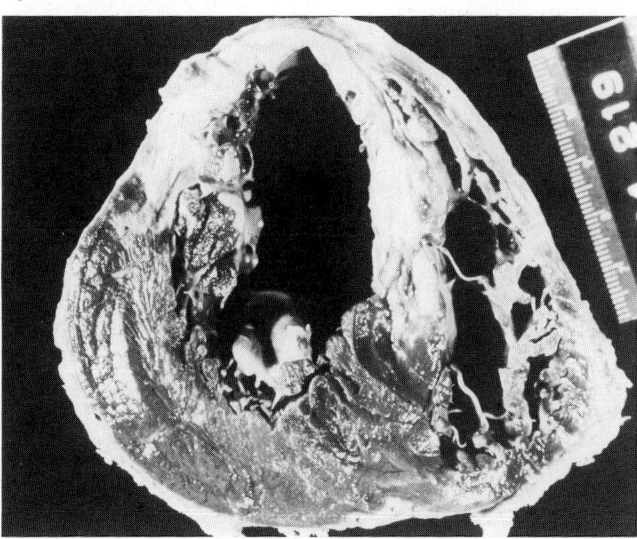

Figure 5–1

**8.** Chronic, ischemic heart disease is characterized by all of the following EXCEPT:

A. Diffuse subendocardial fibrosis
B. Diffuse myocardial atrophy
C. Stenosing coronary atherosclerosis
D. Diffuse interstitial fibrosis
E. Large irregular myocardial scars

**9.** Compensated hypertensive heart disease is associated with all of the following features EXCEPT:

A. Concentric thickening of the left ventricular wall
B. Increased myocardial oxygen demand
C. Normal cardiac silhouette by chest radiograph
D. Absence of clinical symptoms
E. Normal electrocardiogram

**10.** Pathologic features of the heart muscle in hypertensive heart disease include all of the following EXCEPT:

A. Increased diameter of myofibers
B. Increased size of myofiber nuclei
C. Synthesis of abnormal proteins by myofibers
D. Increased number of capillaries between myofibers
E. Increased fibrous tissue between myofibers

**11.** Cardiac disorders associated with aging include all of the following EXCEPT:

A. Calcific aortic stenosis
B. Mitral stenosis
C. Mitral annulus calcification
D. Cardiac amyloidosis
E. Brown atrophy of the heart

**12.** Common complications of prosthetic heart valves include all of the following EXCEPT:

A. Hemolytic anemia
B. Infective endocarditis
C. Mechanical malfunction of the prosthesis
D. Arrhythmias
E. Thromboembolism

**13.** Sterile cardiac valvular vegetations are associated with all of the following disorders EXCEPT:

A. Mitral valve prolapse
B. Systemic lupus erythematosus
C. Underlying adenocarcinoma
D. Indwelling pulmonary artery (Swan-Ganz) catheter
E. Rheumatic fever

**14.** All of the following statements about isolated aortic valvular stenosis are true EXCEPT:

A. Rheumatic heart disease is the underlying cause in most cases.
B. Congenital bicuspid valves are a risk factor.
C. Concentric left ventricular hypertrophy characteristically is produced.
D. Symptomatic disease develops only when cardiac decompensation occurs.
E. Heart failure is the most common cause of death in untreated disease.

**15.** The sinoatrial node (the cardiac pacemaker) sends impulses directly to:

A. The atrioventricular node
B. The bundle of His
C. The atrioventricular bundle
D. The right bundle branch
E. The left bundle branch

**16.** Major causes of infectious myocarditis include all of the following organisms EXCEPT:

A. Coxsackie A virus
B. *Trypanosoma cruzi* (Chagas' disease)
C. *Corynebacterium diphtheriae* (diphtheria)
D. *Staphylococcus aureus*
E. *Borrelia burgdorferi* (Lyme disease)

**17.** All of the following features commonly are associated with hypertrophic cardiomyopathy EXCEPT:

A. A disproportionately enlarged ventricular septum
B. Aortic valve thickening
C. Myofiber disarray in the affected myocardium
D. Small left ventricular volume
E. Large left atrial volume

**18.** Cardiac toxicity is known to be produced by all of the following chemical agents EXCEPT:

A. Alcohol
B. Cyclophosphamide
C. Bleomycin
D. Adriamycin
E. Cocaine

**19.** All of the following disorders predispose to cor pulmonale EXCEPT:

A. Pulmonary embolism
B. Pickwickian syndrome
C. Emphysema
D. Patent ductus arteriosus
E. Cystic fibrosis

**20.** All of the following statements correctly describe cardiac transplantation EXCEPT:

A. It is frequently used to treat dilated cardiomyopathy.
B. Endomyocardial biopsy is required for early diagnosis of allograft rejection.
C. Fewer than 33% of transplant recipients survive 5 years.
D. Development of lymphoma is a long-term complication.
E. Silent myocardial infarction is a long-term complication.

**21.** All of the following statements correctly describe cardiac myxomas EXCEPT:

A. They are the most common primary tumor of the heart in adults.
B. They tend to be malignant in the pediatric age group.
C. They occur most frequently in the left atrium.
D. They often are associated with syncopal attacks.
E. Their production of interleukin-6 causes fever.

**22.** All of the following factors exacerbate ischemic heart disease EXCEPT:

A. Pregnancy
B. Advanced lung disease
C. Severe anemia
D. Tachycardia
E. Postmenopausal estrogen replacement

**23.** In a patient with myocardial hypertrophy, the diagnosis of systemic hypertensive heart disease cannot be made in the presence of any of the following conditions EXCEPT:

A. No prior history of hypertension
B. Cardiac amyloidosis
C. Coarctation of the aorta
D. Takayasu's arteritis
E. Aortic stenosis

**24.** The subendocardial region of the ventricular wall is at highest risk of ischemic injury for all of the following reasons EXCEPT:

A. The subendocardial muscle has a higher metabolic demand than the rest of the myocardium.
B. The intermuscular vascular bed is compressed, with the greatest force in this area.
C. This region is less likely to have a collateral vascular supply.
D. The intermuscular arteries in this region more often are affected by stenosing atherosclerosis.
E. This region is too distant from the endocardium to receive oxygen directly from the lumen.

**25.** Complications of the disease shown in Figure 5–2 include all of the following problems EXCEPT:

A. Pancarditis
B. Myocardial abscesses
C. Glomerulonephritis
D. Acute valvular insufficiency
E. Meningitis

**26.** Myocardial infarction in the ABSENCE of coronary atherosclerosis is associated with all of the following factors EXCEPT:

A. Cocaine abuse
B. Coronary arteritis
C. Diabetes mellitus
D. Vegetative endocarditis
E. Coronary artery trauma

**27.** Consequences of rupture of necrotic cardiac muscle following a transmural infarction include all of the following EXCEPT:

A. Cardiac tamponade
B. Acute mitral valvular insufficiency
C. Left-to-right shunt
D. Acute aortic valvular insufficiency
E. Hemopericardium

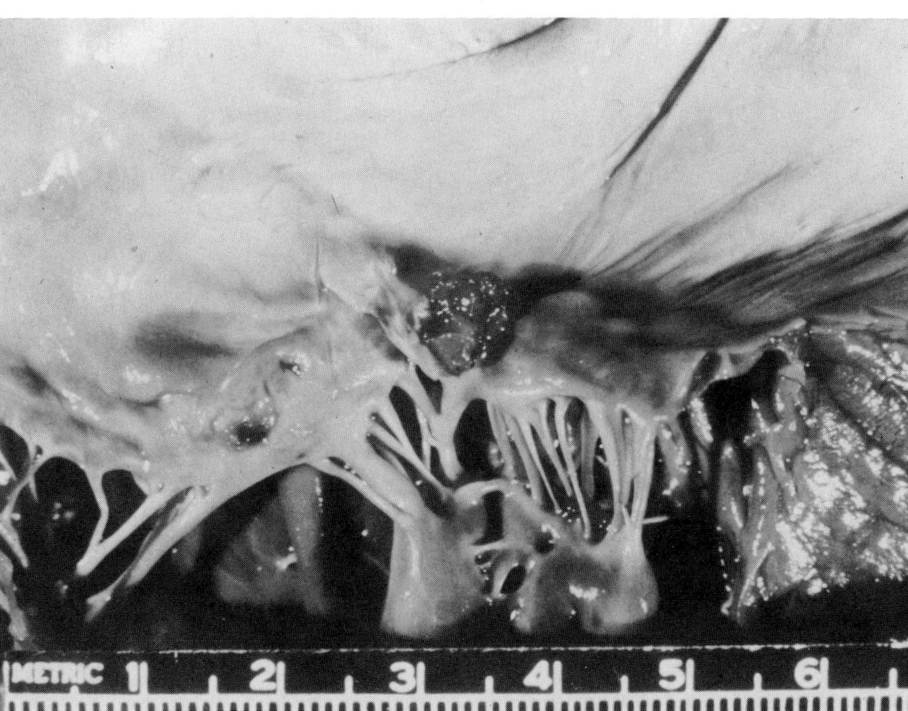


**Figure 5–2**

**DIRECTIONS:** For Questions 28 through 48, you are to decide whether EACH choice is TRUE or FALSE.

For each of the statements about ischemic heart disease (IHD) listed below, choose whether it is TRUE or FALSE.

**28.** In the United States, more people die of IHD every year than of all forms of cancer collectively.
**29.** Only a minority of cases are associated with widespread, severe coronary atherosclerosis.
**30.** Improved therapy has contributed to a declining mortality from IHD.
**31.** Women are protected from IHD during reproductive life.
**32.** Physical conditioning (exercise) is associated with a reduction in the rate of fatal myocardial infarction.

For each of the following statements about rheumatic fever (RF), choose whether it is TRUE or FALSE.

**33.** Rheumatic fever is caused by systemic infection and tissue invasion by group A $\beta$-hemolytic streptococcus.
**34.** Rheumatoid arthritis is a late complication of previously involved joint tissues.
**35.** Rheumatic heart disease is a late complication of previously involved heart tissues.
**36.** Rheumatic fever is more common in children than in adults.
**37.** Culture-positive streptococcal pharyngitis is usually present at the onset of a rheumatic attack.
**38.** Prompt antibiotic therapy of streptococcal pharyngitis is a major factor in the declining incidence of acute RF.
**39.** Group A streptococcal infections of the skin are more likely to cause acute glomerulonephritis than to cause acute RF.
**40.** There is no correlation between the severity of the initial streptococcal infection and the likelihood of developing RF.
**41.** An individual who has once had acute RF is more vulnerable to developing the disease again.
**42.** In the absence of cardiac involvement, complete recovery without residual pathologic changes is the rule.
**43.** Prophylactic long-term antistreptococcal therapy is required for patients who have had RF.
**44.** Genetic predisposition is suggested by the high incidence of HLA-B27 antigens in affected individuals.

For each of the following statements about carcinoid heart disease, choose whether it is TRUE or FALSE.

**45.** The disease is unlikely to develop in association with intestinal carcinoid tumors unless liver metastases are present.
**46.** The disease predominantly affects the left side of the heart.
**47.** The characteristic lesion is an endocardial plaque rich in elastic fibers.
**48.** The disease usually produces insufficiency of the affected valves.

**DIRECTIONS:** For Questions 49 through 92, the set of lettered headings is followed by a list of numbered words or phrases. For each numbered word or phrase choose:
A—if the item is associated with (A) only
B—if the item is associated with (B) only
C—if the item is associated with *both* (A) and (B)
D—if the item is associated with *neither* (A) nor (B)

For each of the features listed below, decide whether it describes atherosclerotic aneurysm, syphilitic aneurysm, both, or neither.

A. Atherosclerotic aneurysm
B. Syphilitic aneurysm
C. Both
D. Neither

**49.** Marked dilation of the aorta is NOT a common feature.
**50.** The thoracic aorta is usually involved.
**51.** Most fatalities occur from rupture.
**52.** Cystic medial degeneration is a characteristic histopathologic change.
**53.** Aggressive antihypertensive therapy is indicated.

For each of the following statements, choose whether it describes acute infective endocarditis, subacute infective endocarditis, both, or neither.

A. Acute infective endocarditis
B. Subacute infective endocarditis
C. Both
D. Neither

**54.** Is produced by *Staphylococcus aureus* in the majority of cases
**55.** Is produced by streptococci in the majority of cases
**56.** Characteristically occurs in previously normal hearts
**57.** Yields positive blood cultures in over 80% of cases
**58.** Is associated with changing cardiac murmurs
**59.** Is associated with intravenous drug abuse

For each of the characteristics listed below, choose whether it describes rheumatic mitral valve disease (mitral stenosis), mitral valve prolapse (myxomatous degeneration of the mitral valve), both, or neither.

A. Rheumatic mitral valve disease (mitral stenosis)
B. Mitral valve prolapse (myxomatous degeneration of the mitral valve)
C. Both
D. Neither

**60.** Occurs more commonly in women
**61.** Predisposes to infective endocarditis
**62.** Is associated with commissural fusion of valve cusps
**63.** Is associated with fibrous thickening of the valve leaflets
**64.** Is associated with ventricular arrhythmias and sudden death
**65.** Eventually requires valve replacement in most cases

For each of the features listed below, choose whether it describes valvular heart disease producing insufficiency, stenosis, both, or neither.

A. Valvular insufficiency
B. Valvular stenosis
C. Both
D. Neither

**66.** Is characterized by failure of the valve to open completely
**67.** Is characterized by failure of the valve to close completely
**68.** Is almost always due to abnormalities of the valve cusps alone
**69.** Is produced by postinflammatory scarring (rheumatic heart disease)
**70.** Is produced by infectious endocarditis
**71.** Commonly occurs in association with rheumatoid arthritis
**72.** Is frequently produced by severe atherosclerosis

For each of the characteristics listed below, choose whether it describes subendocardial myocardial infarction, transmural myocardial infarction, both, or neither.

A. Subendocardial myocardial infarction
B. Transmural myocardial infarction
C. Both
D. Neither

**73.** Severe atherosclerosis of multiple extramyocardial coronary vessels is usually present.
**74.** Stenosing atherosclerosis of penetrating intramyocardial arterial vessels is usually present.
**75.** Involvement is limited to the left ventricle in most cases.
**76.** Acute coronary thrombosis is present in most cases.
**77.** Pericarditis usually develops as a consequence.
**78.** It is frequently seen at autopsy in patients who suffer sudden cardiac death.

For each of the following cardiac regions, choose whether it usually receives its blood supply from the left coronary artery, the right coronary artery, both, or neither.

A. Left coronary artery
B. Right coronary artery
C. Both
D. Neither

**79.** Interventicular septum
**80.** Anterior wall of the left ventricle
**81.** Posterior wall of the left ventricle
**82.** Mitral valve
**83.** Anterior wall of the right ventricle
**84.** Posterior wall of the right ventricle
**85.** Endocardium of the left lateral wall

For each of the following features, choose whether it is commonly associated with left-sided heart failure, right-sided heart failure, both left and right heart failure, or neither.

A. Left-sided heart failure
B. Right-sided heart failure
C. Both left and right heart failure
D. Neither

**86.** Is caused by ischemic heart disease
**87.** Is caused by valvular heart disease
**88.** Is caused by chronic obstructive pulmonary disease
**89.** Produces pulmonary edema
**90.** Produces aldosterone-induced sodium retention
**91.** Produces prerenal azotemia
**92.** Produces centrilobular necrosis of the liver

**DIRECTIONS:** Questions 93 through 128 are matching questions. For each numbered item, choose the most likely associated letter item from those provided. Each numbered item has ONLY ONE answer. Within each group, each lettered item may be the answer to one, more than one, or none of the numbered items.

For each of the characteristics listed below, choose whether it corresponds to a transmural myocardial infarction less than 4 hours old, 4 to 24 hours old, 1 to 2 days old, 3 to 7 days old, or 8 to 14 days old.

A. Less than 4 hours old
B. 4 to 24 hours old
C. 1 to 2 days old
D. 3 to 7 days old
E. 8 to 14 days old

**93.** Peak levels of lactate dehydrogenase in the serum
**94.** Peak tissue infiltration of infarcted muscle by neutrophils seen histologically
**95.** Normal appearance of myocardium on gross examination
**96.** Earliest detection of increased myocardial creatine phosphokinase (CPK-MB) in the serum
**97.** Prominent granulation tissue at the periphery of the infarct seen histologically
**98.** Maximum coagulative necrosis of infarcted muscle seen histologically
**99.** Beginning of electrocardiographic abnormalities
**100.** Maximum risk of cardiac rupture

For each of the features of vasculitis listed below, choose whether it is characteristic of polyarteritis nodosa, giant cell arteritis, Kawasaki's disease, Buerger's disease, or none of these.

A. Polyarteritis nodosa
B. Giant cell arteritis
C. Kawasaki's disease
D. Buerger's disease
E. None of these

**101.** Young children and infants are affected most often.
**102.** The disease is rare under age 50.
**103.** Cigarette smoking is an etiologic factor.
**104.** Cardiac involvement is very common.
**105.** Kidney involvement is very common.
**106.** Gangrene of the extremities often is produced.
**107.** Lymph node enlargement is an associated finding.
**108.** Response to steroids alone is excellent.

For each of the conditions listed below, choose the type of pericarditis it is most likely to produce.

A. Serous pericarditis
B. Hemorrhagic pericarditis
C. Purulent pericarditis
D. Serofibrinous pericarditis
E. Caseous pericarditis

**109.** Cardiopulmonary resuscitation
**110.** Postinfarction (Dressler's) syndrome
**111.** Scleroderma
**112.** Chest radiation
**113.** Cardiac surgery

For each of the statements listed below, choose whether it describes stable angina only, unstable angina only, Prinzmetal's angina only, both stable and unstable angina, both unstable and Prinzmetal's angina, or all of these.

A. Stable angina only
B. Unstable angina only
C. Prinzmetal's angina only
D. A and B
E. B and C
F. All of these

**114.** Is associated with coronary atherosclerosis
**115.** Occurs at rest
**116.** Is induced by exertion and relieved by rest
**117.** Most commonly is accomapnied by S-T segment elevation on electrocardiogram
**118.** Most commonly is accompanied by S-T segment depression on electrocardiogram
**119.** Frequently causes reversible injury to myocardial cells
**120.** Is associated with a very high risk of myocardial infarction

Match each of the therapeutic alternatives for treatment of acute myocardial infarction listed below with the most important rationale for its use.

A. Reduction of myocardial oxygen demand
B. Prevention of coronary thrombosis
C. Coronary thrombolysis
D. Reduction of coronary vasospasm
E. Relief of pain
F. None of these

**121.** Phenobarbital
**122.** Verapamil
**123.** Streptokinase
**124.** Morphine
**125.** Enforced activity restriction
**126.** Propranolol
**127.** Lidocaine
**128.** Tissue type plasminogen activator

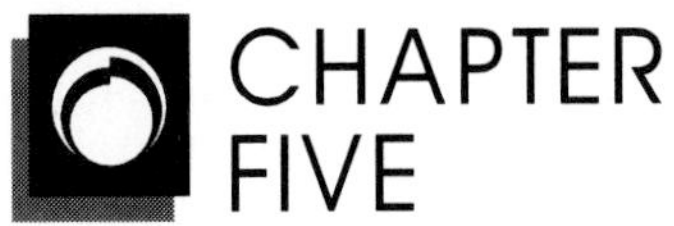

CHAPTER FIVE

# The Cardiovascular System

## ANSWERS

**1. (C)** Cardiac hypertrophy is produced by a compensatory increase in myocyte size and sarcomere content (myocyte hypertrophy) in response to an increased workload (most commonly, the increased peripheral vascular resistance of systemic hypertension). The response is analogous to that of skeletal muscle with weight-bearing exercise (pumping iron). Because cardiac muscle cells cannot divide, no hyperplasia (increase in cell number) occurs. Myocardial hypertrophy results in an overall increase in cardiac size and muscle mass (weight). The degree of cardiac hypertrophy is most accurately determined by the weight of the heart, because a number of superimposed variables (such as the degree of dilation in the failing heart or the contractile state of the ventricles) can alter the heart "size" (i.e., overall diameter or ventricular wall thickness). The histologic appearance of the left ventricular myocardium also may be altered by these factors. Measurement of heart size by cardiac silhouette on chest radiograph is the least accurate way to assess myocardial hypertrophy. A markedly hypertrophied heart may have a normal cardiac silhouette size. Only when the hypertrophied heart begins to fail and undergo dilation will the cardiac silhouette increase in size. Although the weight of the heart varies with the stature of the individual, the range of normal heart weight for the average female is 250 to 300 gm and for the average male 300 to 350 gm. In hypertensive heart disease with left ventricular hypertrophy, the heart weight may exceed 500 gm. *(pp. 521; 541)*

**2. (E)** Acute myocardial infarction (MI) is seldom without complications. In fact, the initial ischemic event proves fatal (sudden cardiac death within 1 to 2 hours) in 20% of patients. Of those who survive, only about 10 to 20% experience no complications. Among the complicated cases, left ventricular congestive failure with pulmonary edema develops in about 60%, but frank cardiogenic shock ("pump failure") occurs in only 10 to 15%. By far the most common complication of MI is the appearance of cardiac arrhythmias (present in 75 to 95% of complicated cases). Arrhythmias are responsible for many sudden deaths related to MI, so control of potentially lethal arrhythmias is one of the primary goals of both mobile and hospital coronary care units. *(pp. 537–539)*

**3. (C)** Systemic hypertension is an extremely common disorder, affecting about 25% of the U.S. population. It is an insidious and treacherous process, remaining asymptomatic until late in its course while producing widespread and often lethal consequences. Hypertensive heart disease (HHD) is the most common consequence of systemic hypertension. HHD is the second most common cause of cardiac disease (ischemic heart disease being the most common), and many patients with untreated systemic hypertension die of complications of HHD (e.g., heart failure, ischemia from hypertension-potentiated coronary artery atherosclerosis, or arrhythmia and sudden cardiac death). However, many other organ systems are affected in systemic hypertension, and their involvement may either dominate the clinical picture or cause the patient's death (or both). Cerebrovascular infarction (stroke), both benign and malignant nephrosclerosis, and vascular complications such as aortic aneurysms are all among the complications of arterial hypertension (which is often accompanied by hypertension-potentiated atherosclerotic vascular disease). Rupture of a berry aneurysm, a relatively uncommon cause of death in general but the most common cause of subarachnoid hemorrhage, frequently is related to systemic hypertension.

Cardiac amyloidosis is not related to hypertension. Deposition of amyloid in the heart may occur as part of the spectrum of disease in any form of systemic amyloidosis. In such cases, the underlying disease is usually an immunocyte dyscrasia, and the amyloid is derived from immunoglobulin light chains. However, in senile amyloidosis (amyloid of aging), amyloid is found only in the heart (isolated organ involvement), and transthyretin is the precursor protein from which the amyloid is derived. This molecule is a normal serum protein involved in the transport of thyroxine and retinol. The reason it deposits in the heart of aged persons is unclear but is not related to hypertension. *(pp. 236; 484–485; 541–542; 976–977; 1312–1313)*

**4. (D)** Figure 5–1 shows a transverse section through the ventricles of a heart with a transmural myocardial infarction (MI) involving the anterior wall of the left ventricle and the anterior aspect of the interventricular septum (the distribution of the anterior descending coronary artery). The neocrotic zone of the left ventricular wall is discolored (pale yellow-tan instead of the normal red-brown color of viable myocardium) and very thinned. Epidemiologic studies have defined clearly a number of key risk factors for MI (the ultimate consequence of ischemic heart disease [IHD] secondary to coronary atherosclerosis). Cigarette smoking substantially increases the risk of MI and is the dominant cause of the increased incidence of MI in women. If smoking is stopped, the increased risk disappears within a few years. Systemic hypertension is also a major risk factor for IHD and MI. The higher the blood pressure, the greater the risk. Both diastolic and systolic hypertension are harmful. Diastolic pressures greater than 70 mm Hg and systolic pressures above 110 mm Hg are associated with increased death rates from IHD.

Numerous prospective studies in well-defined population groups have identified hyperlipidemia as a major risk factor predisposing to IHD. Of particular significance is the level of low-density lipoproteins, which contain about 70% of the total plasma cholesterol and are strongly correlated with atherosclerosis. In addition, hypertriglyceridemia, with increased concentrations of very-low-density lipoproteins, also appears to increase the risk of IHD. In contrast, the serum levels of high-density lipoproteins are inversely related to risk of IHD. Diabetes mellitus is also a major risk factor for IHD, in part as a result of susceptibility of diabetics to hyperlipidemia and hypertension. The incidence of MI in diabetics is twofold greater than that in nondiabetics.

The association between obesity and heart disease is not as clearly defined. Obesity predisposes to other conditions that are associated with increased death rates from MI, such as hyperlipoproteinemia, hypertension, and diabetes mellitus, but only a small increased risk can be ascribed to obesity alone. Thus, obesity is considered a minor rather than a major risk for IHD. *(pp. 473–476; 524; 529; 921)*

**5. (E)** The immediate consequences of acute cardiac ischemia are varied and include: (1) reversible ischemic injury producing classic substernal chest pain known as angina pectoris; (2) sudden death without infarction related to ischemia-induced arrhythmias; (3) irreversible transmural myocardial damage (transmural infarction); and (4) less commonly, no clinical symptomatology (silent ischemia). Diabetes mellitus may be associated with asymptomatic ischemic heart disease ("silent myocardial infarction" [MI]), because diabetic neuropathy sometimes interferes with the sensory preception of ischemic pain. Overall, silent MI occurs in about 1% of patients with MI.

Cardiac rupture does not occur as an immediate consequence of ischemic damage, however. It is an uncommon event (occurs in 1 to 5% of cases of complicated MI) that occurs many days (typically 4 to 7) after an acute transmural MI during the period of peak muscle necrosis, when weakening and thinning of the infarcted wall is most pronounced. *(pp. 528; 535–541)*

**6. (C)** Sudden cardiac death is defined as unexpected death from cardiac causes in the absence of or soon (usually within an hour) after the onset of symptoms. In the vast majority of cases, it occurs as a complication of ischemic heart disease, with the ultimate event being a lethal arrhythmia. Less commonly it occurs as a consequence of marked aortic stenosis, hereditary or acquired conduction system abnormalities, or electrolyte derangements. Cocaine and crack may produce sudden death by a variety of mechanisms: (1) lethal arrhythmia without infarction (direct effect of the drug); (2) myocardial infarction (with or without coronary atherosclerosis) and lethal arrhythmia secondary to ischemic injury; (3) rupture of the aorta, presumably related to hypertension; or (4) dilated myocardopathy with lethal arrhythmia. The latter (cocaine-associated myocardopathy) itself may be related to muscle injury from a variety of sources, including direct drug toxicity, hypersensitivity reactions to the drug, drug-induced vasospasm and ischemia, and/or intercurrent infection. *(pp. 395; 541)*

**7. (A)** There are two basic aims of therapy for acute myocardial infarction: (1) acute intervention to improve immediate survival and to reduce or limit the size of the infarction, and (2) long-term intervention to improve survival during the first year or two following the acute infarction. Clinical studies have shown that the long-term prognosis is improved by treatment with drugs that act to prevent precipitation of myocardial ischemia. For example, $\beta$ adrenergic blocking agents and calcium channel blocking agents (e.g., nifedipine, verapamil) decrease cardiac contractility and reduce oxygen demand. Antiplatelet drugs, such as aspirin, prevent the atheroma-induced aggregation and activation of platelets, which contribute to thrombosis, vasospasm, and other events in myocardial ischemia. When myocardial ischemia cannot be controlled adequately by these medical therapies, surgical revascularization via coronary artery bypass is frequently successful.

Administration of tissue-type plasminogen activator (tPA) in an attempt to restore perfusion to ischemic muscle, however, is only useful in the immediate postinfarction period (within 4 hours of onset). Its beneficial effect results from immediate plasmin-mediated thrombolysis in the occluded vessel(s). If flow is restored within 15 to 20 minutes of coronary occlusion, myocardial necrosis may be averted altogether. Reperfusion after a longer interval can "rescue" the muscle at the edge of an infarct from irreversible injury. Once the damage is done and ischemic cell death has occurred, there is no rationale for tPA administration. Thus, tPA is not useful for long-term therapy. *(pp. 529–530; 535–536)*

**8. (A)** Chronic ischemic heart disease is characterized by insidious ischemic atrophy of the myocardium leading to heart failure, with or without a previous history of overt angina or myocardial infarction. Histologically, diffusely atrophic myofibers are seen within diffusely fibrotic interstitial connective tissue. Scars from healed previous infarcts are usually present, and severe stenosing atherosclerosis of the coronary arteries is invariably present. As more and more myofibers undergo ischemic atrophy, cardiac decompensation and heart failure ensue. Although some patients have anginal attacks or acute myocardial infarctions during the course of their disease, chronic ischemic heart disease may be entirely asymptomatic until heart failure develops. The mural endocardium is usually normal because its oxygen supply comes directly from the lumen, not the stenotic coronary vessels. *(pp. 540–541)*

**9. (E)** Hypertensive heart disease is characteristically insidious in its onset. It develops over a period of time during which the left ventricle undergoes hypertrophy in order to maintain a normal cardiac output in the face of increased peripheral resistance. During this period of compensation. the patient is usually free of clinical symptoms. Myocardial hypertrophy (characteristically concentric in configuration) leads to a significant increase in heart weight (see Question 1) and myocardial oxygen demand. During this compensated phase of hypertensive heart disease, however, the size of the heart, as measured by chest radiograph, is not significantly increased. Only when the heart can no longer compensate and dilation of the failing heart ensues does the cardiac silhouette on chest radiograph show a significant increase. Characteristic electrocardiographic changes are usually present in hypertensive heart disease, even during the asymptomatic phase, and may aid in the diagnosis. *(pp. 520–522; 541–542)*

**10. (D)** A host of gross microscopic, physiologic, electromechanical, and biochemical/molecular changes occur in the heart as a result of the prolonged hemodynamic overload in systemic hypertension. The microscopic changes of myocardial hypertrophy in hypertensive heart disease are subtle. No architectural changes in the tissue are seen, but the cytologic features of the myofibers change as a reflection of their increased workload. In short, the myofibers hypertrophy, and both their cell diameter and nuclear size increase. Nuclear hyperchromatism and pleomorphism also may be seen in advanced stages, and increased amounts of fibrous tissue may be found between myofibers. The myocytes not only look abnormal, their gene expression and protein production are abnormal as well. They synthesize abnormal and possibly dysfunctional proteins. Several different classes may be involved, including those related to contractile elements, to excitation-contraction coupling, and to energy utilization. Although the myocardial oxygen demand is increased, there is no detectable change in the number or distribution of capillaries in the hypertensive heart. The decreasing capillary-to-myocyte ratio is an important element in the evolution to cardiac failure in hypertensive heart disease. *(pp. 520–521; 541–542)*

**11. (B)** A number of cardiac changes are associated with aging, although their etiologies remain largely unknown. One such senile change is calcific aortic stenosis, a fibrotic and calcific deformity of the aortic valve. In some cases, calcific aortic valve stenosis may be related either to a congenitally deformed valve or to a healed infective endocarditis, but in most instances no such associations are present. Thus, the process has been ascribed to age-related degenerative changes alone. Equally obscure in its etiology is calcification of the mitral annulus, which occurs almost exclusively in elderly individuals, especially women. In contrast to calific aortic valve stenosis, calcification of the mitral annulus generally does not affect valve function.

Amyloidosis of aging refers primarily to isolated cardiac involvement by amyloidosis (see Question 3). In this condition, the amyloid is derived from aggregation and proteolysis of transthyretin (TTR), a normal serum transport protein for thyroxine and retinol. In senile cardiac amyloidosis, the amyloid-precursor TTR is a structurally normal (not mutant) protein, and the reason it deposits in the heart of aged persons is unclear.

Brown atrophy refers to the organ shrinkage (atrophy) and lipofuscin accumulation that sometimes are seen in the heart and/or liver of elderly patients. It is regarded as a benign degenerative process.

Mitral stenosis is usually the result of injury from rheumatic heart disease, but it may also be produced by healed infective endocarditis. Unlike aortic stenosis, it does not occur simply as an aging phenomenon. *(pp. 28; 232–237; 519; 544–545; 547)*

**12. (D)** Surgical replacement of diseased heart valves with mechanical or porcine bioprosthetic valves is a common therapeutic approach in all valvular heart disease. Although they are often lifesaving, prosthetic valves are not without their own dangers. They are associated with numerous complications, and about 60% of prosthetic heart valve recipients have a serious complication within 10 years. Hemolytic anemia develops from the mechanical destruction of erythrocytes passing through the prosthesis, especially one that is degraded from wear. Partial separation of the suture line anchoring the valve (dehiscence) occurs uncommonly. The paravalvular leaks that result are usually insignificant but also may cause hemolysis as blood is forced through the narrow channel of the dehiscence.

The major problems associated with prosthetic valves are infection, thromboembolism, and valve deterioration with mechanical dysfunction. Thrombus-related complications are more common with mechanical than bioprosthetic valves. Thrombi may give rise to emboli (most often to the brain, producing stroke or death), become infected and produce infective endocarditis, or produce valve malfunction through mechanical interference. Infective endocarditis develops when the prosthesis becomes seeded by blood-borne bacteria (most often at the suture line). This occurs in about 6% of patients within 5 years of valve replacement. Prosthesis-associated infective endocarditis is a serious complication and can be fatal. Deterioration with valve dysfunction can occur with mechanical valves but is most common with bioprostheses. At least 30% of procine valves require replacement within 10 years because of sterile tissue degeneration. Mechanical malfunction of the valve also may result from nonstructural causes, including such problems as tissue overgrowth (entrapment) or paravalvular leaks.

Whereas arrhythmias occasionally occur in the postoperative period following valve replacement, they are not otherwise commonly associated with prosthetic valves installed by experienced cardiac surgeons. *(pp. 556–557)*

**13. (A)** Sterile thrombotic vegetations are the hallmark of nonbacterial thrombotic endocarditis (NBTE). They may form on either normal or abnormal valves, involve either side of the heart, and tend to be small (1 to 5 mm). NBTE occurs in a variety of clinical conditions, many of which are associated with a hypercoagulable state (e.g., underlying adenocarcinoma). Because NBTE is often associated with chronic debilitating disease, such as malignancy, renal failure, or chronic sepsis, it has been called "marantic" (i.e., "wasting") endocarditis. However, it also may occur in the young and the well nourished who have conditions associated with hypercoagulability (e.g., hyperestrogenemic states). Iatrogenic endocardial trauma (indwelling catheters) is also a well-known predisposing factor. Other specific conditions that produce bland (devoid of organisms or pus) valvular vegetations include rheumatic fever and systemic lupus erythematosus (SLE). In specific, endocardial involvement in SLE is known as Libman-Sacks disease. The major significance of all sterile thrombotic vegetations is their embolic potential.

Mitral valve prolapse is a valvular abnormality that is associated with an increased risk of infectious endocarditis but has no independent association with NBTE. *(pp. 545–546; 549; 554–555)*

**14. (A)** Although aortic stenosis may occur in rheumatic heart disease, either alone or in combination with mitral involvement, most isolated calcific aortic stenoses are nonrheumatic in origin. In the vast majority of cases of isolated aortic stenosis, the lesion is an age-related degenerative phenomenon (see Question 11). It can involve normal valves, but congenitally deformed (e.g., bicuspid) valves represent a significant risk factor. Concentric left ventricular hypertrophy occurs, with obstruction to left ventricular outflow, but is usually asymptomatic for many years. Symptomatic disease (syncope, angina, or congestive heart failure) develops only when cardiac decompensation occurs. Once symptoms occur, the prognosis is poor unless treated by surgical valve replacement. Without treatment, heart failure and death usually ensue within 2 to 3 years. In contrast, valve replacement commonly results in dramatic improvement. *(pp. 544–545)*

**15. (C)** The conduction system of the heart is composed of specialized cardiac muscle fibers called Purkinje cells that conduct action impulses faster than contractile myofibers. The conduction system regulates the rate and rhythm of the heart. The impulse originates in the sinoatrial node (the pacemaker of the heart) in the posterior wall of the right atrium beside the opening of the superior vena cava. It travels through the atrioventricular (A-V) bundle to the A-V node, located where the median wall of the right atrium joins the interventricular septum. From the A-V node, the impulse is propagated along the interventricular septum toward the apex through the bundle of His. At the apex, the bundle of His splits to form the right and left bundle branches that carry the impulse laterally to the two ventricles. *(p. 518)*

**16. (D)** A multitude of microorganisms may cause infectious endocarditis, including viruses, chlamydia, bacteria, fungi, and metazoans. Viruses are the most common cause of myocarditis, producing over half of all cases. Coxsackie A and B, echovirus, poliovirus, and influenza A and B viruses are the most frequently encountered viral agents. Among the causative bacterial agents are *Corynebacterium diphtheriae* (the diphtheria bacillus actually causes exotoxin-mediated myocardial injury rather than direct infection), meningococcus, and *Borrelia burgdorferi*, the spirochete that causes Lyme disease. Myocarditis occurs in about 66% of patients with Lyme disease. Although Chagas' disease is uncommon in the United States, *Trypanosoma cruzi* is a common cause of myocarditis in endemic regions (Mexico, Central America, and South America). *Staphylococcus aureus*, although a common cause of endocarditis, rarely causes myocarditis. *(pp. 562–563)*

**17. (B)** Hypertrophic cardiomyopathy (HCM), also known as idiopathic hypertrophic subaortic stenosis, is characterized by cardiac enlargement and massive myocardial hypertrophy. The hypertrophy may be either symmetrical (10% of cases) or asymmetrical (classic pattern), with disproportionate thickening of the septal wall. Microscopically, a characteristic pattern of myofiber disarray (random rather than parallel orientation) is seen in the involved portions of the myocardium. The thickened wall causes a reduction in the volume of the left ventricular cavity in 90% of the cases and a dilated left atrium in virtually every case (atrial fibrillation is a major complication of HCM). When the subaortic region of the septal wall is involved markedly, outflow obstruction may occur that mimics aortic valvular stenosis. However, the aortic valve is characteristically normal in HCM and does not contribute to the outflow obstruction. *(pp. 644–646)*

**18. (C)** A number of chemical agents are known to produce toxic injury to heart muscle. Some of these substances are widely used and easily available, such as alcohol. Others, such as arsenic and carbon monoxide, might be more likely to be associated with nefarious (suicide or murder) or accidental exposure. Recreational drugs (such as cocaine and crack) cause catecholamine-induced cardiac damage. A similar mechanism of cardiac injury is produced by large amounts of vasopressor agents (e.g., dopamine) administered iatrogenically. Other cardiotoxic agents used frequently in medical treatment include lithium and the chemotherapeutic agents cyclophosphamide, Adriamycin (doxorubicin), and daunorubicin. Bleomycin is associated with diffuse alveolar damage in the lung but not cardiac toxicity. *(pp. 562t; 564–565)*

**19. (D)** Cor pulmonale, or pulmonary heart disease, refers to right ventricular enlargement secondary to hypertension in the pulmonary vascular tree caused by disorders of lung structure or function. Pulmonary hypertension may result from primary (idiopathic) disease in the pulmonary vasculature or from pulmonary parenchymal disease with secondary vascular changes (chronic obstructive pulmonary diseases such as emphysema and chronic bronchitis, diffuse interstitial fibrosis, or cystic fibrosis). Occasionally, pulmonary hypertension may be produced by inadequate function of the chest bellows (e.g., Pickwickian syndrome of marked obesity with secondary respiratory problems) or inadequate ventilatory drive from the respiratory centers in the brain. In addition, acute cor pulmonale may develop from massive pulmonary embolization.

By definition, cor pulmonale is limited to right heart overload caused by lung-related disease and excludes right ventricular enlargement caused by left heart disease or congenital heart disease (e.g., patent ductus arteriosus). *(pp. 427; 542–543)*

**20. (C)** Transplantation of cardiac allografts is now a relatively commonplace therapy for otherwise hopeless cases of severe, intractable heart failure. It is most commonly performed for dilated cardiomyopathy and ischemic heart disease, but appropriate patients with heart diseases of diverse etiologies are treated by this method. Even with current methods of immunosuppression using cyclosporine A, steroids, and azathiaprine, acute allograft rejection is a major postoperative problem. Suppression of rejection is managed most successfully when the process is recognized early, before the onset of clinical signs and symptoms (when substantial myocardial damage already has occurred). Early diagnosis of rejection requires endomyocardial biopsy to look for interstitial lymphocytic inflitration with or without myocyte injury (the characteristic histopathologic findings in allograft rejection).

Even with control of rejection episodes and of supervening infections related to immunosuppression, other life-threatening problems may complicate the postoperative course. For example, malignancies, especially lymphomas related to Epstein-Barr virus infection, may develop as a complication of long-term immunosuppressive therapy. The major limitation to the long-term success of cardiac transplantation, however, is progressive stenosing arteriosclerosis of the coronary arteries of the allograft. This problem is all the more insidious because the resultant ischemia produces no symptoms in the denervated allograft. Thus, silent myocardial infarction with sudden death or congestive heart failure is a major cause of mortality in transplant recipients. Despite all these potential problems, the outcome is usually positive. More than 70% of all transplant recipients survive the first postoperative year, and more than 60% survive 5 years. *(p. 580)*

**21. (B)** Cardiac myxomas are connective tissue tumors of the endocardium. They are the most common primary tumors of the heart in adults (in infants and children, rhabdomyosarcomas are more common). Myxomas usually have the gross appearance of a soft, translucent, pedunculated mass and are composed predominantly of abundant mucopolysaccharide ground substance in which small round myxoma (stromal) cells, smooth muscle cells, and endothelial cells are embedded. Myxomas may arise in any chamber, but 90% occur in the atria. When they occur in the left atrium (the predominant location), they can be associated with intermittent ball valve obstruction of the mitral valve orifice, producing syncopal attacks. Constitutional symptoms, such as fever and malaise, may occur as a consequence of cytokine production (principally interleukin-6) by some tumors.

Cardiac myxomas are benign tumors in all age groups. Their major morbidity and mortality is associated with the above-mentioned ball valve obstruction that may lead to acute cardiac insufficiency or even sudden death. Fragmentation and embolization of papillary tumors also is encountered. *(p. 569)*

**22. (E)** Ischemic heart disease is exacerbated by processes that create an imbalance between myocardial oxygen supply and demand. Either diminished oxygen-carrying capacity of the blood (severe anemia) or decreased ability to oxygenate blood (advanced lung disease) would have the effect of reducing myocardial oxygen supply. Increased muscle mass (myocardial hypertrophy), increased contractile activity (tachycardia), or increased cardiac output states (pregnancy) all increase myocardial oxygen demand. Any of these factors may be superimposed on coronary atherosclerosis and contribute significantly to the production of myocardial ischemia. In contrast to these factors, postmenopausal estrogen replacement would not exacerbate ischemic heart disease in any way. On the contrary, postmenopausal estrogen replacement is associated with a reduced risk of ischemic heart disease because of its antiatherogenic effect. *(p. 524)*

**23. (B)** Two criteria must be met in order to make the diagnosis of hypertensive heart disease (HHD): a prior history of hypertension and left ventricular hypertrophy as an isolated finding. The diagnosis of HHD cannot be made in the presence of other cardiovascular abnormalities, which might themselves lead to increased left ventricular pressure or volume overload with subsequent compensatory hypertropy. Examples of such processes would include: (1) diseases of the aorta, such as coarctation or Takayasu's arteritis; (2) cardiac valvular disease, such as aortic stenosis; and (3) myocardial disease, such as hypertrophic cardiomyopathy. Takayasu's arteritis ("pulseless disease") is a granulomatous vasculitis of unknown etiology that produces fibrous thickening of the aortic arch and stenosis of aortic tributaries. Systemic hypertension may be produced either as a primary effect of aortic disease or as a secondary effect of renal arterial stenosis with renal ischemia and stimulation of renin production. The presence of cardiac amyloidosis would not preclude a diagnosis of HHD in a patient with left ventricular hypertrophy because amyloidosis itself does not cause cardiac hypertrophy. Cardiac amyloidosis is a restrictive disorder, interfering with distensibility of the ventricular walls, not a hypertrophic disorder. *(pp. 493; 541; 561)*

**24. (D)** For several anatomic and physiologic reasons, the subendocardial region is the area of the heart at highest risk of infarction. Its position relative to the oxygen supply is critical. It is at the distal end of the oxygen supply system (the coronary arteries penetrate inward from the pericardial surface to the endocardial surface), but it is too far from the endocardial surface to be oxygenated by blood in the ventricular lumen. Furthermore, the subendocardial region has a higher metabolic demand (oxygen requirement) than the outer zone of the myocardium because it contracts with greater force, and it is less well perfused because the contraction exerts a greater compressive force on its own vascular bed. In addition, the collateral vascular supply to the subendocardial region is less abundant than that in peripheral zones of the myocardium. However, atherosclerosis of intramyocardial arteries is virtually never encountered in any zone of the cardiac wall and is not a contributing factor to subendocardial ischemia. *(pp. 518–519; 529)*

**25. (A)** Figure 5–2 shows vegetations on the mitral valve of a heart with infective endocarditis. This is a hazardous disease caused by colonization or infection of the heart valves or the mural endocardium by a microbial agent (usually a bacterium), leading to the formation of large, friable endocardial surface vegetations (masses of fibrin, inflammatory cells, and organisms). The process is associated with numerous grave complications. Primary among these are cardiac complications, embolic infarction, metastatic infection, and immune complex–related disease. Fragmentation and embolization of septic vegetations may produce either infarction and/or metastatic abscesses in the tissue where the embolus lodges. When the valves of the left heart are involved (the most common pattern), embolization and/or abscess formation may involve almost any organ, including the heart, kidneys, spleen, brain, and meninges. Lung abscesses may occur with right-sided bacterial endocarditis, the form often seen with intravenous drug abuse. Immunologic responses to the infecting organism may lead to immune complex formation and subsequently to (membranous) glomerulonephritis or vasculitis. Local complications of infectious endocarditis involve valvular dysfunction. Rarely, large vegetations cause stenosis or occlusion of the valve orifice. More commonly, tissue destruction from invasive organisms causes valvular incompetence. Acute valvular insufficiency, especially of the aortic valve, is life threatening and requires emergent surgical intervention (valve replacement).

In contrast to infective myocarditis, infective endocarditis does not produce widespread infection or inflammation of heart muscle (pancarditis). Involvement of heart muscle typically is limited to foci directly subjacent to the affected endocardium (direct extension) or scattered foci of metastatic abscess formation caused by septic embolism through the coronary arterial system. *(pp. 550–553; 562–563)*

**26. (C)** About 10% of transmural myocardial infarctions are not associated with atherosclerotic thrombosis of the coronary arteries. In these cases, other mechanisms of coronary injury and/or thrombosis often are implicated in the pathogenesis. Cocaine abuse, with or without underlying coronary atherosclerosis, induces myocardial infarction by mechanisms believed to be related to vasospasm and superimposed thrombosis. Arteritis involving the coronary arteries (e.g., polyarteritis nodosa, Kawasaki's disease, or infectious arteritis) or direct mechanical trauma can cause local injury and thrombosis. Another mechanism of occlusion is embolism. Emboli may originate from mitral or aortic valvular vegetations in either infective endocarditis or nonbacterial thrombotic endocarditis, left atrial or ventricular mural thrombi, or even fragments of an atrial myxoma. Paradoxical emboli from the venous system or the right heart can occur if an abnormal communication between the right and left heart is present (e.g., patent foramen ovale).

Diabetes mellitus is associated with a high risk of myocardial infarction precisely because it is a major risk factor for atherosclerotic vascular disease. Thus, myocardial infarction in a diabetic in the absence of atherosclerosis would be unlikely (even if one of the above factors were also present). *(pp. 529–530)*

**27. (D)** The consequences of necrotic muscle rupture following transmural myocardial infarction (median time to rupture: 4–5 days) depend largely on the site of the involvement. Rupture of the left ventricular free wall results in hemopericardium and acute cardiac tamponade (almost always fatal). Rupture of the interventricular septum produces a left-to-right shunt. The function of the mitral valve depends on both the anchorage of its free margins to the ventricular wall (via chordae tendinae) and the coordinated contraction of the papillary muscles during systole; therefore, papillary muscle rupture causes acute mitral valvular insufficiency. In contrast, aortic valve function is not dependent on muscular contraction or tethering and is not made insufficient by muscle rupture. *(p. 609)*

**28. (True); 29. (False); 30. (True); 31. (True); 32. (True)**

**(28)** Ischemic heart disease (IHD) is the leading cause of death in the United States and other industrialized nations. In the United States, about 600,000 deaths from IHD occur annually (about 80% of all cardiac mortality and 33% of all deaths), more than all forms of cancer collectively.

**(29)** The vast majority of cases of IHD are associated with severe, widespread atherosclerosis of the coronary arteries, underscoring the primary importance of coronary atherosclerosis in the pathogenesis of myocardial infarction (MI).

**(30)** Although the present mortality rate from IHD is still very high, it represents a decline in recent years resulting, in part, from improved therapy of IHD (mainly MI). An equally important factor contributing to the declining death rate is improved lifestyles that lessen the risk of IHD.

**(31)** Except for those having some disorder predisposing to atherosclerosis (e.g., diabetes mellitus or hyperlipidemia), females of reproductive age are at significantly lower risk of dying from IHD than their male counterparts. After age 45, the difference in risk diminishes considerably.

**(32)** A number of variables are believed to influence the risk and/or outcome of MI. Coincident with the current interest in physical fitness, a number of studies have shown that regular exercise reduces the rate of fatal MI. *(pp. 474–476; 528–529)*

**33. (False); 34. (False); 35. (True); 36. (True); 37. (False); 38. (True); 39. (True); 40. (False); 41. (True); 42. (True); 43. (True); 44. (False)**

**(33)** Rheumatic fever is a postinfectious immunologic disease process. It is the result of an immunologic response to pharyngeal (not cutaneous) infection by group A $\beta$ hemolytic streptococci in immunogenetically susceptible individuals. The tissue damage in this disease is mediated not by the organisms but by the generation of antistreptococcal antibodies that cross-react with native tissue antigens.

**(34)** Although involvement of the heart has the most dire consequences, other organs are affected as well. The large joints may be targeted, producing a migratory polyarthritis known as rheumatic arthritis (not to be confused with rheumatoid arthritis). Rheumatic arthritis is a transitory process and always resolves without sequelae. Rheumatoid arthritis, in contrast, is a chronic systemic inflammatory disease that produces a progressive crippling deformity of involved joints. There is no known etiologic connection between the two diseases, despite their similar names and the fact that they each result from an immune response to a microbial agent in an immunogenetically susceptible host. In rheumatoid arthritis, the identity of the inciting pathogen(s) remains unknown, although the Epstein-Barr virus is a prime suspect.

**(35)** The most significant consequence of rheumatic fever is injury to the cardiac tissues. Although inflammation and injury may be produced in any layer of the heart from epicardium to endocardium, rheumatic valvulitis produces the most dire long-term complications. Injured valves undergo progressive fibrous scarring and permanent deformity that result in valve dysfunction and often necessitate surgical repair (replacement with an artificial valve).

**(36)** Although acute rheumatic fever occurs most often in children between the ages of 5 and 15 years, about 20% of cases occur in adults. **(37)** The latent period between the streptococcal pharyngitis and the onset of acute rheumatic fever is 1 to 5 weeks. At the time of the rheumatic attack, throat cultures are usually negative. Evidence of immunologic response to streptococcal antigens in the form of anti-streptolysin O, anti-hyaluronidase, anti-streptokinase, or anti-NADase antibodies is almost always present, however.

**(38)** Prompt antibiotic therapy of streptococcal pharyngitis reduces the incidence of injurious immune responses and is a major factor responsible for the declining incidence of acute rheumatic fever. Other factors include improved socioeconomic living conditions and some apparent overall reduction the virulence of the causative organisms.

**(39)** Streptococcal sepsis occurring through other portals of entry, such as the skin (impetigo), is not usually followed by rheumatic fever. Streptococcal skin infections, like streptococcal infections elsewhere in the body, tend to induce an immune response that causes immune complex–mediated glomerulonephritis. In fact, acute rheumatic fever and acute poststreptococcal glomerulonephritis rarely occur together and do so only coincidentally. It is believed that the nephritogenic strains of streptococci lack the antigens to which the cross-reacting antibodies of rheumatic fever are directed.

**(40)** There is a strong correlation between the severity and duration of the initial streptococcal pharyngitis and the likelihood of developing subsequent rheumatic fever. **(41)** Furthermore, an individual who has once had an initial attack of rheumatic fever is more vulnerable to recurrence of the disease with subsequent bouts of streptococcal pharyngitis. If the initial attack of rheumatic fever produces carditis, subsequent attacks usually produce increasingly severe recurrences of this process. Even in the absence of reactivation, however, rheumatic carditis generally produces postinflammatory fibrocalcific valvular deformity as a late consequence. **(42)** In the absence of cardiac involvement, however, the patient often recovers completely from rheumatic fever and is spared recurrences or chronic sequelae. **(43)** In order to prevent recurrent attacks in the rheumatic patient with cardiac involvement, long-term prophylactic antistreptococcal therapy is the rule.

**(44)** Only 3% of individuals with acute streptococcal pharyngitis ever develop rheumatic fever. Individual susceptibility to rheumatic fever is likely to be related to genetic factors, probably immune response genes to streptococcal antigens. However, the susceptibility to rheumatic fever is not sex-linked, nor is there a defined HLA profile in susceptible individuals. *(pp. 547–550; 1251)*

**45. (True); 46. (False); 47. (False); 48. (True)**

**(45)** Involvement of the heart is one of the major pathologic consequences of the carcinoid syndrome. This syndrome is produced by neuroendocrine (carcinoid) tumors that release a variety of bioactive products into the bloodstream. These substances include serotonin (5-hydroxytryptamine), kallikrein, bradykinin, histamine, prostaglandins, and tachykinins, but it is not clear which of them is/are responsible for producing the syndrome or the cardiac disease. The principal manifestations of the syndrome include: (1) vasomotor disturbances (flushing of the skin); (2) intestinal hypermotility (diarrhea, cramps, and vomiting); and (3) bronchoconstriction (asthma-like symptoms of dyspnea and wheezing). The cardiac involvement of the carcinoid syndrome, like the syndrome itself, is unlikely to develop in association with intestinal carcinoid tumors unless liver metastases are present. With metastatic disease, tumor products escape degradation (deamination) by the liver and enter the systemic venous circulation (via the hepatic venous system). However, extraintestinal tumors occurring in organs that are not drained by the portal system may produce the carcinoid syndrome in the absence of liver metastases.

**(46)** The characteristic cardiac lesion associated with the syndrome occurs mainly on the right side of the heart and **(47)** consists of sclerotic, endocardial plaques that, unlike atherosclerotic plaques, do not contain elastic fibers.

**(48)** The plaques typically occur on the pulmonary valve, although the tricuspid valve and mural endocardium may be involved. The affected valve leaflets become thickened and fused, producing valvular insufficiency. Although the pathogenesis of these lesions is still uncertain, it is believed that they are most likely due to elevated blood levels of tumor-derived serotonin and tachykinins (neuropeptide K and substance P). *(p. 639)*

**49. (D); 50. (B); 51. (C); 52. (D); 53. (D)**

**(49)** There are three major types of aortic aneurysms: (1) atherosclerotic aneurysms; (2) syphilitic (luetic) aneurysms; and (3) dissecting aneurysms (which involve structurally abnormal aortas with underlying mural degeneration). Only dissecting aneurysms fail, in most cases, to produce the marked dilation of the aorta that is the hallmark of atherosclerotic and syphilitic aneurysms.

**(50)** Syphilitic aneurysms almost always involve the thoracic aorta, usually the ascending and transverse portions. Atherosclerotic aneurysms, in contrast, usually occur in the distal abdominal aorta, although they occasionally may involve the descending portion of the aortic arch.

**(51)** Rupture of the dilated, weakened wall of an atherosclerotic or syphilitic aneurysm is a catastrophic, all too common event that constitutes the major cause of mortality associated with these lesions. Death from congestive heart failure is also common with those syphilitic aneurysms that produce either dilation and incompetency of the aortic valve or narrowing of the coronary ostia.

**(52)** All aortic aneurysms are caused by processes that destroy the structural integrity of the arterial wall. In aortic atherosclerosis, the aortic wall eventually is weakened by the progressive tissue destruction and replacement by plaque. Syphilis causes an obliterative endarteritis of the vasa vasorum of the aorta and ischemic destruction of the aortic wall, with fibrous scarring of the media. Cystic medial degeneration is the underlying defect in dissecting aortic aneurysms. This lesion is characterized by accumulations of basophilic mucoid material within the wall (between individual muscle cells and elastic fibers). The resultant mural weakening allows blood to dissect into the wall at a point of intimal rupture. Both the initial intimal tear and the subsequent extension of dissecting hemorrhage within the weakened vessel wall are believed to be consequences of hypertension. **(53)** Thus, aggressive antihypertensive therapy is often effective in limiting the extent of dissection in dissecting aneurysms but would be of little value in either atherosclerotic or syphilitic aneurysms. For any aneurysm suspected of rupture, evidencing acute expansion, or complicated by embolic phenomena, immediate surgical repair is the only effective therapy. *(pp. 499–504)*

**54. (A); 55. (B); 56. (A); 57. (C); 58. (A); 59. (A)**

**(54 and 56)** Bacterial infective endocarditis (IE) is a life-threatening condition caused by colonization or invasion of heart valves or mural endocardium by a microbial agent. Characteristically, large friable masses of fibrin, inflammatory cells, and organisms known as vegetations form on the affected endocardial surfaces, most commonly on the edges of the valve leaflets. Acute bacterial endocarditis, the more pernicious of the two forms of IE (acute and subacute), is associated with abrupt onset and rapid valvular destruction. It usually occurs in previously normal hearts and typically is caused by virulent organisms, most commonly *Staphylococcus aureus*.

**(55)** Subacute IE, in contrast, characteristically occurs on abnormal valves, either congenitally deformed (more commonly) or rheumatic valves. This form of IE is often insidious in onset, and the most common causative organisms tend to be of relatively low virulence. Most cases are caused by various species of streptococci.

**(57)** In both acute and subacute IE, the causative agent can be identified from blood cultures when repeated sufficiently, often in 80 to 95% of cases.

**(58)** Changing cardiac murmurs are associated with acute IE. The murmurs represent valvular function and flow abnormalities produced by the characteristically bulky vegetations. They change suddenly when vegetations fragment and embolize.

**(59)** It is the acute form of IE that frequently is associated with intravenous drug abuse. The cardiac lesions in drug addiction are distinctive, however, because they tend to affect normal, *right-sided* heart valves, especially the tricuspid valve. *(pp. 550–554)*

**60. (C); 61. (C); 62. (A); 63. (C); 64. (B); 65. (A)**

Mitral valve disease that is rheumatic in origin typically produces markedly thickened, inflexible valve cusps and a narrowed mitral orifice, the predominant result being mitral stenosis (although valvular insufficiency also may be present) (see Questions 66 through 72 below). In contrast, mitral valve prolapse (myxoid degeneration of the mitral valve) usually produces enlarged, floppy valve leaflets that, if they become symptomatic at all, result in mitral insufficiency, not stenosis. **(60)** There is no sexual predominance in rheumatic carditis. Once the disorder occurs, however, women are more prone to the subsequent development of mitral stenosis than men (reason unknown). Mitral valve prolapse is primarily a disorder of females.

**(61)** Both rheumatic mitral valve disease and mitral valve prolapse predispose to infective endocarditis and require antibiotic prophylaxis for procedures known to induce bacteremias (e.g., dental extractions).

**(62)** One of the most characteristic gross pathologic features of rheumatic mitral valve disease is fibrous bridging across the valvular commissures (commissural fusion), producing the characteristic "fish mouth" stenotic deformity. In mitral valve prolapse, pronounced interchordal ballooning (hooding) of the leaflets is seen grossly, but commissural fusion is characteristically absent.

**(63)** Fibrosis and thickening of the valve leaflets occurs in both disorders but is typically more pronounced and deforming in rheumatic mitral valve disease.

**(64)** Although myocarditis occurring during an acute attack of rheumatic fever may cause fatal arrhythmias, subsequent (postinflammatory) rheumatic mitral valve disease typically is associated only with atrial fibrillation, which develops with atrial dilation late in the clinical course. Mitral valve prolapse, in contrast, occasionally is associated with both atrial and ventricular arrhythmias, particularly ventricular tachycardia and fibrillation, and even sudden death (happily, this is uncommon).

**(65)** Mitral stenosis from rheumatic valve disease is one of the most significant causes of late morbidity and mortality in rheumatic patients; thus most patients eventually require valve replacement. Although severe isolated mitral regurgitation may complicate mitral valve prolapse and require valvular replacement, overall this is quite uncommon. Nevertheless, in some major medical centers, mitral valve prolapse has become the most common cause of isolated mitral regurgitation severe enough to require valve replacement. *(pp. 545–550)*

**66. (B); 67. (A); 68. (B); 69. (C); 70. (A); 71. (D); 72. (D)**

Valvular heart disease encompasses a number of disorders whose primary features are cardiac valvular damage and dysfunction. Although the causes are numerous and often produce fairly distinctive morphologic changes in the valves, the functional deficits produced tend to fall into only two categories: (1) valvular insufficiency and (2) valvular stenosis. In certain conditions, both insufficiency and stenosis may be present.

**(66)** Valvular stenosis is characterized by a failure of the valve to open completely, impeding flow through the valve. **(67)** Valvular insufficiency implies a failure of the valve to close completely, producing regurgitant flow. **(68)** Although valvular insufficiency may result from damage to either valve cusps or supporting structures (such as papillary muscles, annular rings, or chordae tendineae), valvular stenosis is almost always due to pathologic changes in the valve cusps.

**(69)** Both types of valvular dysfunction may occur in valves damaged by rheumatic heart disease, which characteristically produces fibrosis, distortion, and dysfunction of the valve cusps and of the supporting structures (chordae tendineae).

**(70)** Infectious endocarditis produces destructive lesions of the valves and supporting structures that can cause perforation of the valve leaflet, erosion of the free margins of the valve, or both. These anatomic changes destroy the competency of the valve and produce valvular insufficiency.

**(71)** Cardiac involvement occurs commonly in rheumatoid arthritis (RA), but it usually takes the form of pericardial disease (occurs in about 40% of cases of RA). Although rheumatoid nodules may form in the myocardium or heart valves, this rarely results in valvular incompetence or stenosis.

**(72)** Although atherosclerotic lesions may be found on heart valves, they are usually of no functional significance. *(pp. 543–544; 569)*

**73. (C); 74. (D); 75. (C); 76. (B); 77. (B); 78. (D)**

According to the extent of the ischemic damage, acute myocardial infarction (MI) may be divided into two basic patterns: subendocardial infarction or transmural infarction. Subendocardial MI typically appears as multifocal areas of necrosis confined to the inner one third to one half of the ventricular wall. Transmural infarction is ischemic necrosis involving the complete or nearly complete thickness of the ventricular wall and is at least 2.5 cm in greatest dimension. Occasionally, the patterns may overlap, and in some cases transmural infarcts begin with subendocardial necrosis that is extended by increasing severity or duration of ischemia.

**(73)** Regardless of the pattern, MI is associated with severe multivessel stenotic atherosclerotic disease in the great majority of cases. **(74)** The atherosclerotic lesions of the coronary vessels virtually always are confined to the extramyocardial arterial segments. Intramyocardial arterial vessels are free of atherosclerotic changes in virtually all forms of ischemic heart disease.

**(75)** Virtually all subendocardial infarctions and the great majority of transmural infarctions are limited to the left ventricular wall alone. In only 15 to 30% of transmural infarction involving the posterior wall and posterior septum is the adjacent right ventricular wall involved. Isolated infarction of the right ventricle is extremely rare.

**(76)** The reported incidence of coronary thrombosis at autospy in patients having died from transmural infarction differs from the incidence of thrombosis observed by angiography within hours of onset of an MI. At autopsy, fewer than 50% of cases may show coronary thrombosis. In contrast, angiography reveals thrombosis in 90% of cases within 4 hours and in 60% within 12 to 24 hours after onset of symptoms. Thus, spontaneous lysis of thrombi apparently occurs with passage of time, but it is clear that the vast majority of transmural MIs are associated with acute coronary thrombosis. Subendocardial infarction, in contrast, is associated with occlusive thrombus at autospy in only about 20% of cases. Documented coincidence of either plaque rupture or coronary thrombosis and subendocardial infarction is uncommon, suggesting the possibility that other mechanisms may be more important in the pathogenesis of the infarction (e.g., increased oxygen demand, vasospasm, or platelet aggregation).

**(77)** Postinfarction pericarditis is a well-recognized complication of transmural infarction. A fibrinous or fibrinohemorrhagic pericarditis usually appears from 1 to 3 days after the MI and often produces an audible friction rub. This complication, as well as ventricular aneurysm and myocardial rupture, generally is associated only with transmural necrosis and rarely follows subendocardial infarction.

**(78)** Because morphologic evidence of myocardial necrosis is not present for hours after irreversible injury has occurred, diagnosis of acute MI is rarely possible in patients who suffer sudden cardiac death (death within 1 hour of a cardiac event). Nevertheless, ischemic heart disease is implicated as the major cause of sudden cardiac death, because severe stenosing coronary atherosclerosis is present in 75 to 95% of victims. Less commonly, myocarditis, mitral valve prolapse, hypertrophic cardiomyopathy, or other disorders are found at autopsy. Whatever the underlying disease, almost all cases of sudden cardiac death are believed to be related to arrhythmias. *(pp. 529–530; 539; 541)*

**79. (C); 80. (A); 81. (B); 82. (D); 83. (C); 84. (B); 85. (D)**

**(79, 80, 81, 83, and 84)** The most common pattern of coronary artery distribution is a right-dominant pattern, in which the right coronary artery supplies the posterior descending arterial system. Thus, the right coronary artery normally supplies the posterior wall of both the right and left ventricles, the posterior half of the interventricular septum, and the anterolateral wall of the right ventricle. The left coronary artery normally supplies the anterior wall of the left ventricle, part of the anterior wall of the right ventricle, and the anterior half of the interventricular septum.

**(82 and 85)** The mitral valve is a thin, endothelium-covered, avascular structure that, like the endocardium of the chambers, receives its oxygen supply directly from the blood within the lumen and does not require coronary arterial supply. *(pp. 518–519)*

**86. (A); 87. (A); 88. (B); 89. (A); 90. (C); 91. (C); 92. (C)**

The right side of the heart, which receives the systemic venous return and supplies the low-pressure pulmonary vascular system, and the left side of the heart, which receives the pulmonary venous return and supplies the high-pressure systemic arterial system, comprise two separate anatomic and functional systems. Failure of one of these systems can be caused either by decreased myocardial contractility or by an increased work load imposed on the system. Often, both are present.

**(86)** Because the left ventricle comprises the bulk of the cardiac muscle, does the greatest amount of work, and has the highest oxygen demand, ischemic heart disease primarily affects the left ventricular function and is most frequently associated with left-sided heart failure.

**(87)** Valvular heart disease most commonly involves the mitral and aortic valves and is most commonly associated with left-sided heart failure.

**(88)** Chronic obstructive pulmonary disease causes secondary abnormalities in the pulmonary vasculature that impose an increased workload on the right side of the heart and may cause right-sided heart failure (cor pulmonale).

**(89)** Pulmonary edema is most commonly the result of left-sided heart failure and increased back-pressure in the pulmonary venous system.

**(90)** Aldosterone-induced sodium retention is produced by both left-sided and right-sided heart failure. Left-sided failure leads to decreased cardiac output and a reduction in renal perfusion, whereas right-sided failure leads to congestion and hypoxia of the kidneys from increased venous pressure. In both of these conditions, the renin-angiotensin-aldosterone system is activated, leading to sodium and fluid retention.

**(91)** The decreased renal blood flow and renal hypoxia induced by either left-sided or right-sided heart failure may lead to impaired excretion of nitrogenous waste products and produce prerenal azotemia.

**(92)** Centrilobular necrosis of the liver may result from either passive congestion in the centrilobular area or ischemia associated with reduced arterial flow. Thus centrilobular necrosis is a common consequence of both left-sided and right-sided heart failure. *(pp. 520–523)*

**93. (D); 94. (C); 95. (A); 96. (B); 97. (E); 98. (C); 99. (A); 100. (D)**

The histopathologic changes associated with an acute myocardial infarction evolve in a relatively predictable progression. This reproducible sequence of histologic changes makes it possible to estimate the age of the infarction by microscopic examination of the tissue. **(95)** During the first few hours after an ischemic event, the myocardium appears grossly and histologically normal. Coagulative necrosis cannot be seen by routine histologic staining for about 4 to 12 hours. **(94 and 98)** Histologically, coagulative necrosis of the myocardium and neutrophilic infiltration of the infarcted area are maximal 24 to 48 hours after the ischemic event. **(97)** Toward the end of the first week, the formation of granulation tissue begins, and, by 10 days, the fibrovascular response is prominent around the periphery of the infarcted area.

**(99)** Clinically, the diagnosis of acute myocardial infarction can best be made on the basis of electrocardiographic changes and temporal patterns of specific serum enzyme elevations. Electrocardiographic changes occur in the majority of cases and are present almost immediately following the ischemic event. Unfortunately they may be nondiagnostic in up to 25% of patients. **(93)** Alterations of serum enzyme levels are the most sensitive and reliable indicators of myocardial infarction. The myocardial isozyme of lactate dehydrogenase is apparent in the serum about 24 hours postinfarction but reaches peak levels in 3 to 6 days. It may not return to normal until the end of the second week. The elevation in this isozyme is found to be about 90% sensitive and 95% specific for acute myocardial infarction. **(96)** The myocardial isozyme of creatine phosphokinase (CPK-MB) appears in the serum within 4 to 8 hours after myocardial damage and may peak within the first day or not for several days after infarction. It generally falls to baseline levels by day 4 postinfarction.

**(100)** Following transmural infarction, the dead muscle undergoes progressive myocytolysis and loses its structural integrity. At 3 to 7 days, when the ischemic focus is maximally soft, scar formation is just beginning and lends no structural support to the tissue. Myocardial rupture occurs most frequently during this period. *(pp. 608–613).*

**101. (C): 102. (B); 103. (D); 104. (C); 105. (A); 106. (D); 107. (C); 108. (B)**

**(101, 104, and 107)** Although the vasculitides are a diverse group of disorders that all result in vascular inflammation and necrosis, they tend to fall into a set of distinctive clinicopathologic syndromes. Kawasaki's disease, for example, is a distinctive disorder of young children and infants manifested by fever, conjunctival and oral erythema and erosion, skin rash, and enlargement of lymph nodes (the constellation is known as the mucocutaneous lymph node syndrome). A severe vasculitis primarily involving the heart (coronary arteries) is the major pathologic feature and major cause of mortality. Kawasaki's disease is the leading cause of acquired heart disease in children in the United States. *(p. 495)*

**(102 and 108)** Giant cell arteritis, in contrast, is a condition that rarely occurs in individuals under the age of 50 (average age 70) and most commonly involves the temporal artery. The disease may be difficult to diagnose and can cause visual impairment if untreated, but the therapeutic response to steroids is excellent. *(pp. 492–493)*

**(103 and 106)** Buerger's disease (thromboangiitis obliterans) is a distinctive vasculitic syndrome, strongly related to cigarette smoking, that causes thrombosis and occlusion of the intermediate and small arteries and veins of the extremities. Vascular insufficiency that often leads to severe pain and gangrene of the extremities is produced. *(p. 498)*

**(105)** Polyarteritis nodosa is the prototypic systemic vasculitis. It may affect any artery of medium or small size in any organ or system of the body. In contrast to the vasculitides mentioned previously, the kidneys commonly (85%) are involved by polyarteritis nodosa. In fact, kidney involvement with renal failure is the most common cause of death in this disorder. This disease most often affects young adults and can be treated effectively in 90% of cases by corticosteroids and cyclophosphamide administration (supportive evidence of an immunologic origin for this disorder). *(p. 494)*

**109. (D); 110. (D); 111. (A); 112. (D); 113. (B)**

The character of pericarditis is often an indication of its etiology. **(109)** Cardiopulmonary resuscitation produces cardiac trauma and acute inflammation that characteristically produces a serofibrinous pericarditis. **(110)** The postinfarction (Dressler's) syndrome, a condition thought to be autoimmune in origin that develops several weeks after a myocardial infarction, is a common cause of serofibrinous pericarditis. **(111)** Scleroderma, like other processes that produce mild noninfectious inflammation, typically causes a serous pericarditis. **(112)** More profound inflammation with leakage of fibrin, such as that produced by chest radiation, more characteristically would produce serofibrinous pericarditis. **(113)** Hemorrhagic pericarditis often follows cardiac surgery and sometimes may be severe, causing tamponade and requiring reoperation. *(pp. 566–568)*

**114. (F); 115. (E); 116. (A); 117. (C); 118. (D); 119. (F); 120. (B)**

**(114, 115 and 116)** All forms of angina pectoris are associated with coronary atherosclerosis. Stable (typical) angina is severe chest pain caused by increased oxygen demand (e.g., exercise) in the face of restricted arterial flow (atherosclerotic narrowing of the coronary arteries). It characteristically is induced by physical exertion or emotional excitement and relieved by relaxation. In contrast to stable angina, both unstable angina and Prinzmetal's angina often occur at rest. Unstable or crescendo angina refers to a deteriorating pattern of previously stable angina, precipitated by less exertion, occurring with greater frequency, and lasting for longer periods. It is known to be caused by coronary vasospasm. However, coronary atherosclerosis also may be present.

**(117 and 118)** Most commonly, only Prinzmetal's angina is associated with S-T segment elevations on an electrocardiogram (indicative of transmural ischemia). Stable angina and unstable angina typically produce S-T segment depressions corresponding to subendocardial ischemia in the left ventricle.

**(119)** All forms of anginal pain are caused by myocardial ischemia, which falls short of producing infarction. Thus the myocardial injury that occurs during a transient anginal attack is usually reversible. The myocardial cells will recover if the balance of oxygen supply and demand are restored relatively quickly.

**(120)** The development of unstable angina, characterized by either prolonged pain, onset of pain at rest in a patient with stable angina, or an increased intensity of exertional anginal pain, is an ominous sign portending myocardial infarction and has thus been dubbed "preinfarction angina." *(p. 528)*

**121. (A); 122. (D); 123. (C); 124. (E); 125. (A); 126. (A); 127. (F); 128. (C)**

**(121)** Phenobarbital, or diazepam often is used in the initial management of acute myocardial infarction to sedate the patient, relieve anxiety, and thereby reduce stress-related increase in cardiac workload (and oxygen demand).

**(122)** Verapamil is a calcium channel blocker that produces vasodilation and is especially useful in reducing the vasospastic component of an acute ischemic event. It also has negative inotropic and chronotropic effects on the heart, which help to reduce myocardial work.

**(123)** Streptokinase is used primarily for its fibrinolytic effects. It may be infused directly into the coronary arteries or into the systemic circulation to lyse coronary thrombi.

**(124)** Although morphine has sedative and sympatholytic effects that may be beneficial in initial treatment, the most important reason for its use is for prompt relief of the severe pain of acute myocardial infarction.

**(125)** Restriction of the patient's physical activities is of primary importance in reducing the work of the heart and minimizing its oxygen demand.

**(126)** Propranolol is a $\beta$-adrenergic blocking agent that reduces heart rate, contractility, and blood pressure. All of these effects tend to reduce oxygen consumption by the myocardium.

**(127)** Lidocaine is a local anesthetic that stabilizes neuronal membranes and prevents the initiation and conduction of nerve impulses. The drug also increases the electrical stimulation threshold of the myocardium during diastole. It sometimes is used intravenously in the management of acute myocardial infarction to control life-threatening arrhythmias of ventricular origin.

**(128)** Tissue-type plasminogen activator is a fibrinolytic agent that is effective in producing coronary thrombolysis and restoring coronary patency if administered within 4 hours of the onset of infarction. *(pp. 535–539)*

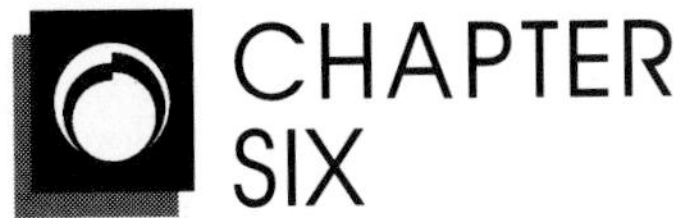

# CHAPTER SIX

# The Respiratory System

**DIRECTIONS:** For Questions 1 through 19, choose the ONE BEST answer to each question.

**1.** All of the following cell types are normal components of alveolar walls EXCEPT:

A. Endothelial cells
B. Type II pneumocytes
C. Lymphocytes
D. Mast cells
E. Neuroendocrine cells

**2.** All of the following commonly contribute to postoperative atelectasis following uncomplicated abdominal surgery EXCEPT:

A. Adult respiratory distress syndrome
B. Diaphragmatic elevation
C. Voluntary suppression of coughing
D. Excessive bronchial secretions
E. Limitation of respiratory movements

**3.** Diffuse alveolar damage (producing adult respiratory distress syndrome) is the major pattern of pulmonary damage produced by all of the following EXCEPT:

A. Oxygen toxicity
B. Narcotic overdose
C. Pneumothorax
D. Cardiopulmonary bypass surgery
E. Septic shock

**4.** Chronic bronchitis is associated with all of the following pathologic changes EXCEPT:

A. Goblet cell hyperplasia in bronchi
B. Goblet cell metaplasia in bronchioles
C. Hypertrophy of bronchial submucosal glands
D. Inflammatory infiltration of bronchioles
E. Inflammatory infiltration of alveolar walls

**5.** Complications of the disease shown in Figure 6–1 include all of the following EXCEPT:

A. Chronic bronchitis
B. Bronchiectasis
C. Pleural fibrosis
D. Metastatic abscess formation
E. Permanent lobar solidification

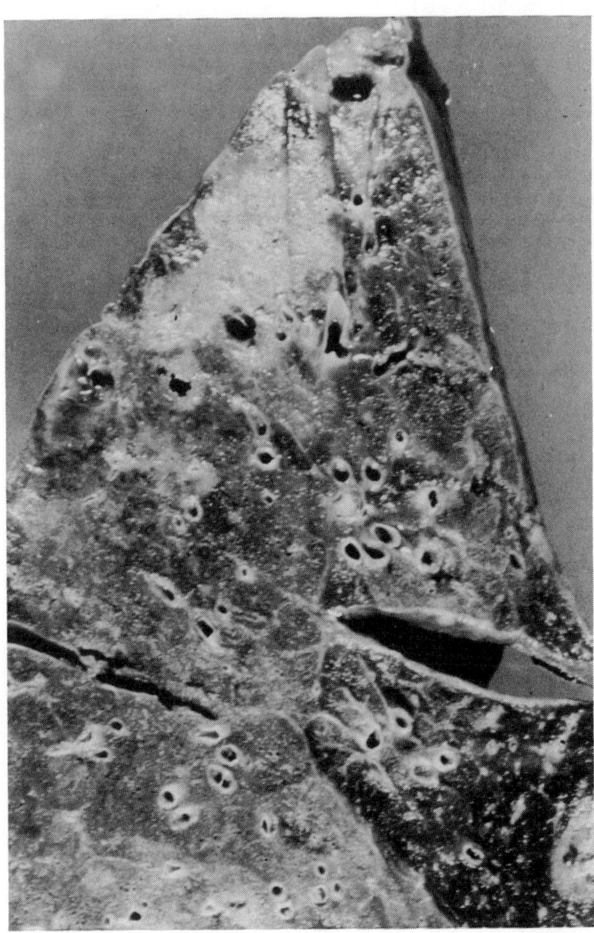

**Figure 6–1**

**6.** All of the following factors commonly predispose to bacterial pneumonias EXCEPT:

A. Viral respiratory tract infections
B. Cigarette smoking
C. Congestive heart failure
D. Bacterial urinary tract infection
E. General anesthesia

**7.** Aspiration of gastric contents produces any of the following types of pulmonary injury EXCEPT:

A. Adult respiratory distress syndrome
B. Lipoid pneumonia
C. Lung abscess
D. Empyema
E. Pulmonary alveolar proteinosis

**8.** Causes of diffuse interstitial (restrictive) lung disease include all of the following EXCEPT:

A. Sarcoidosis
B. Asbestos
C. Rheumatoid arthritis
D. Cigarette smoke
E. Bleomycin

**9.** Eosinophilic infiltrates characterize all of the following disorders EXCEPT:

A. Pneumocystis infection
B. Löeffler's syndrome
C. Allergic bronchopulmonary aspergillosis
D. Bronchial asthma
E. Pigeon breeders' lung

**10.** Which of the following statements correctly describes the adult respiratory distress syndrome?

A. It usually develops suddenly in an otherwise healthy individual.
B. Lymphocytes are the major mediators of the alveolar injury.
C. Interstitial infiltrates on chest radiograph precede the onset of dyspnea.
D. The overall mortality rate is very low.
E. The underlying cause usually cannot be determined from biopsy alone.

**11.** Cigarette smoke contributes to the pathogenesis of the disease shown in Figure 6–2 by all of the following mechanisms EXCEPT:

A. Attracting neutrophils into the lung
B. Stimulating release of neutrophil elastase
C. Inhibiting the ability of pulmonary leukocytes to clear bacteria
D. Directly inhibiting $\alpha_1$-antitrypsin
E. Stimulating macrophage elastase activity

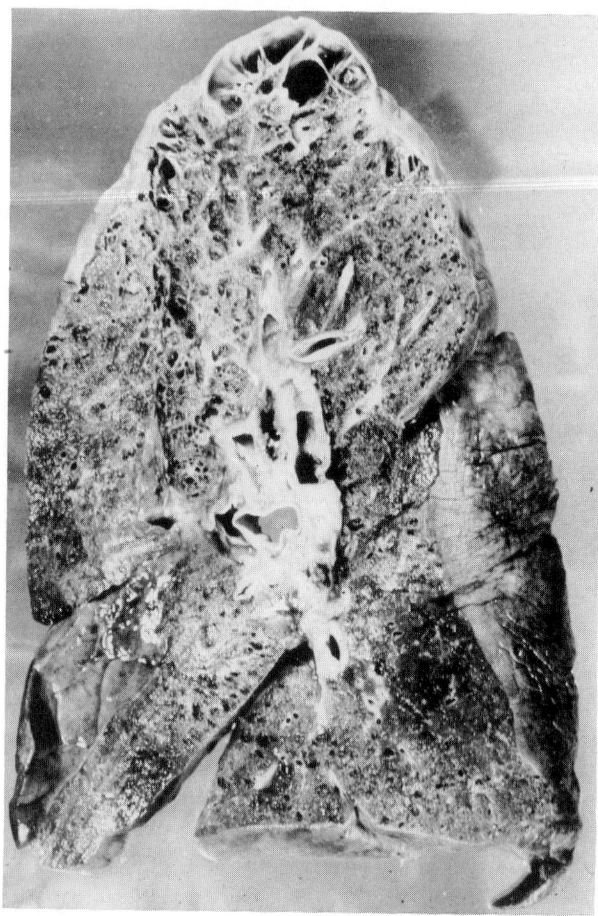

**Figure 6–2**

**12.** The type of pulmonary lesion pictured in Figure 6–3 is produced by all of the following diseases EXCEPT:

A. Chronic berylliosis
B. Silicosis
C. Sarcoidosis
D. Histoplasmosis
E. Tuberculosis

**13.** Primary pulmonary hypertension:

A. Is associated strongly with cigarette smoking
B. Often is associated with pulmonary embolism
C. Usually is associated with chronic obstructive lung disease
D. Produces atherosclerosis of the pulmonary arteries
E. Occurs in individuals who drink "bush tea"

**14.** An air bronchogram and a chest radiograph in a 15-year-old girl who has suffered from repeated pulmonary infections all her life show bilateral bronchiectasis. Which of the following disorders is this patient least likely to have?

A. Cystic fibrosis
B. Immunoglobulin A immunodeficiency
C. Kartagener's syndrome
D. Congenital bronchiectasis
E. Chronic granulomatous disease

**15.** A patient with lymphoma being treated with systemic chemotherapy suddenly develops dyspnea and pulmonary infiltrates. Which of the following causes is the LEAST likely cause of these respiratory problems?

A. *Pneumocystis carinii* infection
B. Drug-induced diffuse alveolar damage
C. Cytomegalovirus infection
D. Lymphomatous infiltrates
E. Goodpasture's syndrome

**16.** In which of the types of vasculitis listed below is the lung the primary target of involvement?

A. Wegener's granulomatosis
B. Polyarteritis nodosa
C. Henoch-Schönlein purpura
D. Essential cryoglobulinemic vasculitis
E. Kawasaki syndrome

**17.** All of the following statements correctly describe mesothelioma EXCEPT:

A. It often resembles an adenocarcinoma histologically.
B. It often resembles a sarcoma histologically.
C. It is causally related to asbestos exposure.
D. It is causally related to cigarette smoking.
E. It has no effective treatment.

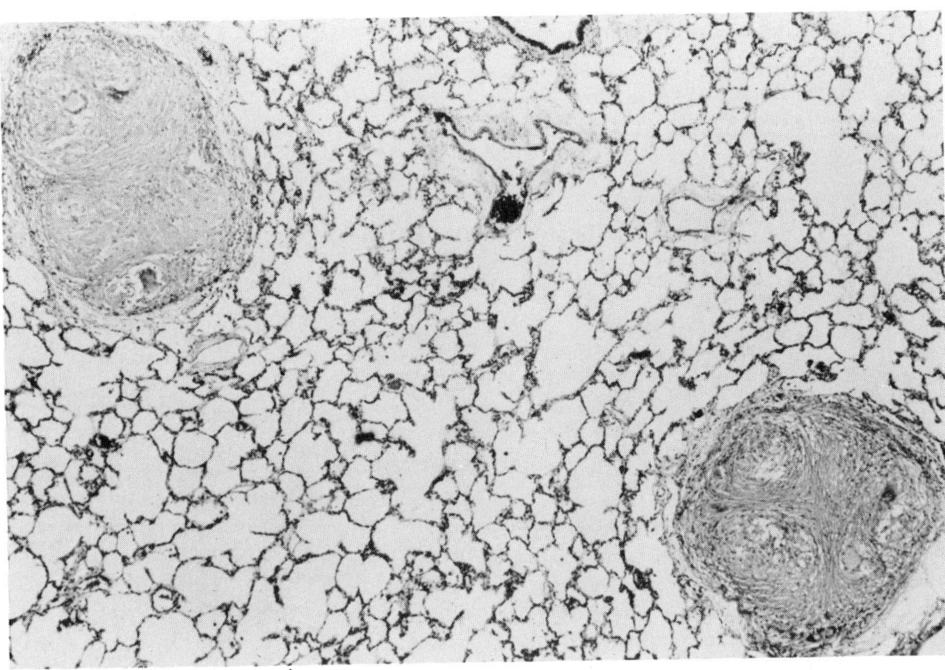

**Figure 6–3**

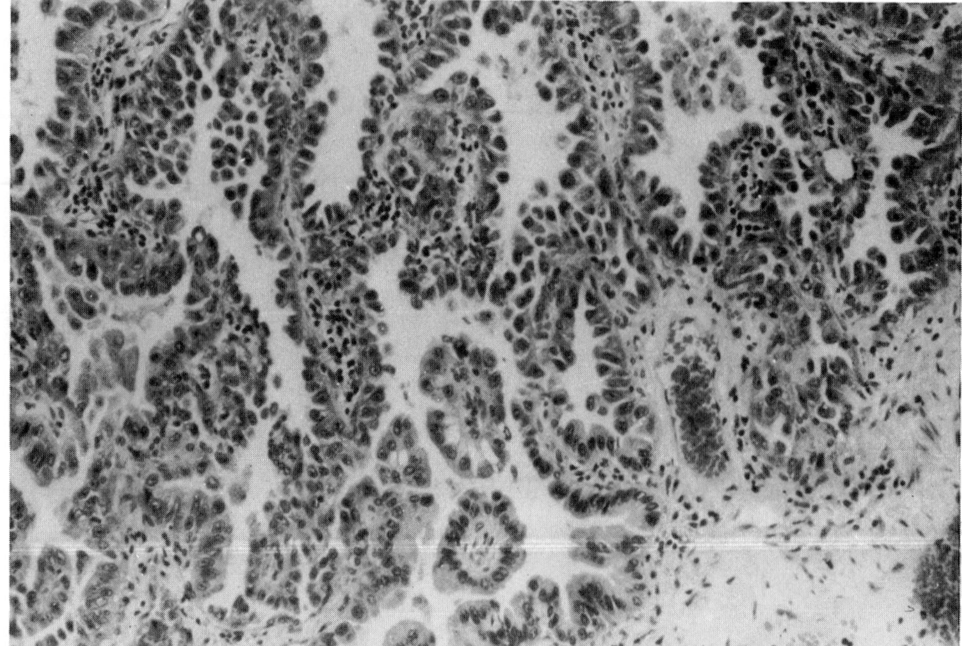

**Figure 6–4**

**18.** Cigarette smoking is causally related to all of the following pulmonary diseases EXCEPT:

A. Chronic bronchitis
B. Centrilobular emphysema
C. Asthma
D. Small airway disease (bronchiolitis)
E. Bronchogenic carcinoma

**19.** The lesion pictured in Figure 6–4 is a tumor that has all of the following characteristics EXCEPT:

A. It does not destroy alveolar architecture.
B. It sometimes mimics diffuse interstitial pneumonitis on chest radiograph.
C. It commonly contains neoplastic Clara cells.
D. It rarely metastasizes.
E. It has a better prognosis than other lung cancers.

**DIRECTIONS:** For Questions 20 through 39, you are to decide whether EACH choice is TRUE or FALSE.

For each of the following statements about pulmonary embolism, choose whether it is TRUE or FALSE.

**20.** The pelvic veins are the most common source of the causative thromboemboli.
**21.** Immobilization is a major risk factor.
**22.** Chest radiography is a sensitive means of rapid diagnosis.
**23.** Small emboli commonly resolve without treatment.
**24.** Large emboli cause sudden death.
**25.** Lung infarction occurs in over 50% of cases.
**26.** Diffuse interstitial fibrosis (honeycomb lung) is a chronic complication.

For each of the following statements about bronchial asthma, choose whether it is TRUE or FALSE.

**27.** Most bronchial asthma is mediated by an immune response producing immunoglobulin E.
**28.** In nearly all patients with asthma, the airways are hyperreactive to bronchoconstrictor agents.
**29.** Infection-induced asthma is usually caused by gram-positive cocci.
**30.** Aspirin-sensitive asthma is caused by the formation of immune complexes.
**31.** Curschmann's spirals are a characteristic histologic finding.

For each of the following statements about pulmonary infection by *Mycobacterium tuberculosis*, choose whether it is TRUE or FALSE.

**32.** The primary focus of infection is most commonly located in the apex of the upper lobe.
**33.** The degree of tissue injury is directly related to the destructive potential of the organism.
**34.** With the most severe tuberculous infections, granulomas frequently fail to form.
**35.** Infected immunodeficient individuals have less severe pulmonary disease than infected immunocompetent individuals.
**36.** Infected immunodeficient individuals are more likely to transmit *M. tuberculosis* to others than infected immunocompetent individuals.
**37.** Reactivation of the primary infection eventually occurs in most untreated (albeit immunocompetent) individuals.
**38.** Miliary dissemination throughout the body is likely to occur if a tuberculous lesion extends into a pulmonary artery.
**39.** Antituberculous chemotherapy is recommended for all otherwise normal individuals developing a newly positive purified protein derivative skin test.

**DIRECTIONS:** For Questions 40 through 51, the set of lettered headings is followed by a list of numbered words or phrases. For each numbered word or phrase choose:
A—if the item is associated with (A) only
B—if the item is associated with (B) only
C—if the item is associated with *both* (A) and (B)
D—if the item is associated with *neither* (A) nor (B)

For each of the characteristics listed below, choose whether it describes bronchogenic cysts, bronchopulmonary sequestrations, both, or neither.

A. Bronchogenic cysts
B. Bronchopulmonary sequestrations
C. Both
D. Neither

**40.** Usually occur singly
**41.** Usually occur in otherwise normal individuals
**42.** Never communicate with the airway system
**43.** Frequently become infected
**44.** Predispose to bronchogenic carcinoma

For each of the characteristics listed below, choose whether it describes Goodpasture's syndrome, idiopathic pulmonary hemosiderosis, both, or neither.

A. Goodpasture's syndrome
B. Indiopathic pulmonary hemosiderosis
C. Both
D. Neither

**45.** Occurs much more often in males than in females
**46.** Produces severe interstitial nephritis in addition to lung disease
**47.** Occurs in adults uncommonly
**48.** Produces necrotizing hemorrhagic interstitial pneumonitis
**49.** Produces pulmonary vasculitis
**50.** Is caused by anti–basement membrane antibodies
**51.** Is associated with high mortality when untreated

**DIRECTIONS:** Questions 52 through 83 are matching questions. For each numbered item, choose the most likely associated item from those provided. Each numbered item has ONLY ONE answer. Within each group, each lettered item may be the answer to one, more than one, or none of the numbered items.

For each of the characteristics listed below, choose whether it describes bronchi, bronchioles, alveoli, all of these, or none of these.

A. Bronchi
B. Bronchioles
C. Alveoli
D. All of the above
E. None of the above

**52.** Contain pores of Kohn
**53.** Contain goblet cells
**54.** Contain Clara cells
**55.** Are coated by surfactant
**56.** Are rich in secretory immunoglobulin
**57.** Contain macrophages in their lumens
**58.** Contain mucus glands
**59.** Contain neuroendocrine cells
**60.** Contain squamous cells
**61.** Contain mast cells

For each of the characteristics listed below, choose whether it describes centriacinar (centrilobular) emphysema, panacinar (panlobular) emphysema, irregular emphysema, interstitial emphysema, or none of these.

A. Centriacinar (centrilobular) emphysema
B. Panacinar (panlobular) emphysema
C. Irregular emphysema
D. Interstitial emphysema
E. None of the above

**62.** Is associated with $\alpha_1$-antitrypsin deficiency
**63.** Occurs most commonly in cigarette smokers
**64.** Occurs in residual lung after lobectomy
**65.** Occurs in children with whooping cough
**66.** Does not produce bullae

For each of the microorganisms listed below, choose the pattern of pulmonary injury with which it is most commonly associated: diffuse alveolar damage, lobar pneumonia, necrotizing bronchopneumonia, lung abscess, or none of these.

A. Diffuse alveolar damage
B. Lobar pneumonia
C. Necrotizing bronchopneumonia
D. Lung abscess
E. None of the above

**67.** Cytomegalovirus
**68.** *Staphylococcus aureus*
**69.** *Streptococcus pneumoniae* (pneumococcus)
**70.** *Bacteroides* species
**71.** Microfilariae
**72.** Thermophilic bacteria
**73.** *Mycobacterium tuberculosis*
**74.** *Mycoplasma pneumoniae*
**75.** *Klebsiella pneumoniae*
**76.** *Legionella* species

For each of the characteristics listed below, choose which type of bronchogenic carcinoma it describes: squamous cell carcinoma, adenocarcinoma, small ("oat")-cell carcinoma, or none of these.

A. Squamous cell carcinoma
B. Adenocarcinoma
C. Small ("oat")-cell carcinoma
D. None of the above

**77.** Is the most common type of lung cancer in women
**78.** Frequently occurs in the periphery of the lung
**79.** Is etiologically unrelated to cigarette smoking
**80.** Contains dense-core neurosecretory granules
**81.** Elaborates parathyroid hormone more frequently than any other lung cancer
**82.** Produces the syndrome of inappropriate antidiuretic hormone secretion more frequently than any other lung cancer
**83.** Is not treated by surgical resection

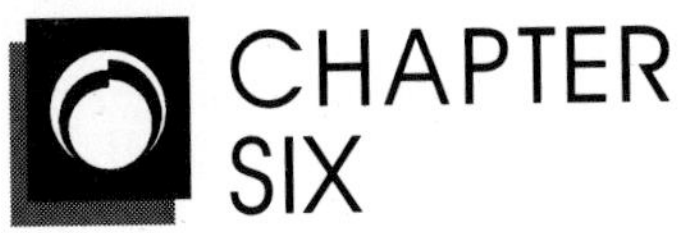

# The Respiratory System

## ANSWERS

**1. (E)** Normal cellular components of the alveolar walls (septa) include only capillary endothelial cells, type I pneumocytes (alveolar lining cells), type II pneumocytes (surfactant-producing secretory cells), and scattered cells found in the interstitial space, such as mast cells, fibroblast-like interstitial cells, smooth muscle cells, lymphocytes, and monocytes. Neuroendocrine cells, along with ciliated epithelial cells and goblet cells, reside in the bronchial epithelium. The neuroendocrine cells of the bronchus, like those of the gastrointestinal tract and skin, are true epithelial cells that have undergone neuroendocrine differentiation during development (i.e., they are not derived from the neural crest). They make a number of small polypeptide hormones, such as serotonin, calcitonin, and gastrin-releasing peptide (bombesin). No neuroendocrine cells are found in the normal alveolus. *(p. 674)*

**2. (A)** Atelectasis is a collapse or an incomplete expansion of alveoli and is characterized by areas of relatively airless pulmonary parenchyma. It may occur in normal lung tissue or as part of a pathologic process. In postoperative abdominal surgery patients, atelectasis is frequently multifactorial. Unless the surgery is complicated by factors that cause lung injury (e.g., shock, infection, aspiration), it occurs in otherwise normal lungs. The compressive form of atelectasis may result from elevated diaphragms secondary to abdominal distention. Compressive atelectasis also occurs in this setting because of patients' voluntary suppression of coughing and/or limitation of respiratory movements as a result of pain. Furthermore, with increased bronchial secretions elicited by general anesthetics, the obstructive form of atelectasis also occurs in these patients.

Although the adult respiratory distress syndrome (adult hyaline membrane disease) produces atelectasis through damage to pneumocytes and loss of surfactant, uncomplicated abdominal surgery would not be associated with this disorder. *(pp. 675–678).*

**3. (C)** Diffuse alveolar damage (DAD) refers to the pattern of pathologic injury in lungs seen in the adult respiratory distress syndrome (ARDS), a life-threatening constellation of respiratory insufficiency, cyanosis, and hypoxemia. Thus, the two terms often are used interchangeably. DAD is characterized by congestion (sometimes with focal hemorrhage), interstitial and intra-alveolar edema, and inflammation. Fibrin and necrotic cellular debris from injured pneumocytes and inflammatory infiltrates form waxy deposits known as "hyaline membranes" that coat the alveolar walls. Hyaline membranes are a characteristic feature of both ARDS and hyaline membrane disease of the newborn (see Chapter 2, Questions 1 and 13) and represent the end result of diffuse damage to the alveolar walls mediated by different mechanisms. In hyaline membrane disease of the newborn, a deficiency of pulmonary surfactant in developmentally immature lungs is the specific underlying cause. In contrast, DAD refers to injury to mature lung tissue caused by any one of a wide variety of insults, including: (1) oxygen toxicity; (2) narcotic overdose; (3) shock associated with sepsis, trauma, hemorrhagic pancreatitis, burns, or complicated surgery, especially cardiac surgery involving extracorporeal cardiac bypass pumps; (4) inhalation of toxins and irritant gases; (5) aspiration of gastric contents; (6) hypersensitivity reactions to organic solvents and drugs; and (7) diffuse pulmonary infections, most commonly caused by viruses or *Pneumocystitis carinii.*

Pneumothorax (filling of the pleural cavity with air) results in compressive atelectasis of the involved lung but not in DAD. DAD involves infectious, toxic, or oxidant injury to the alveolar endothelium and epithelium, whereas compressive atelectasis simply causes collapse of normal lung tissue. *(pp. 675–678)*

**4. (E)** Chronic bronchitis, a major form of chronic obstructive pulmonary disease, is defined clinically as a condition causing persistent cough with sputum production for at least 3 months in at least two consecutive years.

The sputum overproduction (productive cough) in chronic bronchitis is caused by mucus hypersecretion in the inflamed bronchi and bronchioles. Histologically, the condition is characterized by hypertrophy and hyperplasia of the mucus-secreting goblet cells of the tracheobronchial tree as well as goblet cell metaplasia in small bronchioles that do not normally contain mucus-producing cells. The submucosal mucous glands of the trachea and bronchi also are enlarged greatly. Although mucus hypersecretion in large airways is the hallmark of well-developed disease, early manifestations center on inflammation and injury in the small airways (small bronchi and bronchioles measuring less than 2 to 3 mm in diameter). In addition to goblet cell metaplasia of bronchioles, inflammatory infiltration of bronchiolar walls, clusters of pigmented alveolar macrophages in lumens, and fibrosis of the alveolar wall all may be seen in early disease. Inflammation of alveolar walls, however, is not a characteristic feature of chronic bronchitis. Alveolar inflammation is seen in various forms of pneumonia and pneumonitis, but alveoli are not direct targets of injury in chronic bronchitis. They may, of course, become inflamed as a result of a pneumonia complicating chronic bronchitis, because excessive secretions impair the clearing mechanisms of the mucociliary transport system of the lung and constitute a risk factor for bacterial pneumonia. In general, processes that produce alveoltis as their primary manifestation are more likely to be associated with restrictive rather than obstructive pulmonary disease. *(pp. 688–689; 696)*

**5. (A)** Figure 6–1 shows the cut surface of a lung with a necrotizing infective bronchopneumonia (cavitating abscesses are seen that clearly indicate a necrotizing process). Organisms that produce this type of pneumonia are capable of tissue destruction. They elaborate extracellular enzymes that allow them to penetrate and destroy normal structures. Additional tissue injury is produced by the liberation of lysosomal enzymes from neutrophils attracted to the site of infection. Thus, the consequences of necrotizing bronchopneumonia can be quite severe. The process may damage airways permanently and result in a postinfective bronchiectasis. Spread to the pleural cavities with resultant empyema formation may organize to form a sheath of pleural fibrosis around the involved lung. Penetration of venous structures and lymphatics by the organism leads to systemic bacteremia and metastatic abscess formation. Organization of the exudate and scarring of the damaged lung may lead to permanent solidification of the lung parenchyma. Chronic bronchitis (see Question 4), however, is not a consequence of bronchopneumonia. It is caused by chronic irritation of airways by inhaled substances (usually cigarette smoke). Microbiologic infections may play a secondary role in maintaining or exacerbating chronic bronchitis, but they do not initiate the process. *(pp. 688; 696–698)*

**6. (D)** Conditions that predispose to bacterial pneumonias are those that impair the natural defense mechanisms of the lung or the resistance of the host in general. Injury to the mucociliary apparatus and interference with phagocytic or bactericidal action of alveolar macrophages are common predisposing factors, because both are produced by cigarette smoke. Viral diseases, inhalation of toxic or hot gases, and inherited defects of cilia structure (i.e., Kartagener's syndrome) are other causes of injury to the mucociliary apparatus. Pulmonary congestion and edema are also predisposing factors and contribute to the development of bronchopneumonia in patients with congestive heart failure. An additional predisposing factor is loss or suppression of the cough reflex, which can occur with general anesthesia, coma, neuromuscular disorders, drugs, or chest pain.

Bacterial infections elsewhere in the body, such as the urinary tract, usually do not lead to bacterial bronchopneumonia by hematogenous spread unless some other predisposing factor is present. For instance, if a bacteremia from a urinary tract infection occurs in a patient with pulmonary edema or bronchial obstruction with accumulation of secretions, the development of bronchopneumonia would be more likely than in a patient with normal lungs. The portal of entry of the organisms in the vast majority of bacterial pneumonias is the respiratory tract. *(p. 696)*

**7. (E)** Diverse types of pulmonary injury may result from aspiration of regurgitated gastric contents. The specific pattern of injury is dependent on the nature of the aspirated material. Aspiration of hydrochloric acid produces a pattern of diffuse alveolar damage and results in the clinical syndrome of adult respiratory distress. If the regurgitated material has a high lipid content (e.g., mineral oil or ice cream), alveolar macrophages ingesting the lipids fill the alveolar spaces. The resultant pattern of foamy macrophages and acute inflammation in alveolar spaces is known as lipoid pneumonia. With the aspiration of infected material, an event most commonly associated with acute alcoholism, coma, anesthesia, sinusitis, gingival dental sepsis, or debilitation, lung abscess formation may result. Anaerobic organisms normally found in the oral cavity (*Bacteroides*, *Fusobacterium*, and *Peptococcus* species) are the most common causative agents. Likewise, aspiration of material containing necrotizing organisms may result in an infection that extends to the pleural cavity and produces an empyema.

Pulmonary alveolar proteinosis (PAP) is unrelated to aspiration injury. Its exact etiology is unknown, but it develops in association with dust or chemical inhalation, immunosuppression, and hematologic malignancies with opportunistic infection, and most likely results from defective macrophage clearance of intra-alveolar accumulations of surfactant. The "proteinosis" in PAP refers to the turbid fluid that characteristically fills the alveolar spaces in this disease. The fluid is endogenously rather than exogenously derived (aspirated). *(pp. 677; 697; 699; 719)*

**8. (D)** Diffuse interstitial pulmonary disease of any etiology is characterized histologically by increased collagen deposition within the normally thin and delicate alveolar walls. This interstitial scarring drastically reduces the normal plasticity and elasticity of the lung (restricts compliance) and acts as a barrier to oxygen diffusion across the alveolar wall. Thus, affected patients have dyspnea and eventually cyanosis, but no wheezing or other stigmata of airway obstruction, the *sine qua non* of chronic obstructive pulmonary disease (see Question 4). Conditions that lead to restrictive lung disease are heterogeneous but they all have the capacity to initiate alveolar injury and inflammation (alveolitis) with the stimulation of immune and inflammatory effector cells. Cytokines generated during this process both mediate persistent tissue injury and stimulate collagen deposition that ultimately leads to fibrosis in the alveolar walls. Although the etiologies are diverse, the disorders tend to produce similar clinical signs, symptoms, radiographic alterations, and pathophysiologic changes that justify their categorization as a group. Among the known causes of restrictive lung disease are infiltrative disorders (e.g., sarcoidosis); inorganic dusts (e.g., asbestos); collagen vascular diseases (e.g., rheumatoid arthritis); drugs and toxins, including chemotherapeutic agents such as bleomycin; and infections (especially viral).

Although cigarette smoke is associated with a multitude of pulmonary diseases, including chronic bronchitis, emphysema, and bronchogenic carcinoma, it is not known to be associated with diffuse interstitial fibrosis. *(pp. 682; 704–705)*

**9. (A)** A number of pathologic entities of the lung are characterized primarily by infiltration with eosinophils and often are accompanied by eosinophilia in the blood. These disorders run the gamut from benign transitory disease to chronic debilitating conditions. Whatever their clinical course or primary etiology, these disorders all are believed to represent immunologically mediated hypersensitivity responses. Löeffler's syndrome is a transient benign condition causing simple interstitial eosinophilia in the lung, most likely an allergic reaction (type I immune response) to an unknown antigen. Allergic bronchopulmonary aspergillosis is an example of a chronic eosinophilic syndrome associated with both type III and type IV hypersensitivity reactions to *Aspergillus* antigens. This is to be contrasted with actual infection by *Aspergillus*, which occurs only in immunosuppressed or debilitated patients. Bronchial asthma is a classic example of a type I immunologic response—usually to environmental antigens—causing bronchoconstriction. In bronchial asthma, the walls of the affected airways are infiltrated by eosinophils (see Questions 27 through 31). Pigeon breeder's lung is an example of a hypersensitivity pneumonitis caused by an allergic response to inhaled proteins from serum, excreta, or feathers of birds. In the acute phase of the disease, pigeon breeders' lung, like other forms of hypersensitivity pulmonary disease, is characterized pathologically by inflammatory infiltrates that include numerous eosinophils.

Although pulmonary eosinophilia is associated with a number of parasitic infections in the lung, it is not produced by the protozoan *Pneumocystis carinii*. This partiular parasite characteristically produces a pattern of diffuse alveolar damage (with diffuse interstitial inflammation). *(p. 355–356; 689–692; 706; 716)*

**10. (E)** Although many diverse conditions may produce the adult respiratory distress syndrome (ARDS), most are dire problems that themselves lead to hospitalization, such as shock, sepsis, drug toxicity, extensive burns, massive trauma, and acute pancreatitis. Thus, ARDS is seen most commonly in patients under treatment for some other predisposing condition who initially may have no respiratory problems. Typically the onset of severe dyspnea heralds the development of ARDS, even though the chest radiograph initially may be normal. The initial pathologic event in ARDS is either capillary endothelial (most often) or (occasionally) alveolar epithelial injury mediated by either neutrophils or macrophages or both, but immune (i.e., lymphocyte-mediated) processes are not involved. Although the process does not necessarily progress in all patients and sometimes may be treated successfully with reversal of the underlying disease and respiratory support therapy, the overall mortality for this syndrome is still about 60%.

Lung biopsy is usually of little diagnostic use in the setting of ARDS both because the underlying etiology is usually evident to the treating physician and because the histopathologic picture is generic and nonspecific. Notable exceptions include ARDS caused by opportunistic infection in the immunocompromised patient. Specifically, *Pneumocystis carinii*, which can be identified by special stain, and viruses such as cytomegalovirus, which produce intracellular inclusions, can be identified by biopsy. *(pp. 676–678)*

**11. (C)** Figure 6–2 shows the cut surface of a lung with emphysema, a chronic obstructive lung disease characterized by the destruction of alveolar walls. The normal architecture of the lung is destroyed, leaving behind irregular cystic spaces that do not function in oxygen exchange. The damage is caused by enzymatic digestion of alveolar structural elements, principally elastic tissue. Neutrophils and macrophages produce elastases that initiate and propagate the injury. These cells are attracted to the lung and are stimulated to release their elastases by cigarette smoke. Neutrophil chemotaxis is induced both directly by nicotine and indirectly via either the release of cytokines from macrophages or the activation of the alternate complement pathway. Normally, the destructive effects of endogenous inflammatory cells are controlled by the antiproteases in serum and interstitial tissue, especially $\alpha_1$-antitrypsin ($\alpha_1$-AT). However, oxidants in cigarette smoke and free radicals produced by neutrophils reduce $\alpha_1$-AT activity. Although cigarette smoke does compromise the ability of pulmonary leukocytes to clear bacteria and thus increases susceptibility to infection, infection does not contribute to the pathogenesis of emphysema. *(p. 686)*

**12. (B)** Figure 6–3 shows noncaseating pulmonary granulomas. Granulomas in the lung are caused by either fungal (e.g., histoplasmosis), mycobacterial (e.g., tuberculosis) or bacterial (brucellosis) infection, foreign body or hypersensitivity responses to inhaled dusts (organic or inorganic–e.g., berylliosis), or idiopathic hypersensitivity responses (sarcoidosis, Wegener's granulomatosis). Although fungal and mycobacterial granulomas often are associated with central necrosis, it should be remembered that all large caseating granulomas come from small noncaseating granulomas. Thus the absence of caseation by no means rules out infectious etiologies.

Silicosis does not produce granulomas but rather collagenous nodules in the lung that may coalesce to form large, calcified fibrous scars. These collagenous nodules are the result of macrophage interactions with the undigestible silica particles, which result in macrophage activation and the elaboration of tumor necrosis factor, interleukin-1, free radicals, and fibrogenic cytokines. *(pp. 324–328; 706; 708–709; 712–714)*

**13. (D)** Primary pulmonary hypertension is a disease process characterized by increased resistance in the pulmonary vascular tree in the absence of any known cause of increased pulmonary pressure (e.g., chronic lung disease; recurrent pulmonary emboli; antecedent heart disease; ingestion of certain drugs or plant products, such as those used to make "bush tea," a tropical concoction brewed from the leguminous plant *Crotalaria spectabilis*). Primary pulmonary hypertension occurs most commonly in young women and occasionally is seen in children. It often is associated with Raynaud's phenomenon, which lends support to the concept that primary pulmonary hypertension is a form of autoimmune collagen vascular disease. Both Raynaud's phenomenon and pulmonary hypertension occur in such disorders as scleroderma, systemic lupus erythematosus, and rheumatoid arthritis. At present, the underlying cause of primary pulmonary hypertension remains unknown. Yet, by definition, it is not associated with any form of chronic obstructive or interstitial lung disease that itself is known to produce (secondary) pulmonary hypertension. Whether primary or secondary, however, pulmonary hypertension produces identical changes in the pulmonary vascular tree, principally characterized by marked thickening of the arterioles and small arteries. The increased pressures in the pulmonary arteries produce atheromatous lesions that, although not as severe, are indistinguishable from those of systemic atherosclerosis. *(p. 681)*

**14. (D)** Bronchiectasis is a permanent dilation of bronchi or bronchioles produced by necrotizing infection in these airways. In children and young adults, bronchiectasis is usually the result of a congenital or hereditary condition, because bronchiectasis following necrotizing pneumonias complicating childhood diseases such as measles, whooping cough, and influenza is no longer common in the United States. Therefore, cystic fibrosis, immunodeficiency states, inherited defects in leukocyte function (e.g., chronic granulomatous disease), immotile cilia syndromes (e.g., Kartagener's syndrome), or congenital bronchiectasis all are associated with bronchiectasis in the pediatric and young adult age group. Overall, these conditions are associated with bronchial mucus plugging (obstruction) or increased susceptibility to bronchial infection, or both. In cystic fibrosis, the characteristic thick, tenacious bronchial secretions obstruct bronchi and frequently become infected with necrotizing bacterial organisms. In the United States, nearly half of the cases of bronchiectasis in children or young adults are attributable to cystic fibrosis.

With immunoglobulin A immunodeficiency, the lung is robbed of one of its most important natural defense mechanisms against microbial invasion. Thus, heightened susceptibility to repeated bacterial infection results and is associated with localized or diffuse bronchiectasis.

The immotile cilia syndrome results from structurally abnormal, dyskinetic, or akinetic cilia. Coordinated ciliary action is essential to effective mucociliary transport for elimination of inhaled particles (such as bacteria), one of the most important of the lung's defense mechanisms against infection, so chronic infection and bronchiectasis are virtually inevitable in the immotile cilia syndrome. In Kartagener's syndrome, a subset of the immotile cilia syndrome, sinusitis and situs inversus are also present.

Chronic granulomatous disease encompasses a group of inherited defects in the genes encoding the several components of NADPH oxidase, which generates superoxide, a key component of the bactericidal system in neutrophils. In the absence of effective neutrophil function, macrophage activation (with granuloma formation) must substitute for neutrophils as the first line of defense. Patients are unusually susceptible to recurrent infections.

Congenital bronchiectasis is caused by a defect in the development of bronchi. Although it is certainly a cause of bronchiectasis in the young, it usually affects either a single lobe or a single lung, but it is not usually diffuse (bilateral). *(pp. 63; 692–694)*

**15. (E)** Patients with lymphoma who are being treated with systemic chemotherapy and are immunosuppressed may develop a variety of life-threatening pulmonary diseases that require rapid diagnosis (often by open lung biopsy) and treatment. Infection by either common pathogens or opportunistic organisms is frequent in immunosuppressed patients such as these. *Pneumocystis carinii*, a ubiquitous protozoan that rarely, if ever, infects immunocompetent individuals, is a relatively common cause of pneumonia in this setting. Opportunistic viral (e.g., cytomegalovirus) pneumonias are also common.

Noninfectious causes of pulmonary disease in lymphoma patients under treatment include chemotherapeutic drug-related injury and involvement of the lung by tumor. Numerous chemotherapeutic drugs are associated with the production of diffuse alveolar damage in the lung. This produces a radiologic picture of diffuse pulmonary infiltrates that is often indistinguishable from viral or *Pneumocystis* pneumonia. The correct diagnosis is of emergent importance in cases such as the one described. Antibiotics would have no effect on drug reactions or lymphomatous infiltrates. Conversely, additional chemotherapy (and further immunosuppression) would be contraindicated in the case of infection or drug reaction but required if the infiltrate were of lymphomatous origin.

Goodpasture's syndrome is also a life-threatening disorder of sudden onset requiring immediate diagnosis and treatment, but it is typically unrelated to malignancy or to treatment modalities of any sort. It is primarily a disease of young males (6:1 male/female ratio) characterized by the simultaneous appearance of rapidly progressive and necrotizing hemorrhagic interstitial pneumonitis. The disease is caused by circulating autoantibodies directed at the $\alpha_3$ chain of type IV collagen in basement membranes. What triggers the antibody formation is unknown, but there is a high prevalence of HLA-DRW 15/DQW6 haplotype in Goodpasture's syndrome, suggesting a genetic predisposition to autoimmunity. *(677; 704; 717; 947)*

**16. (A)** In only two vasculitic syndromes is the lung the primary target of involvement: Wegener's granulomatosis and the Churg-Strauss syndrome (allergic granulomatosis and angitis, not mentioned as a choice in this question). Wegener's granulomatosis produces the classic triad of (1) necrotizing granulomas of the upper and lower respiratory tract, (2) focal necrotizing vasculitis of the lungs, and (3) necrotizing glomerulitis. Unlike Wegener's granulomatosis, the Churg-Strauss syndrome lacks respiratory tract granulomas and glomerulonephritis. The Churg-Strauss syndrome is associated strongly with bronchial asthma and eosinophilia and only rarely involves the kidneys.

Polyarteritis nodosa rarely, if ever, produces pulmonary vasculitis. In fact, sparing of pulmonary vessels is a highly characteristic feature of polyarteritis nodosa. Similarly, the Kawasaki syndrome and Henoch-Schönlein purpura also typically spare the lung. The Kawasaki syndrome is a vasculitic syndrome in infants and children involving large arteries (often the coronaries) and accompanied by a desquamative skin rash and cervical lymph node enlargement. Henoch-Schönlein purpura, another vasculitis occurring most commonly in children, characteristically involves small vessels in the skin, gastrointestinal tract, and kidneys. Essential cryoglobulinemic vasculitis (leukocytoclastic angitis) may involve virtually any organ, including the lung, but has no particular predilection for producing pulmonary disease. *(pp. 491t; 494–497; 718; 960)*

**17. (D)** Mesotheliomas are uncommon tumors that arise from either the visceral or the parietal pleura. They may present diagnostic difficulties because they manifest several different histologic patterns. The tubular pattern resembles adenocarcinoma histologically and can be difficult to differentiate from a peripheral bronchogenic adenocarcinoma that has involved the pleura secondarily. Alternatively, mesotheliomas may exhibit a spindle cell growth pattern and resemble a sarcoma. For these reasons, their correct identification may require immunohistochemical studies or electron microscopic examination. Mesotheliomas are causally related to heavy asbestos exposure, and the lifetime risk of developing this tumor in heavily exposed individuals is as high as 7 to 10%. The tumor has a dismal prognosis. There is no effective therapy, and 50% of patients die within the first year after diagnosis. Few survive longer than 2 years.

Cigarette smoking does not seem to be related causally to mesothelioma, because asbestos workers who smoke appear to be at no greater risk than their nonsmoking cohorts. However, asbestos workers who smoke are at much greater risk of developing bronchogenic carcinoma than nonsmoking asbestos workers. *(pp. 730–732)*

**18. (C)** Cigarette smoking is causally related to all of the forms of chronic obstructive pulmonary disease except asthma (which has either immunologic or undefined causes of hyper-reactive airways) and all forms of bronchogenic carcinoma. In short, if cigarettes disappeared, a great deal of pulmonary disease (including chronic bronchitis, centrilobular emphysema, small airway disease [bronchiolitis], and the leading cancer killer in the Western world) undoubtedly would follow. *(pp. 683t; 685–686; 688; 690; 720–721)*

**19. (E)** Figure 6–4 is a micrograph of a bronchoalveolar carcinoma. Although clearly malignant tumors, these are distinctive because they do not destroy alveolar architecture. Instead, they use the alveolar wall as a scaffold for growth. This growth pattern sometimes gives them the appearance of diffuse interstitial pneumonitis rather than that of a tumor on chest radiograph and even on gross examination of the resected lung. Bronchoalveolar carcinomas originate from terminal airways and contain mucin-producing bronchiolar cells and/or Clara cells, the specialized secretory cells of the bronchioles that produce a watery, mucus-poor protein. Rarely, type II pneumocytes are also present. These tumors are also distinctive among other forms of lung cancer in their tendency to metastasize late and in their overall better prognosis (25% overall 5-year survival rate for bronchoalveolar carcinoma versus 9% for other forms of lung cancer). Although metastases are not large or widely disseminated, they eventually occur in 45% of cases. Of interest is the fact that the association with cigarette smoking is less well defined for bronchoalveolar carcinoma (and other adenocarcinomas) than for squamous cell carcinoma of the lung. *(pp. 723; 725–726)*

**20. (False); 21. (True); 22. (False); 23. (True); 24. (True); 25. (False); 26. (False)**

**(20 and 21)** Pulmonary emboli are by far the most common cause of thrombotic occlusion of the pulmonary artery. *In situ* thrombosis is rare. Pulmonary embolism usually occurs in patients suffering from some underlying disease (e.g., cardiac disease or cancer) or in those immobilized for long periods of time. Risk is also increased in any hypercoagulable state. However, because immobilization is not only a major risk factor but one that is more readily reversible than most others, much attention is devoted to prevention, such as early ambulation after surgery or delivery or isometric exercises for the bed-ridden. Ninety-five percent of pulmonary thromboemboli orginate from the deep veins of the lower extremities, elastic stockings commonly are used to prevent pooling of blood in the extremities.

**(22)** Unfortunately, pulmonary embolism is quite elusive on the chest radiograph. If infarction has occurred, a wedge-shaped infiltrate may appear on the chest radiograph 12 to 36 hours later. In the absence of infarction, however, the chest radiograph of a patient with pulmonary embolism may be entirely normal, and ventilation-perfusion scans using radioactive tracers may be needed to establish the diagnosis. **(23)** Happily, small emboli often resolve completely after the initial acute insult without medical treatment, especially in younger patients. The embolus initially contracts like all thrombi and subsequently is reduced in size by the serum thrombolytic activity. Total lysis of the clot usually ensues.

**(24)** Large emboli, however, may cause instantaneous death by completely occluding blood flow to the lungs. **(25)** With emboli of lesser size, occlusion of lobar or segmental arteries may cause regional infarction of the lung but not sudden death. Because of its dual blood supply, infarction from pulmonary emboli occurs more readily in patients with a compromised bronchial arterial system. Thus, pulmonary infarction tends to develop in elderly patients with severe systemic atherosclerosis. Overall, less than 10% of pulmonary emboli actually cause infarction.

**(26)** Unresolved multiple small pulmonary emboli eventually may lead to pulmonary hypertension and pulmonary vascular sclerosis with cor pulmonale (see Chapter 5, Question 19) but do not cause diffuse interstitial lung disease. Diseases causing diffuse interstitial fibrosis of the lung all produce alveolitis (not vascular occlusion) as the primary insult. *(pp. 679–680; 704)*

**27. (True); 28 (True); 29. (True); 30. (False); 31. (True)**

**(27)** Bronchial asthma is a chronic obstructive pulmonary disease characterized by hyper-reactivity of the tracheobronchial tree, producing paroxysmal episodes of bronchospasm with severe dyspnea. Asthma has been divided into two basic types according to the precipitating factor and the pathogenetic mechanism: (1) atopic or extrinsic asthma (type I hypersensitivity reactions) triggered by environmental antigens (dust, pollen, foods, and so forth) and mediated by immune responses leading to the production of immunoglobulin E (IgE) and (2) nonatopic or intrinsic asthma, usually triggered by respiratory tract infection but not clearly associated with a hypersensitivity immune response. Specific subtypes of atopic asthma include occupational asthma (involving inhalation of fumes, chemicals, or dusts) and allergic bronchopulmonary aspergillosis (see Question 9). Most bronchial asthma is atopic (allergic) in type. On re-exposure to the antigen, presensitized IgE-coated mast cells and basophils release a host of chemical mediators that cause bronchoconstriction, increase venular permeability, and increase bronchial secretions. **(28)** However, no matter what the type of asthma—extrinsic or intrinsic—the airways are hyper-reactive to stimuli that would have little or no effect on the airways of nonasthmatics. Indeed, hyper-reactivity of airways is a universal feature of asthma and is part of the very definition of the disease.

**(29)** Although hypersensitivity to microbial antigens possibly may play a role in triggering the intrinsic type of asthma produced by some respiratory tract infections, the organism involved is usually a virus (e.g., rhinovirus, parainfluenza virus). Gram-positive cocci are associated more commonly with bronchopneumonia than with bronchial asthma.

**(30)** Aspirin-sensitive asthma, in contrast to other types of asthma, is thought to be related to the drug's ability to inhibit the cyclo-oxygenase pathway of arachidonic acid metabolism without affecting the lipo-oxygenase route. In this situation, the elaboration of the bronchoconstrictor leukotrienes is favored, and asthma ensues. The pathogenetic mechanism of aspirin-sensitive asthma does not appear to involve an immunologic response of any sort; no antibodies or immune complexes are formed.

**(31)** Histologically, the most striking feature in bronchial asthma is the occlusion of bronchi and bronchioles by thick mucus plugs that contain whorls of shed epithelium known as Curschmann's spirals. Within the bronchiole, numerous eosinophils are also present that contain characteristic inclusions known as Charcot-Leyden crystals. *(pp. 690–692)*

**32. (False); 33. (False); 34. (True); 35. (False); 36. (True); 37. (False); 38. (False); 39. (True)**

After a long period of relatively low incidence rates of tuberculosis in the United States, *Mycobacterium tuberculosis* infections and deaths have been increasing since the mid-1980s as a result of both infection in patients with acquired immunodeficiency syndrome (AIDS) and the emergence of drug-resistant strains. **(32)** The lungs are by far the most common target of infection by *M. tuberculosis*. The initial pulmonary infection has a characteristic pattern of involvement that consists of a focus of caseating granuloma formation in the pulmonary parenchyma plus involvement of the lymph nodes draining that area (the Ghon complex). The location of the parenchymal focus is characteristically either just above or just below the interlobar fissure between the upper and lower lobes. This is the region of the lung in which air flow is the greatest and, consequently, where the greatest number of organisms are likely to be carried. The apices of the lung are the sites of highest oxygen tension, and it is here that secondary foci of reactivated tuberculosis are most likely to occur.

**(33)** *Mycobacterium tuberculosis* produces no known endotoxins, exotoxins, or tissue-destructive proteolytic enzymes. Thus, the tissue injury produced during infection is primarily related to the immune response to the organism rather than the organism itself. The immune response to *M. tuberculosis* involves both CD4+ T-cell activation of macrophages and CD8+ T-cell cytotoxic attack on mycobacterially infected macrophages. The end result is the formation of caseating granulomas, the hallmark of the disease. **(34)** In highly susceptible, highly sensitized individuals, however, this common pattern of involvement may not be seen. Instead, infection tends to produce overwhelming disease with a diffuse necrotizing bronchopneumonia, traditionally referred to as "galloping consumption."

**(35 and 36)** With diminished T-cell function (e.g., in AIDS), the response to *M. tuberculosis* also is altered. Persons with AIDS develop infection at much higher rates than healthy individuals, have more abundant pulmonary disease, and are more likely to transmit *M. tuberculosis* to others than infected immunocompetent individuals. Infection in patients with AIDS usually results in granulomas that are poorly formed, are more frequently necrotic, and contain more abundant acid-fast organisms. Most primary tuberculosis is asymptomatic. It is only in the secondary form of the disease (chronic pulmonary tuberculosis) that symptoms usually are produced.

**(37)** Most cases of secondary pulmonary tuberculosis develop from reactivation of an old, sometimes subclinical primary infection. Fortunately, however, reactivation occurs in no more than 5 to 10% of cases of untreated primary infection in immunocompetent individuals. **(38)** Once reactivation has occured, however, the subsequent course of the disease is somewhat unpredictable. With erosion of caseous lesions into vascular structures, widespread hematogenous dissemination may occur. With erosion into the pulmonary artery, miliary spread throughout the lungs would occur. Systemic dissemination, however, would occur with erosion into a pulmonary vein. **(39)** Only about 3 to 5% of recent tuberculin converters develop active disease in the first year, but 5 to 15% may progress to active disease within 5 years. The consequences of secondary pulmonary tuberculosis may be severe, so eradication of the primary disease is warranted in all cases. Thus, any patient who has recently developed a positive purified protein derivative (PPD) skin test (indicating recent infection) requires antituberculous chemotherapy (i.e., isoniazid) for at least 1 year. *(pp. 324–327; 700–703)*

**40. (C); 41. (C); 42. (B); 43. (C); 44. (D)**

The two most commonly encountered developmental defects of the lung are bronchogenic congenital cysts and bronchopulmonary sequestrations. Bronchogenic cysts develop from a detached fragment of primitive foregut that forms a cystic structure lined by bronchial-type epithelium. "Bronchopulmonary sequestration" refers to an abnormal lobe of lung tissue located within the normal lung but having its own blood supply from the aorta. **(40 and 41)** Both bronchogenic cysts and sequestrations usually occur singly in otherwise normal individuals. **(42)** Unlike bronchogenic cysts, which may or may not communicate with the normal airway system of the involved lung, bronchopulmonary sequestrations never communicate with a main bronchus. **(43)** Because they tend to fill with proteinaceous secretions, both defects are prime sites for the development of infection, **(44)** but neither is associated with neoplastic transformation. *(p. 675)*

**45. (A); 46. (D); 47. (B); 48. (C); 49. (D); 50. (A); 51. (C)**

Goodpasture's syndrome and idiopathic pulmonary hemosiderosis (IPH) are two distinctive interstitial diseases of the lung that both produce intrapulmonary hemorrhage as their major manifestation. **(46)** In contrast to IPH, Goodpasture's syndrome is characterized by the simultaneous development of a necrotizing hemorrhagic interstitial pneumonitis and rapidly progressing glomerulonephritis (not interstitial nephritis). **(45 and 47)** Goodpasture's syndrome has a striking predominance among males, usually in the second or third decade of life. In contrast, IPH has no male predominance and occurs most commonly in children and adolescents, although some adult cases are seen.

**(48 and 49)** Both Goodpasture's syndrome and IPH produce necrotizing hemorrhagic interstitial pneumonitis; neither produces vasculitis. Vasculitis-associated pulmonary disease encompasses a separate and unrelated category of disorders, including the Churg-Strauss syndrome and Wegener's granulomatosis. **(50)** In IPH, the cause of injury is unknown. In Goodpasture's syndrome, the destructive process is caused by autoantibodies directed against the capillary basement membranes in glomeruli and alveolar septa (see Question 15). No autoantibodies have been identified in IPH.

**(51)** Both Goodpasture's syndrome and IPH (especially that occurring in childhood) are devastating disease processes with significant mortality. Untreated Goodpasture's syndrome is more rapidly lethal than IPH, however. Immediate treatment with intensive plasmapheresis and immunosuppressant chemotherapy has improved the previously dismal survival rate in this disease. Although the course of IPH in any given patient is unpredictable, there is no proven effective treatment for the disease and the childhood form has a mean survival of about 3 years. *(pp. 717–718; 947–948)*

**52. (C); 53. (A); 54. (B); 55. (C); 56. (B); 57. (C); 58. (A); 59. (A); 60. (E); 61. (D)**

**(53, 58, and 59)** The distinctive histologic features of different components of the pulmonary parenchyma correspond to their physiologic roles. The bronchi are characterized by their submucosal mucus-secreting glands, mucosal goblet cells, mural cartilage, and content of mucosal neuroendocrine cells. The mucus produced by submucosal glands and goblet cells coats the bronchial surface, entraps inhaled particles, and is swept toward the oropharynx by ciliary action, where it is swallowed or expectorated. This mucociliary transport is the major defense mechanism of the tracheobroncial tree. Mural cartilages prevent total luminal occlusion when the smooth muscle of the wall is constricted. Neuroendocrine cells produce serotonin, calcitonin, and bombesin (gastrin-releasing hormone). Bronchial stem cells with potential for neuroendocrine differentiation may give rise to neuroendocrine tumors (bronchial carcinoids).

**(54 and 56)** In contrast to bronchi, bronchioles are devoid of goblet cells and mucus glands. They normally are coated with a watery proteinaceous material made by mucosal Clara cells that is rich in secretory immunoglobulin contributed by mucosal B lymphocytes and plasma cells. Bronchioles contain no cartilage and are capable of complete luminal occlusion on constriction of their mural smooth muscle (in an asthmatic attack, for example).

**(52, 55, and 57)** Alveoli are unique in the production of surfactant by type II pneumocytes in their walls. Surfactant is critical for maintaining low surface tension in the alveoli and, hence, compliance to expansion on inspiration. Adjacent alveoli are interconnected by mural passages known as pores of Kohn. They provide a pathway by which bacteria and exudate can spread through neighboring alveoli during the course of a bronchopneumonia. Alveoli normally contain macrophages within their lumens that are the basis for alveolar defense against inhaled bacteria and small particulate matter.

**(60 and 61)** Mast cells are ubiquitous in the lung; they are found in the walls of bronchi, bronchioles, and alveoli. Thus, mast cells can participate in hypersensitivity responses at any level of the pulmonary tree. In contrast, squamous cells are never present in the normal lung. When found, they represent a metaplastic response to injury. Metaplastic squamous cells may go on to become dysplastic and/or neoplastic with continued injury (e.g., cigarette smoking). Thus, squamous cell carcinoma is the most common type of lung cancer, even though the normal lung contains no squamous mucosa. *(pp. 673–674; 723)*

**62. (B); 63. (A); 64. (E); 65. (D); 66. (D)**

Emphysema is a chronic obstructive pulmonary disease characterized by abnormal permanent enlargement of the air spaces distal to the terminal bronchioles, accompanied by destruction of their walls but without obvious fibrosis. Several types of emphysema have been defined on the basis of their particular pathologic and clinical patterns. **(62)** One of the most clinically distinctive types is panacinar (panlobular) emphysema. This type is associated with $\alpha_1$-antitrypsin deficiency and is characterized pathologically by uniform enlargement of the acini from the level of the respiratory bronchioles to the terminal alveolar sacs. **(63)** Centriacinar (centrilobular) emphysema is the type that occurs most commonly in cigarette smokers. As its name implies, centriacinar emphysema is characterized by enlargement of the central or proximal structures of the acini (the respiratory bronchioles) with sparing of the distal alveoli.

**(64)** Although hyperinflation of the residual lung occurs after surgical removal of the lobe, the process does not involve any pulmonary parenchymal destruction and cannot be classified as an emphysematous process even though it is known by the unfortunate term "compensatory emphysema." Enlargement of air spaces without destruction of their walls is properly termed overinflation. **(65)** Likewise, it should be recognized that the process known as "interstitial emphysema" is similarly misnamed because it involves no permanent tissue destruction. Interstitial emphysema refers to the entrance of air into the connective tissue stroma of the lungs, mediastinum, or subcutaneous tissue from tears in the alveolar walls. Usually alveolar tears occur when pressures in the alveolar sacs are sharply increased by a combination of coughing and some form of bronchiolar obstruction (such as occurs in children with whooping cough). **(66)** Thus, because it is not a form of pulmonary emphysema or chronic obstructive pulmonary disease, interstitial edema would not be associated with bullous disease, an end-stage form of true emphysema of any type. Bullae (balloon-like sacs measuring >1 cm in diameter when inflated) or blebs (smaller than bullae) form when extensive alveolar destruction has occured. *(pp. 683–688)*

**67. (A); 68. (C); 69. (B); 70. (D); 71. (E); 72. (E); 73. (E); 74. (A); 75. (C); 76. (C)**

Although not totally predictable in every case, specific microorganisms tend to produce characteristic patterns of pulmonary injury. **(67 and 74)** Diffuse alveolar damage is a pattern of injury most commonly seen in viral and *Mycoplasma* pneumonias. **(69)** Bronchopneumonia involving an entire lobe (lobar pneumonia) most commonly is caused by *Steptococcus pneumoniae* (pneumococcus) but may be caused by other non-necrotizing bacteria. **(68, 75, and 76)** Necrotizing bronchopneumonia is the characteristic pattern of injury produced by such virulent organisms as *Staphylococcus aureus, Klebsiella pneumoniae,* and *Legionella* species. Although any necrotizing bronchopneumonia may progress to abscess formation, this is a relatively infrequent complication. **(70)** *Bacteroides* species and other anaerobic organisms, however, are associated more commonly with lung abscess formation than with any other pattern of pulmonary injury. Pulmonary abscesses from anaerobic organisms are usually the result of aspiration.

**(72)** Thermophilic bacteria, such as those that infect heated water reservoirs in humidifiers or air conditioners, are of low virulence and do not cause direct pulmonary injury. Instead, thermophilic bacteria elicit a hypersensitivity immune response (both type I and type IV immune reactions). The result is a pneumonitis ("hypersensitivity pneumonitis") characterized by interstitial inflammatory infiltrates of mononuclear cells and eosinophils and scattered, noncaseating granulomas. **(73)** *Mycobacterium tuberculosis* is an organism of low virulence. In the immunocompetent host, it elicits a type IV immune response, producing granulomas that are the hallmark of this type of infection (see Questions 32 through 39).

**(71)** Microfilariae produce a distinctive reaction in the lung characterized by patchy interstitial and intra-alveolar inflammatory infiltrates comprised predominantly of eosinophils. Thus, the disease is known as tropical pulmonary eosinophilia. *(pp. 324–327; 352–353; 373–374; 696–699)*

**77. (B); 78, (B); 79. (D); 80. (C); 81 (A); 82. (C); 83. (C)**

In industrialized nations, bronchogenic carcinoma accounts for the highest number of cancer deaths. **(77)** Among the histologic types of lung cancer, squamous cell carcinoma and adenocarcinoma are the most common, each accounting for 25 to 40% of all bronchogenic malignancies. Adenocarcinoma is the type most commonly seen in women, whereas most squamous cell carcinomas occur in men.

**(78)** Unlike squamous cell carcinoma or small-cell carcinoma, which both occur more frequently in a central location in the lung in association with the major bronchi, adenocarcinoma often occurs in a peripheral location. **(79)** Although adenocarcinoma is associated less frequently with a history of cigarette smoking than squamous cell or oat cell carcinomas, none of the major forms of bronchogenic carcinoma can be said to be etiologically unrelated to cigarette smoking. **(80)** Small-cell carcinomas are distinctive in several ways, one being their tendency toward neuroendocrine differentiation. This is evidenced by the finding of dense-core neurosecretory granules in their cytoplasm on electron microscopic examination.

**(81)** Bronchogenic carcinomas occasionally produce and secrete hormones that are not responsive to normal feedback regulatory mechanisms. One of the most characteristic ectopic hormonal syndromes associated with a specific tumor type is the production of parathyroid hormone by squamous cell carcinoma of the lung. The other major histologic types of bronchogenic carcinoma rarely, if ever, produce parathyroid hormone. **(82)** Small-cell carcinoma of the lung, in contrast, is the most common type of malignancy to be associated with the syndrome of inappropriate antidiuretic hormone production.

**(83)** Small-cell carcinoma of the lung is the only type of lung tumor for which surgical resection is ineffective. This type of lung cancer is treated more often with radiotherapy and chemotherapy. Even with treatment, however, the overall mean survival time for treated small-cell carcinoma is only about 1 year. For the other histologic types, early diagnosis with lobectomy or pneumonectomy is the best chance for cure of the disease. Unfortunately, most bronchogenic carcinoma is discovered in clinically advanced (unresectable) stages, accounting for the poor prognosis of the disease (overall 5-year survival rate of about 9%). *(pp. 720–725)*

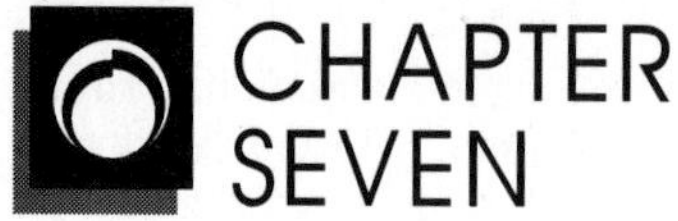

CHAPTER SEVEN

# The Hematopoietic and Lymphoid Systems

**DIRECTIONS:** For Questions 1 through 18, choose the ONE BEST answer to each question.

**1.** All of the following statements correctly describe hereditary spherocytosis EXCEPT:

A. Red blood cells lack the membrane-associated protein spectrin.
B. A mutation in the ankyrin gene is present in most cases.
C. Hemolytic crisis is an occasional complication.
D. An aplastic crisis is an occasional complication.
E. Splenectomy is invariably therapeutic.

**2.** Features of megaloblastic anemias include all of the following EXCEPT:

A. Hypersegmented neutrophils
B. Giant platelets
C. Increased intramedullary hemolysis
D. Increased extramedullary hemolysis
E. Epithelial atypia of the gastric mucosa

**3.** Functions of the normal spleen include all of the following EXCEPT:

A. Generation of immune responses
B. Destruction of abnormal erythrocytes
C. Storage of erythrocytes
D. Production of erythrocytes
E. Storage of platelets

**4.** All of the following statements correctly describe aplastic anemia EXCEPT:

A. Production of all hematopoietic bone marrow elements is reduced.
B. Chemical/drug exposure is the most common cause.
C. Fanconi's anemia represents an inherited form of the disease.
D. No underlying etiology is evident in 50% of cases.
E. Splenomegaly is a characteristic clinical finding.

**5.** All of the following statements correctly describe disseminated intravascular coagulation EXCEPT:

A. Widespread thromboses are characteristic.
B. Widespread hemorrhages are characteristic.
C. It most often presents as a primary (idiopathic) condition.
D. The brain is the organ most often involved.
E. It is associated with mucin-secreting adenocarcinomas.

**6.** Multiple myeloma is associated with all of the following features EXCEPT:

A. Hypercalcemia
B. Renal failure
C. Amyloidosis
D. Increased susceptibility to viral infections
E. Rouleau formation on peripheral smear

**7.** Osmotic fragility characterizes the erythrocytes in:

A. Fanconi's anemia
B. Sickle cell anemia
C. Glucose-6-phosphate dehydrogenase deficiency
D. Hereditary spherocytosis
E. Pernicious anemia

**8.** Hematologic disorders occurring mainly in populations in the Middle East (Mediterranean region) include all of the following EXCEPT:

A. Glucose-6-phosphate dehydrogenase deficiency
B. Factor IX deficiency (Christmas disease)
C. Thalassemia major
D. Thalassemia minor
E. α-Chain disease

**9.** Microangiopathic hemolytic anemia is encountered in association with all of the following factors EXCEPT:

A. Cold agglutinins
B. Thrombotic thrombocytopenic purpura
C. The hemolytic-uremic syndrome
D. Malignant hypertension
E. Prosthetic heart valves

**10.** Iron-deficiency anemia is commonly associated with all of the following factors EXCEPT:

A. Colon cancer
B. Lung cancer
C. Gastrectomy
D. Normal menses
E. Pregnancy

**11.** Polycythemia vera is a proliferative disorder of stem cells that:

A. Has an X-linked recessive mode of transmission
B. Is associated with high levels of erythropoietin
C. Produces abnormalities in the red cell series only
D. Is rapidly fatal if untreated
E. Is compatible with a normal life span if treated

**12.** A cell surface antigen common to all leukocytes is:

A. CD2
B. CD7
C. CD14
D. CD19
E. CD45

**13.** Inceased blood viscosity (hyperviscosity syndrome) is a major complication of all of the following disorders EXCEPT:

A. Polycythemia vera
B. Immunoglobulin A myeloma
C. Hairy-cell leukemia
D. Waldenström's macroglobulinemia
E. Sickle cell anemia

**14.** All of the following statements correctly describe nodular non-Hodgkin's lymphomas EXCEPT:

A. They often are associated with a predictable chromosomal translocation.
B. They have a better prognosis than diffuse lymphomas.
C. They are characterized by cells with irregular nuclear contours.
D. They are always composed of neoplastic B cells.
E. They are highly responsive to chemotherapy.

**15.** All of the following features are characteristic of myeloid metaplasia with myelofibrosis EXCEPT:

A. Clonal proliferation of marrow fibroblasts
B. Giant platelets in the peripheral blood
C. Teardrop-shaped red cells in the peripheal blood
D. Elevated leukocyte alkaline phosphatase levels in the serum
E. Massive splenomegaly

**16.** Transformation to acute leukemia occurs as a complication of all of the following disorders EXCEPT:

A. Paroxysmal nocturnal hemoglobinuria
B. Myeloid metaplasia with myelofibrosis
C. Aplastic anemia
D. Hairy-cell leukemia
E. Polycythemia vera

**17.** Intermediate grade lymphomas include all of the following EXCEPT:

A. Follicular, predominantly large-cell lymphoma
B. Follicular, predominantly small cleaved cell lymphoma
C. Diffuse, small cleaved cell lymphoma
D. Diffuse, mixed small- and large-cell lymphoma
E. Diffuse large-cell lymphoma

**18.** Chronic myelogenous leukemia is characterized by all of the following features EXCEPT:

A. Lack of alkaline phosphatase in circulating neutrophils
B. Extreme splenomegaly
C. Transition to acute leukemia
D. Philadelphia chromosomes in stem cells
E. Excellent response to chemotherapy

**DIRECTIONS:** For Questions 19 through 25, you are to decide whether EACH choice is TRUE or FALSE.

For each of the following statements about Hodgkin's disease, choose whether it is TRUE or FALSE.

**19.** The Reed-Sternberg cell is the malignant cellular element of Hodgkin's disease.
**20.** Mixed cellularity is the most common subtype of Hodgkin's disease.
**21.** All subtypes of Hodgkin's disease spread by serial progression from one contiguous lymph node group to another.
**22.** A leukemic phase is common in the lymphocyte-predominant subtype of Hodgkin's disease.
**23.** The subtype of Hodgkin's disease is the most important prognostic indicator.
**24.** Patients with infectious mononucleosis have an increased risk of developing Hodgkin's disease.
**25.** Patients successfully treated for Hodgkin's disease have an increased risk of developing lung cancer.

**DIRECTIONS:** For Questions 26 through 55, the set of lettered headings is followed by a list of numbered words or phrases. For each numbered word or phrase choose:
A—if the item is associated with (A) only
B—if the item is associated with (B) only
C—if the item is associated with *both* (A) and (B)
D—if the item is associated with *neither* (A) nor (B)

For each of the features listed below, choose whether it is characteristic of warm antibody hemolytic anemia, cold agglutinin immune hemolytic anemia, both, or neither.

A. Warm antibody hemolytic anemia
B. Cold agglutinin immune hemolytic anemia
C. Both
D. Neither

**26.** Antibodies to red cells are usually complement-fixing immunoglobulin G.
**27.** Antibodies to red cells are usually monoclonal immunoglobulin M.
**28.** The disorder often is caused by drugs.
**29.** The disorder occurs in association with lymphoma.
**30.** Splenomegaly commonly is produced.
**31.** Complement-mediated intravascular hemolysis occurs.

For each of the statements listed below, choose whether it describes acute lymphocytic leukemia, acute myelogenous leukemia, both, or neither.

A. Acute lymphocytic leukemia
B. Acute myelogenous leukemia
C. Both
D. Neither

**32.** The disease most commonly occurs in the elderly.
**33.** Leukemic cells have chromosomal abnormalities in the vast majority of cases.
**34.** Leukemic cells commonly contain Auer rods.
**35.** The presence of the Philadelphia chromosome in tumor cells is associated with a poor prognosis.
**36.** Leukemic cells suppress normal hematopoiesis.
**37.** Patients treated for Hodgkin's disease with chemotherapy and irradiation have an increased risk of developing the disease.
**38.** Generalized lymphadenopathy is present.
**39.** Bleeding of gums secondary to thrombocytopenia is common.
**40.** Infiltration of gums by leukemic cells is common.
**41.** Soft tissue chloromas are characteristic.
**42.** Bone pain is a common symptom.
**43.** Intensive chemotherapy is curative in over 60% of cases.

For each of the features listed below, choose whether it describes idiopathic thrombocytopenic purpura, thrombotic thrombocytopenic purpura, both, or neither.

A. Idiopathic thrombocytopenic purpura
B. Thrombotic thrombocytopenic purpura
C. Both
D. Neither

**44.** Produces an abnormal bleeding time
**45.** Produces splenomegaly
**46.** Is associated with antiplatelet antibodies
**47.** Is caused by activation of the coagulation system
**48.** Is associated with microangiopathic hemolytic anemia
**49.** Is associated with systemic lupus erythematosus
**50.** Is associated with a high mortality rate

For each of the statements below, choose whether it describes acute lymphocytic leukemia, chronic lymphocytic leukemia, both, or neither.

A. Acute lymphocytic leukemia
B. Chronic lymphocytic leukemia
C. Both
D. Neither

**51.** The disease is often asymptomatic.
**52.** The malignancy is usually of B cell origin.
**53.** Hyperdiploidy is a favorable prognostic feature.
**54.** Prognosis correlates with the clinical stage of disease.
**55.** Most cells express immunoglobulin light chains on their surfaces.

**DIRECTIONS:** Questions 56 through 94 are matching questions. For each numbered item, choose the most likely associated lettered item from those provided. Each numbered item has ONLY ONE answer. Within each group, each lettered item may be the answer to one, more than one, or none of the numbered items.

For each of the following features of hemolytic anemia, choose whether it is characteristic of $\beta$-thalassemia, paroxysmal nocturnal hemoglobinuria, sickle cell anemia, glucose-6-phosphate dehydrogenase deficiency, or none of these.

A. $\beta$-Thalassemia
B. Paroxysmal noctural hemoglobinuria
C. Sickle cell anemia
D. Glucose-6-phosphate dehydrogenase deficiency
E. None of these

**56.** Antimalarial drugs cause hemolytic crises.
**57.** Splenic hypofunction predisposes to infections.
**58.** The cells are unusually sensitive to lysis by endogenous complement.
**59.** Heinz bodies appear within red cells.
**60.** Hypoxia causes hemolytic crises.
**61.** Platelets are abnormal.
**62.** Granulocytes are abnormal.
**63.** Transformation to acute myelogenous leukemia occasionally occurs.
**64.** It commonly leads to death before age 20.
**65.** Red cell precursors characteristically are destroyed within the marrow.
**66.** Expansion of the erythron within the bone marrow does not occur.
**67.** Autoantibodies to red cells contribute to the hemolysis.

For each of the conditions or situations associated with hemorrhagic diatheses listed below, choose whether the major cause is vascular fragility, thrombocytopenia, defective platelet function, a clotting factor defect, or disseminated intravascular coagulation.

A. Vascular fragility
B. Thrombocytopenia
C. Defective platelet function
D. Clotting factor defect
E. Disseminated intravascular coagulation

**68.** Cushing's syndrome
**69.** Hereditary hemorrhagic telangiectasia
**70.** Von Willebrand's disease
**71.** Massive transfusions
**72.** Henoch-Schönlein purpura
**73.** Rickettsial infection
**74.** Promyelocytic (M3) leukemia
**75.** Scurvy
**76.** Folate deficiency
**77.** Acquired immunodeficiency syndrome

For each of the drugs and chemicals listed below, choose whether the hematologic defect with which it is associated is immune hemolytic anemia, aplastic anemia, neutropenia, all of these, or none of these.

A. Drug-related immune hemolytic anemia
B. Drug-related aplastic anemia
C. Drug-related neutropenia
D. All of these
E. None of these

**78.** Penicillin
**79.** $\alpha$-Methyldopa
**80.** Thiouracil
**81.** Quinidine
**82.** Benzene
**83.** Aminopyrine
**84.** Phenacetin

For each of the diseases listed below, choose whether it is characterized by increased circulating numbers of neutrophils, lymphocytes, eosinophils, or none of these.

A. Elevated neutrophil count
B. Elevated lymphocyte count
C. Elevated eosinophil count
D. None of these

**85.** Tuberculosis
**86.** Bronchial asthma
**87.** Infectious mononucleosis
**88.** Myocardial infarction
**89.** Eosinophilic granuloma

For each of the features listed below, choose whether it is characteristic of acute disseminated Langerhans' cell histiocytosis (Letterer-Siwe syndrome), multifocal Langerhans' cell histiocytosis (Hand-Schüller-Christian disease), unifocal Langerhans' cell histiocytosis (eosinophilic granuloma), all of these, or none of these.

A. Acute disseminated Langerhans' cells histiocytosis (Letterer-Siwe syndrome)
B. Multifocal Langerhans' cell histiocytosis (Hand-Schüller-Christian disease)
C. Multifocal Langerhans' cell histiocytosis (eosinophilic granuloma)
D. All of these
E. None of these

**90.** Diabetes insipidus is a classic manifestation.
**91.** The disease commonly occurs before the age of 3.
**92.** The mortality rate is 100% in untreated disease.
**93.** Infiltrating Langerhans' cells contain pentalaminar inclusion bodies.
**94.** A skin rash is characteristically absent.

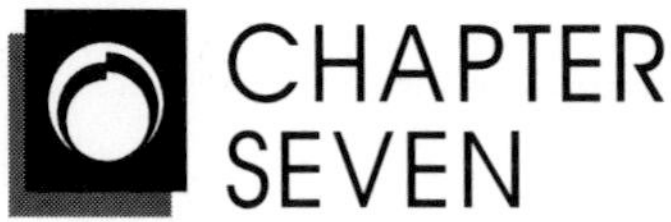

CHAPTER SEVEN

# The Hematopoietic and Lymphoid Systems

## ANSWERS

**1. (A)** Hereditary spherocytosis (HS) is an inherited structural defect of red blood cell (RBC) membranes that renders erythrocytes spheroidal, less flexible, and more prone to splenic sequestration and destruction. In 75% of cases, it is an autosomal dominant disorder. The abnormality is related to a deficiency of spectrin, the major protein in the cell membrane–associated filamentous network responsible for maintenance of RBC shape. The spectrin content of RBCs in HS varies from 60 to 90% of normal (correlating with severity of disease) but is not absent altogether. The molecular basis of the spectrin deficiency in HS is varied. In some cases, a primary defect in the spectrin molecule is present, but, more commonly, the primary defect is a mutation of the ankyrin gene. Ankyrin is a spectrin-associated protein that links spectrin to the inner surface of the cell membrane. A mutation-related reduction in ankyrin production occurs that, in turn, results in decreased spectrin assembly along the RBC membrane. In either case, the defect results in abnormally shaped cells that stagnate in the spleen because their inflexibility makes it difficult for them to leave the cords of Billroth and enter the sinusoids. The consequence of their prolonged contact with splenic macrophages is engulfment and degradation. The premature destruction of RBCs produces a chronic extravascular hemolytic anemia with an accumulation of hemoglobin breakdown products (producing a mild jaundice with unconjugated hyperbilirubinemia and sometimes pigment cholelithiasis as well) and a concomitant increase in erythropoiesis in the bone marrow. The cardinal role of the spleen in producing the HS-associated anemia is underscored by the invariable correction of the anemia, despite the persistence of spherocytes, by splenectomy. The stability of the disease may be punctuated with acute crises, often triggered by intercurrent infections. Either a hemolytic crisis (sudden onset of massive hemolysis with fever, abdominal pain, jaundice, and even shock) or an aplastic crisis (temporary suppression of RBC production in the bone marrow) may occur. These crises require blood transfusions to support the patient until the crisis remits. *(pp. 589–591)*

**2. (B)** Megaloblastic anemias, resulting from either vitamin $B_{12}$ or folate deficiency, are characterized by defective DNA synthesis in all hematopoietic cells. The impairment of DNA synthesis leads to the production of cytologically abnormal red cells and leukocytes and an overall decrease in the production of all cell lines. Although DNA synthesis is impaired in megaloblastic anemia, synthesis of RNA and protein is unaffected. Thus, asynchrony between nuclear and cytoplasmic maturation develops during hematopoiesis. This results in macrocytic erythrocytes, giant neutrophils with hypersegmented nuclei, and large, bizarre megakaryocytes. Defective erythropoiesis leads to increased intramedullary hemolysis of the abnormal precursors. Increased extramedullary hemolysis of defective red cells occurs as well, augmented by a poorly characterized plasma factor produced in this disease. Although the impact on the hematopoietic system is most profound, the acquired defect in DNA synthesis affects all rapidly proliferating cells in the body. Therefore, the intestinal mucosa (especially the gastric epithelium) also suffers from nuclear-cytoplasmic asynchrony and develops megaloblastic cytologic changes.

Although giant megakaryocytes are seen in megaloblastic anemia, giant platelets are not a feature of this disease. Giant platelets usually are seen either in myeloproliferative disorders such as myeloid metaplasia or in the absence of a spleen (e.g., postsplenectomy or autoinfarction). *(pp. 603–605; 662)*

**3. (D)** The normal spleen is the filter for the bloodstream and has both immunologic and hematologic functions. It is the "lymph node" of the circulatory system; that is, it traps circulating antigens in the periarteriolar lymphoid sheaths, where they come in contact with effector lymphocytes. The spleen also traps defective and/or obsolete circulating erythrocytes. Half of the normal daily effete red cell clearance occurs in the spleen, and in disease states, virtually all of the destruction of structurally abnormal (e.g., spherocytes) or antibody-coated red cells occurs there. The spleen also functions as a reservoir pool and storage site for erythrocytes and platelets. Normally, stored elements can be extruded on demand. In disease states with splenomegaly and hypersplenism, the spleen traps and hoards blood cells of all types, leading to peripheral cytopenias.

Although the spleen functions as a hematopoietic organ in fetal life and in disease states that compromise or replace bone marrow, hematopoiesis does not normally take place in the spleen. *(pp. 172; 584; 668–669; 587–588)*

**4. (E)** Aplastic anemia is a condition caused by hematopoietic stem cell failure or suppression and is characterized by inadequate production or release of all differentiated cell lines. The condition occurs without any definable underlying cause in about 50% of cases (idiopathic aplastic anemia). However, it most often occurs as a result of stem cell injury from a variety of chemical agents (the most common cause), physical agents, or infections. Whatever the cause, the diagnosis is made by the characteristic findings on examination of the peripheral blood (pancytopenia) and the bone marrow (marked hypocellularity). Splenomegaly is characteristically absent and, if present, would make a diagnosis of aplastic anemia highly questionable.

Among the physical agents that can cause aplastic anemia, whole-body irradiation is the prototype. Infections that are known to induce aplastic anemia are largely, if not exclusively, viral in origin and include infectious mononucleosis, cytomegalovirus infection, varicella zoster infection, and hepatitis C. Chloramphenicol is one of many drugs that can cause aplastic anemia, but curiously, it is the only one that is known to do so in either a dose-related or an idiosyncratic manner. Aplastic anemia also occurs as part of a rare autosomal recessive disorder known as Fanconi's anemia, which is characterized by defects in DNA repair. Little presently is known about the specific pathogenetic mechanisms by which aplastic anemia is produced in these different settings. There is also recent evidence that some cases of aplastic anemia can be treated effectively by immunosuppression, suggesting that the stem cell suppression may be immunologically mediated (by suppressor T cells).

The outcome in aplastic anemia is quite unpredictable. In some cases caused by chemicals or drugs, withdrawal of the toxic agent may result in spontaneous recovery, but idiopathic disease has a poor prognosis. Whatever the cause, aplastic anemia often can be treated effectively by bone marrow transplantation to replace the defective stem cell population. However, some forms of marrow injury causing aplastic anemia appear to result in genetic alterations that later are manifested as acute leukemia. *(pp. 613–615)*

**5. (C)** Disseminated intravascular coagulation (DIC) is an acquired thrombohemorrhagic disorder characterized by activation of the coagulation cascades via either the extrinsic pathway (triggered by the release of tissue thromboplastin), the intrinsic pathway (triggered by factor XII activation), or both. The result is widespread thrombosis and hemorrhage (a consequence of depletion of the elements required for homeostasis). Although any organ can be affected, the brain is involved most often (followed in order of frequency by the heart, lungs, kidneys, adrenals, spleen, and liver). DIC occurs in association with a variety of disorders that involve release of thromboplastic tissue-derived substances into the circulation and/or produce widespread endothelial injury. The principal causes include systemic sepsis, major trauma, obstetric conditions, and malignancy. In particular, mucin-secreting adenocarcinomas frequently are associated with DIC, because they release a variety of thromboplastic substances, including tissue factors, proteolytic enzymes, and mucin, all of which are thrombogenic. It is important to recognize that DIC always occurs as a secondary complication of some other underlying condition and does not occur as a primary process. *(pp. 623–626)*

**6. (D)** Multiple myeloma is a malignancy of plasma cells that originates in the bone marrow and involves the skeleton at multiple sites. The neoplastic cells bear surface markers of plasma cells (e.g., PCA-1), but they also may express antigens associated with other hematopoietic cell lines, suggesting origin from a pluripotential stem cell with differentiation primarily along the B cell/plasma cell pathway. In 99% of cases, myeloma cells secrete immunoglobulins or their components, which are detectable either by immunoelectrophoretic analysis of blood or by the appearance of light chains (Bence Jones proteins) in the urine. Typically, multiple myeloma forms osteolytic lesions that have a characteristic "punched-out" appearance on radiographs. The associated bone resorption frequently leads to hypercalcemia. Renal failure is common in patients with multiple myeloma and is second only to bacterial infection as the leading cause of death in this disease. The most significant factor leading to renal failure is the toxic effect of the filtered immunoglobulin light chains on the renal tubular epithelium, although infiltration of the interstitium by tumor cells also occurs. Amyloidosis of immunologic origin occurs in about 10% of patients with multiple myeloma and also may contribute to renal failure. Coating of erythrocytes with circulating immunoglobulins causes a rouleau formation characteristically seen on peripheral smear.

Bacterial infection is a common complication of multiple myeloma. Recurrent infections with bacteria such as *Streptococcus pneumoniae*, *Staphylococcus aureus* and *Escherichia coli* not only pose major clinical problems but constitute the leading cause of death among patients with this disease. The susceptibility to bacterial infection is due to severe depression of normal immunoglobulin production. However, because cellular immunity is relatively unaffected in multiple myeloma, susceptibility to viral infections is not increased significantly. *(pp. 663–665)*

**7. (D)** Osmotic fragility is a property of the red blood cells (RBCs) in hereditary spherocytosis and forms the basis of a common laboratory test used in confirming the diagnosis of this disease (see Question 1). This test measures the ability of RBCs to swell in a graded series of hypotonic solutions. Spherocytes, already rotund and "swollen," are osmotically fragile because they can tolerate less swelling than normally shaped (slender, discoid) RBCs before they hemolyze.

In the hereditary form of aplastic anemia (see Question 4), known as Fanconi's anemia, RBC production is reduced drastically, but the structural properties of the erythrocytes in this disease are not abnormal. In sickle cell anemia, RBCs characteristically undergo structural deformation in environments of lowered oxygen tension. Therefore, common diagnostic tests for sickle cell anemia are based on mixing a blood sample with an oxygen-consuming reagent such as metabisulfite to induce sickling. Red cells in glucose-6-phosphate dehydrogenase deficiency are characterized by their sensitivity to oxidative injury and will undergo hemolysis when exposed to oxidant drugs. In pernicious anemia, the deficiency of vitamin $B_{12}$ caused by destruction of intrinsic factor-producing gastric parietal cells results in defective DNA synthesis in hematopoietic cells, but synthesis of RNA and protein is unaffected. Thus, nuclear and cytoplasmic maturation are not synchronized, and affected cells appear enlarged and abnormally formed (the precise basis of these morphologic changes is not fully understood as yet). These cells are apparently structurally (as well as morphologically) abnormal, because they undergo autohemolysis in the bone marrow more readily than normal cells and are more avidly phagocitized by macrophages. However, none of the above disorders is characterized by changes in the surface-volume ratio of the RBCs that would render them osmotically fragile. *(pp. 591; 595; 604; 614)*

**8. (B)** A number of hematologic disorders occur predominantly in populations in the Mediterranean area or in patients of Middle Eastern heritage. Principal among these are two hereditary hemolytic anemias, a severe form of glucose-6-phosphate dehydrogenase (G6PD) deficiency and $\beta$-thalassemia (thalassemia major), and an unusual B cell lymphoma of the small intestine (Mediterranean lymphoma or immunoproliferative small intestinal disease). The Mediterranean form of G6PD deficiency ("G6PD Mediterranean") is characterized by both a severely impaired synthesis and a reduced stability of this enzyme. The resultant abnormalities in glutathione metabolism render the red blood cells extremely susceptible to oxidant injuries. This leads to hemolysis on exposure to oxidant drugs or during events in which the generation of oxidant free radicals by macrophages is increased. The prevalence of the mutant G6PD gene in Mediterranean populations is believed to be related to the fact that G6PD deficiency protects against malaria, caused by *Plasmodium falciparum*.

$\beta$-Thalassemia results from a defect in the production of the $\beta$-globin chains of hemoglobin, with unimpaired production of $\alpha$-globin chains. The $\beta$-thalassemia genes are most frequent in and the disease most prevalent in Mediterranean countries. Several different mutant genes have been defined: (1) promotor region mutations that reduce RNA polymerase binding and reduce gene transcription by 75 to 80%; (2) chain terminator mutations that prematurely terminate mRNA translation and generate nonfunctional fragments of gene product; and (3) splicing mutations (the most common) resulting in the production of abnormal mRNA that is degraded in the cell nucleus. Only with the promotor region mutation is any normal gene product synthesized ($\beta^+$ talassemia). The other mutations lead to a total absence of $\beta$-globin chains ($\beta^0$ thalassemia). In general, those individuals homozygous for $\beta^0$ or $\beta^+$ genes have a severe, transfusion-dependent anemia (thalassemia major), and those heterozygous for these genes (having one normal gene) have milder or asymptomatic disease (thalassemia minor or thalassemia intermedia).

$\alpha$-Chain disease, also known as immunoproliferative small intestinal disease or Mediterranean lymphoma, is a third disorder that occurs most commonly in Mediterranean populations, typically in children and young adults. It is an unusual form of B cell lymphoma with an immunoglobulin A–producing monoclonal gammopathy. It is characterized histologically by massive infiltration of the intestinal mucosa with plasma cells and with smaller numbers of lymphocytes and histiocytes. The infiltrate also produces a severe malabsorption syndrome, a prominent feature of this disorder. Like other monoclonal gammopathies, the disease is progressive and fatal.

Christmas disease, or hemophilia B, is a rare but severe coagulopathy resulting from a deficiency of coagulation factor IX. This disease has an X-linked recessive mode of transmission but has no increased incidence among Mediterranean populations. *(pp. 591; 598; 623; 666; 821)*

**9. (A)** Hemolysis caused by narrowing or obstruction in the microvasculature is known as microangiopathic hemolytic anemia. The disorder is always secondary to some vascular lesion that physically traumatizes and fragments red cells. In thrombotic thrombocytopenic purpura, a disorder characterized by widespread platelet microthrombi in arterioles, capillaries, and venules, microangiopathic hemolytic anemia is produced by a narrowing or obstruction in the microvasculature through which red cells must pass (see Questions 44 through 50). Similarly, in the hemolytic-uremic syndrome, glomerular capillaries and afferent arterioles are occluded by microthrombi that create the intravascular shear forces leading to red cell injury. In malignant hypertension, red cells are damaged while passing through the markedly narrowed, constricted arterioles. Prosthetic heart valves, especially aortic valves, create turbulent blood flow and abnormal pressure gradients that produce red cell injury.

In contrast to the causes of physical injury to erythrocytes mentioned above, cold agglutinins produce immunologic injury to red cells. Cold agglutinins are immunoglobulin M antibodies produced either during the recovery phase of certain infections (e.g., mycoplasma pneumonia or infectious mononucleosis) or in lymphoproliferative disorders that bind avidly to red cells at low temperatures (0 to 4° C). This leads to red cell agglutination, complement fixation, and finally, hemolysis. *(pp. 602–603)*

**10. (B)** Although dietary deficiency is the most common cause of iron-deficiency anemia worldwide, chronic blood loss and increased requirements for iron are by far the most common causes of this disorder in the Western world. Chronic blood loss often occurs in benign or malignant diseases of the gastrointestinal tract, which cause bleeding into the lumen and subsequent loss of blood in the stool. In fact, patients with colon cancer may present first to the clinician with symptoms of iron-deficiency anemia. Increased requirements for iron are present during childhood (active growth), menstruation, and pregnancy. Economically deprived women having frequent, multiple pregnancies are at particular risk for iron deficiency. Iron deficiency also may develop as a result of impaired iron absorption. This is a common occurrence following gastrectomy because gastric acid is important to iron absorption. Furthermore, gastrectomy reduces transit time through the duodenum, the principal site of iron absorption. Unlike anemias resulting from folate or vitamin $B_{12}$ deficiency, iron-deficiency anemia affects only red cell hemoglobin production and does not produce abnormalities in any of the other hematopoietic cell lines.

With the exception of malignancies of the gastrointestinal tract, female genital tract, and urinary tract, hemorrhage produced by other malignancies (such as lung cancer) usually occurs within the tissues and does not lead to iron loss. *(p. 612)*

**11. (D)** Polycythemia vera is a myeloproliferative disorder of hematopoietic stem cells in which erythropoietin-hypersensitive erythrocyte precursors predominate. Although more common in males and whites than in females or blacks, polycythemia vera has no well-defined mode of genetic transmission. The disease characteristically produces a striking elevation in the total red cell mass (mostly progeny of the defective stem cells) that suppresses erythropoietin output and normal red cell production. Although the predominant manifestation of polycythemia vera is excessive proliferation of the erythroid series, the granulocytic and megakaryocytic cell lines also are affected to a lesser degree. The concomitant elevation in the granulocyte and platelet count is supportive evidence that polycythemia vera is a disorder of pluripotent myeloid stem cells. The disease has a variable course, but it is usually fatal within months after diagnosis if left untreated. However, even if the red blood cell mass is controlled by regular phlebotomy (with or without myelosuppressive chemotherapy), the median survival time is about 10 years. With long-term survival, many patients develop a "spent phase" with myeloid metaplasia and myelofibrosis. Another terminal complication is the transformation to acute myeloblastic leukemia, which occurs in 15% of patients treated with chemotherapy and in 2% of those treated with phlebotomy alone. *(pp. 658–660)*

**12. (E)** The lineage of white cells and the stage of their maturation can be determined by analysis of the cell surface proteins (termed cluster designation or "CD" proteins) that are expressed characteristically (and sometimes exclusively) during different stages of their development. These molecules usually play direct or accessory roles as surface receptors that are essential to cell function. Identification of specific CD molecules on the surfaces of tumor cells by immunohistochemical staining methods using monoclonal antibodies aids in both the diagnosis and the classification of leukocyte neoplasms. CD proteins 1 through 8 are all primarily T-cell–associated antigens. Specific and mutually exclusive expression of CD4 by helper T cells and CD8 by cytotoxic or suppressor T cells definitively differentiates these two T-cell subsets, whereas CD2 and CD7 are expressed on all T cells. CD 19, CD10 (also known as CALLA), CD20, CD21, and CD22 are primarily B-cell–associated antigens. CD14 is a monocyte antigen. Only CD45 and CD11a are present on all leukocytes, irrespective of their lineage. Thus, these antigens would allow the differentiation of a tumor of hematopoietic origin from a carcinoma or sarcoma with similar histopathologic features. *(pp. 172; 637)*

**13. (C)** Increased serum viscosity causes circulatory impairment, particularly in the central nervous system and retina, yielding symptoms such as headache, dizziness, or visual impairment. A hyperviscosity syndrome is a common consequence of hematologic disorders that significantly increase either the number of circulating cellular elements or serum protein levels. Thus, hyperviscosity frequently complicates plasma cell dyscrasias and monoclonal gammopathies, such as immunoglobulin A myeloma and Waldenström's macroglobulinemia, that are characterized by high serum protein levels (massive amounts of immunoglobulin). It is also responsible for the major symptomatic manifestations of polycythemia vera, which greatly increases the circulating erythrocyte number (progeny of aberrant stem cells). The same phenomenon may occur in acute leukemias with very high blast counts. In sickle cell anemia, increased blood viscosity is caused by the inelasticity of sickled red cells. Hyperviscosity in turn contributes to the relative hypoxia that favors further sickling of red cells upstream, eventually leading to complete vascular occlusion and infarction.

In hairy-cell leukemia, the neoplastic B cell proliferation is confined largely to the bone marow, liver, and spleen and the peripheral blood is usually pancytopenic. Leukocytosis is not a common feature and, even when it occurs (in 25% of patients), is not of a magnitude sufficient to produce hyperviscosity. *(pp. 594–599; 656–660; 663–666)*

**14. (E)** Irrespective of their specific cellular subtype, non-Hodgkin's lymphomas with nodular growth patterns have several notable similarities. They are always composed of neoplastic B cells, and their nodularity is a recapitulation of lymphoid follicle formation (denoting differentiated cell function). The cells of nodular lymphomas typically have cleaved or folded nuclear contours, another reflection of their B cell lineage. (B lymphocytes inside normal germinal [follicular] centers have similar nuclear irregularities). In about 85% of cases, the tumor cells of low-grade nodular lymphomas contain a characteristic chromosomal abnormality, a t(14;18) translocation. Follicular lymphomas are all slowly progressive tumors with a long natural history that is largely unaffected by treatment. Thus, although they are low grade, they are relentless and impossible to eradicate. *(pp. 637–638)*

**15. (A)** Myeloid metaplasia with myelofibrosis is a myeloproliferative syndrome characterized by fibrous replacement of the bone marrow and the proliferation of neoplastic myeloid stem cells in extramedullary sites. The spleen is the major site of the neoplastic extramedullary hematopoiesis (myeloid metaplasia) and is usually enlarged enormously, weighing up to 4000 gm. The blood elements produced in this disease have numerous cytologic abnormalities. Particularly characteristic are teardrop-shaped erythrocytes and giant platelets. Myeloblasts, myelocytes, and metamyelocytes typically constitute a small fraction of the white cell population on the peripheral smear in myelofibrosis, so the disease sometimes can be difficult to differentiate from chronic myelogenous leukemia. In myeloid metaplasia, however, leukocyte alkaline phosphatase levels often are elevated, whereas in chronic myelogenous leukemia they are characteristically low.

The fibroblast populations responsible for the marrow fibrosis in myelofibrosis are neither clonal proliferations nor progeny of the neoplastic stem cells. They represent reactive proliferations that are responding to inappropriate production of growth factors by neoplastic megakaryocytes. *(pp. 660–662)*

**16. (D)** Paroxysmal nocturnal hemoglobinuria (see Questions 56 through 67), myeloid metaplasia with myelofibrosis (see Question 15), aplastic anemia (see Question 4), and polycythemia vera (see Question 11) are all myeloid stem cell disorders. Although their etiologies and manifestations are completely different, they have one unfortunate feature in common—predisposition to acute leukemia. In each disease, a small but well-defined proportion of cases is complicated by terminal transformation to acute leukemia. Hairy-cell leukemia is a rare B-cell neoplasm (not a stem cell disorder) and has no predisposition to evolve into acute leukemia. *(pp. 602; 614; 656–660)*

**17. (B)** The Working Formulation for Clinical Usage is a widely used classification of lymphomas based on survival statistics. It has three grades; low, intermediate, and high, with average 10-year survival rates of 45%, 26%, and 23%, respectively. Each grade includes several morphologically defined categories. Lymphomas with the most favorable prognosis (low grade) include: (1) small lymphocytic lymphoma; (2) follicular, predominantly small cleaved cell lymphoma; and (3) follicular, mixed small cleaved and large-cell lymphoma. Intermediate-grade lymphomas include: (1) follicular, predominantly large-cell lymphoma; (2) diffuse small cleaved cell lymphoma; (3) diffuse mixed small- and large-cell lymphoma; and (4) diffuse large-cell lymphoma. Three high-grade lymphomas are defined: (1) large-cell immunoblastic lymphoma; (2) lymphoblastic lymphoma; and (3) small noncleaved cell lymphoma, including Burkitt's lymphoma. Although it may not appear so, the Working Formulation actually represents a simplified approach to this complex group of malignancies and to numerous previous classification schemes that were even more complex. *(pp. 634–641)*

**18. (E)** Chronic myelogenous leukemia (CML) represents a clonal neoplastic proliferation of multipotent myeloid stem cells. CML is unique among the myeloid stem cell disorders because the affected stem cells and their progeny have a characteristic chromosomal abnormality, the Ph (Philadelphia) chromosome (representing a reciprocal translocation between chromosomes 9 and 22), in more than 90% of cases. Although the abnormal stem cells of CML give rise to erythroid, granulocytic, and megakaryocytic precursors, the granulocytic series predominantes. In contrast to the situation in acute myelogenous leukemia, granulocyte maturation is not blocked, and a vast number of mature leukemic cells fill the bone marrow and peripheral blood. Although they look identical to normal neutrophils, leukemic neutrophils of CML can be distinguished by their near-total lack of alkaline phosphatase. Another characteristic feature of CML is extreme splenomegaly. Chemotherapy is an unsatisfactory method of treatment for CML and does not alter the median survival time. The inevitable course of the disease is terminal transition to an acute leukemic phase known as "blast crisis." *(pp. 654–655)*

**19. (True); 20. (False); 21. (True); 22. (False); 23. (False); 24. (True); 25. (True)**

Hodgkin's disease (HD) long has been classified separately from the non-Hodgkin's lymphomas on the basis of its numerous unique features. **(19)** Hodgkin's disease is characterized by a proliferation of giant neoplastic cells of probable lymphoid lineage known as Reed-Sternberg (RS) cells. The RS cell is the only malignant element in Hodgkin's disease. In each of the histologic subtypes of Hodgkin's disease, RS cells are associated with a variable number of other leukocytes, but these so-called background cells are reactive rather than neoplastic in nature. RS cells are always lymphocytic in origin, but the lineage may be either T cell or B cell in any given case. Only in the nodular form of lymphocyte-predominant Hodgkin's disease is the RS always of B-cell origin.

**(20)** The most common subtype of Hodgkin's disease is nodular sclerosis, representing about 40% of cases. Mixed cellularity, lymphocyte-predominant, and lymphocyte-depleted subtypes of Hodgkin's disease follow in descending order of frequency. **(21)** No matter what the subtype, Hodgkin's disease almost always spreads by contiguity from one chain of lymph nodes to the adjacent group, a feature rarely associated with non-Hodgkin's lymphoma. **(22)** In further contrast to most non-Hodgkin's lymphomas, Hodgkin's disease (of any type) rarely manifests a leukemic state.

**(23)** Although the subtypes of Hodgkin's disease, based on the relative numbers of RS cells and background cells, are associated with differences in clinical behavior, they are far less important than clinical staging as indicators of prognosis.

**(24)** Although the pathogenesis of Hodgkin's disease is still obscure, it has been suggested that it may represent a consequence of delayed infection with a common viral agent. Usually cited in support of this hypothesis is the resemblance of the RS cell to a virally transformed cell and the increased incidence (two- to threefold) of Hodgkin's disease in young adults with Epstein-Barr virus infection (infectious mononucleosis). Moreover, Epstein-Barr virus genomes (in clonal patterns) can be identified in the RS cells in 40 to 50% of cases of Hodgkin's disease.

**(25)** Although the modern aggressive modes of therapy largely have obliterated the prognostic differences between the various subtypes of Hodgkin's disease and significantly improved survival, it appears that this has not happened without a cost. Long-term survivors of combined chemotherapy and radiotherapy have a significantly increased risk of secondary cancers, including acute nonlymphocytic leukemia and lung cancer (most frequently) as well as non-Hodgkin's lymphoma, breast cancer, gastric cancer, and malignant melanoma. *(pp. 643–648)*

**26. (D); 27. (B); 28. (A); 29. (C); 30. (A); 31. (B)**

Immunohemolytic anemias are characterized by the production of anti–red cell antibodies that either directly produce hemolysis or indirectly lead to increased red cell destruction. The type of antibody generated determines to a large extent the nature of the resultant disorder and forms the basis of the classification of these disorders.

**(26 and 27)** In cold agglutinin immune hemolytic anemia (IHA), the antibodies produced are primarily monoclonal complement-fixing immunoglobulin M. Although the antibodies in warm antibody IHA are usually immunoglobulin G, they do not appear to be of monoclonal origin nor do they usually fix complement.

**(28)** Warm antibody IHA often occurs in association with drugs. The drug acts as a hapten in inducing an immune response to red cells (e.g., penicillin, quinidine, and phenacetin) or may initiate directly the production of antibodies that are directed against intrinsic red cell antigens such as the Rh blood group antigens (e.g., α-methyldopa). **(29)** In contrast to drug-associated IHA, lymphoma-associated IHA may be of either the warm antibody or cold agglutinin type.

**(30)** In warm antibody IHA, most of the red cell destruction is not due to intravascular hemolysis. Instead, antibody-coated red cells are bound to Fc receptors on monocytes and splenic macrophages and undergo spheroidal transformation as parts of their cell membrane are ingested by the phagocytes to which they are attached. The spherocytes (like those that occur in the hereditary spherocytosis—see Question 1) then are susceptible to splenic sequestration and destruction. Thus, splenomegaly is a common feature of warm antibody IHA. In cold agglutinin IHA, both intravascular hemolysis and extravascular destruction occur, and splenomegaly does not typically occur.

**(31)** Only in cold agglutinin IHA does intravascular hemolysis occur with frequency. The agglutinating antibodies bind to red cells, fix complement, and induce hemolysis at low temperatures (e.g., in the extremities). However, at core body temperatures, the bound antibodies are released, leaving only bound complement (specifically C3b) on the cell membrane. These complement-coated cells are then susceptible to phagocytosis in the spleen and liver. *(pp. 601–602)*

**32. (D); 33. (C); 34. (B); 35. (C); 36. (C); 37. (B); 38. (C); 39. (C); 40. (B); 41. (B); 42. (C); 43. (A)**

Acute leukemias are dramatic neoplastic proliferations of white blood cell precursors that do not undergo normal maturation (i.e., the cells are arrested at early stages of maturation). The acute leukemias are characterized by markedly increased numbers of circulating immature white cells ("blasts"). Although they have many overlapping features, acute leukemias of lymphocytic origin differ from those of nonlymphocytic origin in both pathologic and clinical behavior.

**(32)** A feature common to both acute lymphocytic leukemia (ALL) and acute myelogenous leukemia (AML) is their occurrence predominantly in the young. ALL is the most frequent type of leukemia in children under 15 years of age, whereas AML occurs mainly in young adults (the 15- to 39-year-old age group). **(36)** Another feature characteristic of both forms of acute leukemia is the suppression of normal hematopoiesis, the combined result of bone marrow replacement by neoplastic cells and tumor-induced humoral inhibition. **(39)** The result is anemia, fever caused by infection in the absence of normal leukocytes, and thrombocytopenia with bleeding (e.g., gingival bleeding, petechiae, epistaxis). **(42)** The marrow expansion in both ALL and AML leads to subperiosteal bone infiltration, bone resorption, and bone pain. **(33)** In both forms of acute leukemia, chromosomal abnormalities are found in the leukemic cells in about 90% of cases. Some of the numerical or structural changes in the chromosomes have prognostic significance. For example, in ALL, hyperploidy is associated with a good prognosis and translocations are associated with a poor prognosis.

**(34)** By routine histologic examination, ALL and AML may be difficult to distinguish from one another, because both are composed of a uniform population of undifferentiated blast elements. However, the cell of origin can be determined by special enzymatic, histochemical, and/or immunohistochemical marker studies. For example, the blasts of ALL express the pan B-cell antigen CD19 in almost every case. In AML, monoclonal antibodies that recognize determinants on various myelomonocytic cells are useful in establishing the diagnosis. Distinguising histologic features of some AML cells include intracytoplasmic azurophilic granules and, in some cases, distinctive red-staining needle-like structures known as Auer rods. Lymphoblasts contain neither cytoplasmic granules nor Auer rods.

**(35)** The Philadelphia chromosome, a reciprocal translocation from a long arm of chromosome 22 to chromosome 9, is a characteristic feature of *chronic* myelogenous leukemia (CML). It is present in more than 90% of cases of CML. However, it sometimes (uncommonly) occurs in acute leukemias as well. When present in either ALL (2- to 5% of childhood cases; 15% of adult cases) or AML (3% of cases), it is associated with a poor prognosis.

**(37)** Patients treated with chemotherapy and radiotherapy for Hodgkin's disease are at increased risk of developing AML and non-Hodgkin's lymphomas. ALL, however, does not occur with increased frequency in these patients (see Question 25).

**(38)** Clinical features are often helpful in differentiating ALL from AML. Generalized lymphadenopathy, splenomegaly, and hepatomegaly are characteristic of both but may be more prominent in ALL. **(40)** Distinctive clinical features of AML include infiltration of gums (in the M4 and M5 classes of AML) and of soft tissues (in the M1 and M3 classes) by tumor cells. **(41)** Tumorous accumulations of AML cells in soft tissues often have a greenish color and are known as "chloromas."

**(43)** The response to treatment is markedly different in ALL and AML. The ability to achieve complete remission in 90% and cure in about 66% of children with ALL represents a triumph of modern chemotherapy. Current treatment modalities for AML, in contrast, achieve 5-year survival in only 15 to 30% of cases. Thus, allogeneic bone marrow transplantation may be a more effective method of treatment in this disease. *(649–654)*

**44. (C); 45. (D); 46. (A); 47. (D); 48. (B); 49. (A); 50. (B)**

**(44)** Idiopathic thrombocytopenic purpura (ITP) and thrombotic thrombocytopenic purpura (TTP) are both hemorrhagic disorders related to reduced platelet number (and, hence, have increased bleeding time). **(47)** The coagulation system is unaffected in these disorders (thus, prothrombin times and partial thromboplastin times are usually normal).

**(46)** ITP is an autoimmune thrombocytopenia associated with antiplatelet antibodies. **(49)** Although ITP usually appears as a primary disease, it sometimes occurs in association with another autoimmune disease, such as systemic lupus erythematosus. **(45)** Antibody-coated platelets are destroyed in the spleen, but the spleen remains normal in size. In the bone marrow, megakaryocytes usually are increased to compensate for the peripheral destruction of platelets. The disease can be treated effectively with steroids and/or splenectomy.

**(48)** TTP is a platelet consumption syndrome of unknown etiology characterized by widespread platelet thrombi throughout the body that cause a microangiopathic hemolytic anemia. **(45)** Neither antiplatelet antibodies nor immunologically mediated splenic platelet destruction occurs in TTP. The injury is thought to be related primarily to an acquired endothelial abnormality or injury predisposing to secondary platelet aggregation. **(50)** This rare disorder is life-threatening and uniformly fatal unless treated aggressively with corticosteroids, platelet aggregation inhibitors, and exchange transfusions. Even with treatment, as many as 20% of patients succumb. *(pp. 618–619)*

**51. (B); 52. (C); 53. (A); 54. (B); 55. (B)**

**(51)** Only chronic leukemias, with their insidious onset and indolent course, may be, for a time, asymptomatic; acute leukemias are characteristically abrupt in onset and highly symptomatic (with fatigue, fever/infection, bleeding). This is the case whether the leukemia is lymphoid or myeloid in origin.

**(52)** The vast majority of lymphocytic leukemias, both acute and chronic, are composed of neoplastic B cells. T-cell leukemias are rare. In acute lymphocytic leukemia (ALL), the prognosis correlates with the degree of differentiation (maturation) of the B cells, as reflected by cell surface markers. For example, early precursor B-cell ALL has the most favorable prognosis. **(53)** The presence of hyperdiploidly (>50 chromosomes) also is associated with a good prognosis.

There is no staging system for acute leukemia. **(54)** In contrast, clinical stage is the most important determinant of prognosis in chronic lymphocytic leukemia (CLL), and cytogenic factors are of less significance. **(55)** Most CLL cells express surface immunoglobulin (monoclonal kappa or lambda light chains) and are more mature than ALL cells. Nevertheless, CLL cells are unable to differentiate into plasma cells. *(pp. 649–650; 655–656)*

**56. (D); 57. (C); 58. (B); 59. (D); 60. (C); 61. (B); 62. (B); 63. (B); 64. (A); 65. (A); 66. (D); 67. (E)**

β-Thalassemia, paroxysmal nocturnal hemoglobinuria (PNH), sickle cell anemia, and glucose-6-phosphate dehydrogenase (G6PD) deficiency are all major forms of hemolytic anemias. The unique pathogenetic defect in each disorder produces distinctive, sometimes pathognomonic, features.

**(56)** G6PD deficiency produces derangements in the hexose monophosphate shunt and glutathione metabolism. Glutathione is essential for red cell protection against oxidant injury, so oxidant substances, such as the antimalarial drugs, trigger red cell injury and hemolysis in affected individuals. **(59)** Heinz bodies (precipitates of denatured hemoglobin) from within the red cells of G6PD-deficient individuals when oxidation of the sulfhydryl group of globin chains occurs. Heinz bodies contribute to the demise of the red cell in two ways: (1) they render the red cell membrane to which they are attached less deformable and more prone to sequestration in the spleen; and (2) when they are "pitted" from the cell by splenic macrophages, the resultant loss of cell membrane produces spherocytes that are themselves more susceptible to splenic sequestration. **(66)** Unlike the other forms of hemolytic anemias that produce chronic continual red cell destruction, G6PD deficiency produces intermittent bouts of acute hemolysis. It does not, therefore, lead to prolonged stimulation of erythropoietic production with expansion of the erythron in the bone marrow.

**(57)** Sickle cell anemia classically produces a unique if somewhat poorly understood depression of splenic function, even while the spleen is enlarged early in the course of the disease. The resultant splenic hypofunction predisposes to blood-borne infections, especially to those caused by *Salmonella* and pneumococci. Later in the course of the disease, the spleen actually may undergo autoinfarction as a result of repeated bouts of sickling in the sinuses, leading to thrombosis, hypoxic injury, and resultant scarring. Predisposition to bacterial infection is a major consequence of splenectomy (functional or surgical) in any individual. **(60)** It is the deoxygenated form of sickle hemoglobin that undergoes polymerization and causes red cell deformation, so hypoxia is the major stimulus to sickling and hemolytic crises.

**(58, 61 and 62)** In contrast to thalassemia, sickle cell anemia, and G6PD deficiency (all of which affect red cell function only), PNH produces functional abnormalities in all hematopoietic cell lines. PNH is a disorder of stem cells that is characterized by a cell membrane defect (deficiency of anchor proteins that link complement-inactivating proteins to the cell membrane) that renders all blood cells more sensitive to complement-mediated lysis. In patients with PNH, the striking predisposition to intravascular thromboses and infection is evidence of the platelet and granulocyte abnormalities, respectively. **(63)** Like other hematopoietic stem cell disorders, PNH may evolve into acute myelogenous leukemia as a terminal event.

**(64)** Although the other forms of hemolytic anemia can be severe and debilitating, $\beta$-thalassemia clearly has the worst prognosis. The disease produces such a profound, transfusion-dependent anemia that most patients die at an early age unless aggessively supported by transfusions. Even with medical therapy, the average age at death is 17 years. Currently, bone marrow transplantation from human leukocyte antigen–identical sibling is the only curative therapy. **(65)** In this disorder, which is caused by a defect in the synthesis of $\beta$-globin chains (see Question 8), red cell precursors characteristically are destroyed within the marrow (a phenomenon known as ineffective erythropoiesis). This occurs because the free $\alpha$-globin chains form unstable intracellular aggregates that are injurious to the red cell precursors. In severely affected patients, it is estimated that 70 to 85% of the marrow normoblasts are destroyed in situ. This contrasts with the other forms of hemolytic anemia, in which red cell destruction is primarily extramedullary.

**(67)** All four of these diseases are the result of an intrinsic defect in the red cell. In contrast to immune hemolytic anemias, which represent acquired disorders of red cells and often are associated with antibodies reactive with erythrocytes, these disorders are not associated with immunologically mediated red cell destruction. *(pp. 591–602)*

**68. (A); 69. (A); 70. (D); 71. (B); 72. (A); 73. (A); 74. (E); 75. (A); 76. (B); 77. (B)**

**(68)** Hemorrhagic disorders occur when an abnormality of vessel walls, platelets, coagulation factors, or a combination of these is present. In Cushing's syndrome, vascular fragility predisposing to skin hemorrhages results from the protein wasting effect of excessive corticosteroids.

**(69)** Likewise, the hemorrhagic diathesis in hereditary hemorrhagic telangiectasia is caused by vascular fragility, but in this disorder, the defect is primary to the vascular walls, which are extremely thin and prone to disruption and bleeding.

**(70)** In von Willebrand's disease, the von Willebrand's factor (vWF) component of the factor VIII-vWF complex is qualitatively or quantitatively defective. Von Willebrand's factor consists of a series of variably sized polypeptide multimers that are linked to the procoagulant protein of factor VIII, the enzymatic portion of the molecule responsible for the activation of factor X in the intrinsic coagulation pathway. The major function of vWF is the facilitation of platelet adhesion to subendothelial collagen. Thus, a prolonged bleeding time (a measure of platelet function) and a marked tendency toward spontaneous bleeding occur in von Willebrand's disease.

**(71)** Blood stored for longer than 24 hours is virtually depleted of platelets, so massive transfusions can produce a hemorrhagic diathesis simply by diluting platelets to thrombocytopenic levels. In the presence of a normal bone marrow, the effect is transient.

**(72)** Widespread weakening of vascular walls, with resultant hemorrhage, is a common feature of hypersensitivity vasculitides. Henoch-Schönlein purpura is a prototypic example of immune complex–mediated vascular damage with a resultant hemorrhagic diathesis.

**(73)** Direct damage to the vascular wall occurs in certain infections caused by organisms that have the ability to invade vessels. Rickettsial infections, for example, classically cause vascular damage and a hemorrhagic diathesis (see Chapter 4, Question 8).

**(74)** Disseminated intravascular coagulation is a well-known complication of promyelogenous leukemia (the M3 subclass of AML). In this disorder, the release of procoagulant substances from the granules of the neoplastic promyelocytes activates the coagulation cascade, producing disseminated coagulation and an attendant hemorrhagic diathesis.

**(75)** Vitamin C is required for cross-linking and other events in normal collagen metabolism, so scurvy causes structural weakness of collagen in connective tissues and blood vessel walls (see Chapter 3, Question 9). Abnormal bleeding is the result of vascular fragility.

**(76)** Folate deficiency causes a megaloblastic anemia with defective production of all hematopoietic elements (see Chapter 3, Questions 49 and 50). Ineffective megakaryocyte production of platelets results in thrombocytopenia and abnormal bleeding.

**(77)** Thrombocytopenia is also one of the most common hematologic manifestations of the acquired immunodeficiency syndrome (AIDS). It is believed to be multifactorial, but contributing mechanisms are immune complex–mediated injury, formation of antiplatelet antibodies, and human immunodeficiency virus suppression of megakaryocytes. *(pp. 616–618)*

**78. (A); 79; (A); 80. (C); 81. (A); 82. (B); 83. (C); 84. (A)**

Drugs and chemicals cause numerous hematologic problems. Although drug-related hematologic disorders are seldom completely predictable, many are associated repeatedly with particular drugs or drug classes. Many of these hematologic effects are among the most important complications of drug therapy.

**(78)** Penicillin is the prototype for drugs which act antigenically as haptens. It combines with the red cell membrane, induces antibody production to the drug–red cell antigen complex, and produces a warm antibody immune hemolytic anemia.

**(79)** $\alpha$-Methyldopa is also a prototype drug associated with immune hemolytic anemia, but in contrast to penicillin, it directly initiates the production of antibodies against intrinsic cell antigens.

**(80)** Thiouracil is one of a small number of drugs that often is associated with agranulocytosis, probably on the basis of decreased production and/or increased destruction of neutrophils. Thiouracil also may cause an immunologically mediated destruction of mature neutrophils.

**(81)** Quinidine is a drug often responsible for the genesis of immune hemolytic anemia. In contrast to both penicillin and $\alpha$-methyldopa, however, the drug serves as a hapten that binds to a plasma protein. The drug-protein complex, in turn, evokes antibody production. It is the attachment of the resultant complement-fixing immune complexes to the red cell membranes that mediates their destruction. **(84)** Phenacetin is another drug associated with the induction of immune hemolytic anemia by this same mechanism.

**(82)** Exposure to benzene is a well-known cause of acquired aplastic anemia. It is one of a number of toxic drugs that cause myeloid stem cell damage in a dose-related manner.

**(83)** Along with thiouracil and certain sulfonamides, aminopyrine is one of the drugs associated with immunologically mediated agranulocytosis. *(pp. 602; 614; 630)*

**85. (B); 86. (C); 87. (B); 88. (A); 89. (D)**

Reactive proliferations of white cells represent a normal host response to inflammatory stimuli. The relative degree of stimulation of each of the white cell series varies with the underlying cause. Certain inflammatory conditions classically stimulate one of the white cell lines much more strongly than the others, a feature that can be helpful in diagnosis.

**(85 and 87)** An elevated lymphocyte count (lymphocytosis) is usually immunologic in origin. It often accompanies chronic inflammatory states with sustained immunologic stimulation, such as tuberculosis. Lymphocytosis is also common in viral infections, such as infectious mononucleosis, in which the primary host response is immunologic and little acute inflammation is produced.

**(86)** Bronchial asthma is a prototypic example of a type I immune response with production of immunoglobulin E that affixes to mast cells and stimulates mast cell degranulation on exposure to the inciting antigen (see Chapter 6, Question 27). Mast cells then release their eosinophil chemotactic factor, and an eosinophilic leukocytosis occurs.

**(88)** Elevated neutrophil counts (polymorphonuclear leukocytosis) characteristically occur in association with acute inflammatory states such as those produced by bacterial infection or tissue necrosis. The muscle necrosis that accompanies acute myocardial infarction classically produces this response.

**(89)** Eosinophilic granuloma is a unifocal proliferative disorder of Langerhans' cells. Eosinophils are a variable, although frequently prominent, feature of the parenchymal lesions that usually involve the bone marrow. However, systemic elevation of eosinophils usually does not occur, and standard hematologic tests tend to be nondiagnostic in this disease. *(pp. 631–632; 667)*

**90. (B); 91. (A); 92. (A); 93. (D); 94. (C)**

**(91 and 92)** Proliferative disorders of Langerhans' cells (bone marrow–derived, antigen-presenting dendritic cells) vary widely in their clinical and pathologic behavior. The Letterer-Siwe syndrome, also known as acute disseminated Langerhans' cell histiocytosis, is an acute systemic proliferation of Langerhans' cells that has an aggressive clinical course. It typically occurs in infants and young children under the age of 3 and is sometimes present at birth. Although untreated disease is uniformly fatal, intensive chemotherapy has dramatically altered the outlook for this disease. The overall 5-year survival is 50%.

**(90)** In contrast to the devastating, diffuse disease of the Letterer-Siwe syndrome, multifocal Langerhans' cell histiocytosis (formerly known as Hand-Schüller-Christian disease) is relatively benign. The lesions spontaneously resolve in half the cases, and in the other half, they are cured by chemotherapy. Multifocal Langerhans' cell histiocytosis is characterized by histiocytic infiltrates in multiple tissues, and, in 50% of patients, involvement of the posterior pituitary stalk of the hypothalamus leads to diabetes insipidus.

**(93)** Like normal Langerhans' cells, the Langerhans' cells in all of these proliferation syndromes contain unique rod-shaped cytoplasmic inclusions called pentalaminar bodies or Birbeck granules that can be seen by electron microscopy.

**(94)** In the Letterer-Siwe syndrome, a diffuse macropapular, eczematous, or purpuric skin rash is often present. A seborrhea-like skin eruption is typically present in Hand-Schüller-Christian disease. Only in unifocal Langerhans' cell histiocytosis (eosinophilic granuloma) is involvement limited to the marrow cavity of the bone; involvement of the skin or of other organ systems is characteristically absent. *(pp. 666–667)*

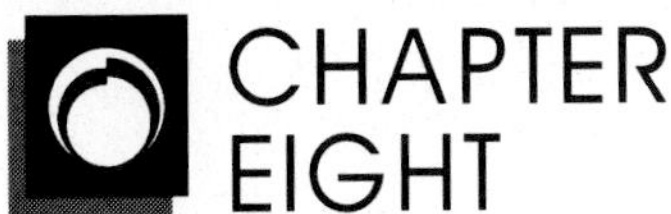

CHAPTER EIGHT

# The Gastrointestinal Tract

**DIRECTIONS:** For Questions 1 through 26, choose the ONE BEST answer to each question.

**1.** The disorder pictured in Figure 8–1 is associated with all of the following features EXCEPT:

A. Autosomal recessive transmission
B. Normal-appearing colon at birth
C. Risk of colon cancer of virtually 100%
D. Multiple osteomas
E. Inherited mutation of a tumor suppressor gene

**2.** Abnormalities associated with achalasia include all of the following EXCEPT:

A. Incomplete relaxation of the lower esophageal sphincter
B. Lack of peristalsis in the esophagus
C. Loss of myenteric ganglion cells in the esophagus
D. Increased basal tone of the lower esophageal sphincter
E. Stenotic muscular hypertrophy of the lower esophageal sphincter

**3.** Cancer patients receiving medical treatment often develop esophagitis from all of the following EXCEPT:

A. Antibiotic toxicity
B. Viral infection
C. Chemotherapeutic agent toxicity
D. Radiation damage
E. Fungal infection

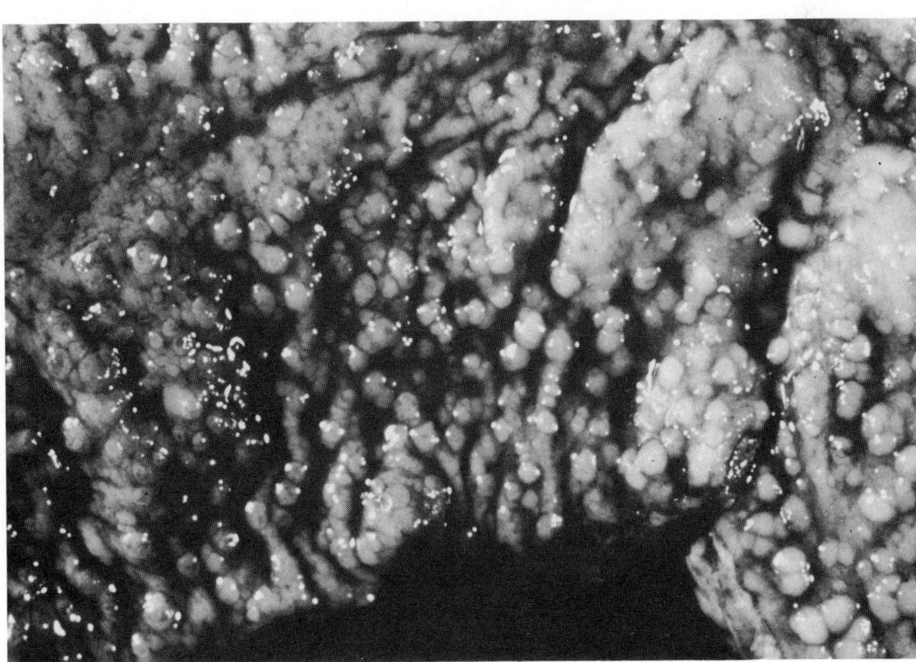

Figure 8–1

**4.** Esophageal disorders that are associated with pulmonary aspiration include all of the following EXCEPT:

A. Esophageal diverticula
B. Achalasia
C. Esophageal involvement by systemic sclerosis (scleroderma)
D. Viral esophagitis
E. Esophageal carcinoma

**5.** The acute gastric ulcerations known as Cushing's ulcers occur in patients who:

A. Ingest nonsteroidal anti-inflammatory drugs
B. Have severe sepsis
C. Have brain tumors
D. Have extensive burns
E. Have Cushing's syndrome

**6.** Mucosal ulceration is a characteristic histologic feature of all of the following causes of infectious enterocolitis EXCEPT:

A. *Entamoeba histolytica*
B. *Salmonella* species
C. *Campylobacter jejuni*
D. *Yersinia enterocolitica*
E. Rotavirus

**7.** All of the following statements about congenital megacolon (Hirschsprung's disease) are true EXCEPT:

A. Both Meissner's and Auerbach's plexuses fail to develop.
B. Involvement of the entire colon is rare.
C. The incidence is higher in patients with Down's syndrome.
D. Massive dilation of the affected bowel segment is characteristic.
E. Surgical excision of the affected segment is curative.

**8.** In the United States, the most likely cause of the form of enterocolitis pictured in Figure 8–2 is:

A. Ingestion of the infectious agent from an exogenous source
B. Reactivation of a previous enteric infection
C. Blood-borne spread from another focus of infection in the body
D. Swallowing of organisms coughed up from a pulmonary source of infection
E. None of these

**9.** All of the following statements about small bowel neoplasms are true EXCEPT:

A. Altogether they account for less than 10% of all gastrointestinal tumors.
B. Malignant tumors and benign tumors occur with nearly equal frequency.
C. Hamartomas occur more frequently than adenomas.
D. Adenocarcinoma occurs more frequently than malignant lymphoma.

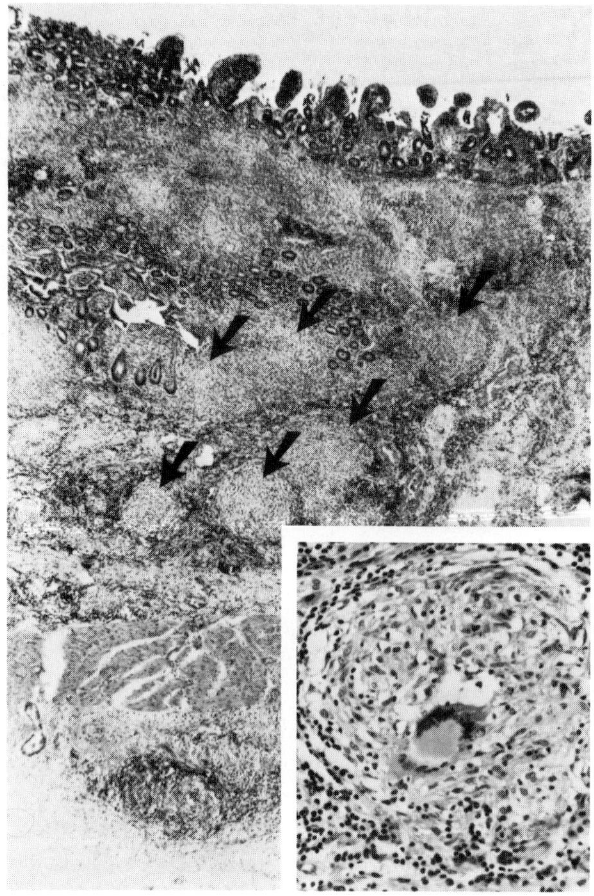

**Figure 8–2**

E. The overall postresection 5-year survival rate in small bowel carcinoma is better than in large bowel carcinoma.

**10.** All of the following statements about celiac sprue are true EXCEPT:

A. It is associated with HLA-DQw2 genotype.
B. Diffuse flattening of mucosal villi is seen histologically.
C. The proximal small bowel is the predominant site of injury.
D. Successful treatment usually requires immunosuppression.
E. The disease is associated with an increased incidence of primary gastrointestinal lymphoma.

**11.** Characteristic gross features of a benign (peptic) gastric ulcer include all of the following EXCEPT:

A. Location on the lesser curvature
B. Small size (less than 2 cm)
C. Irregular margins
D. A smooth base
E. Radial arrangement (puckering) of surrounding mucosal folds

Figure 8–3

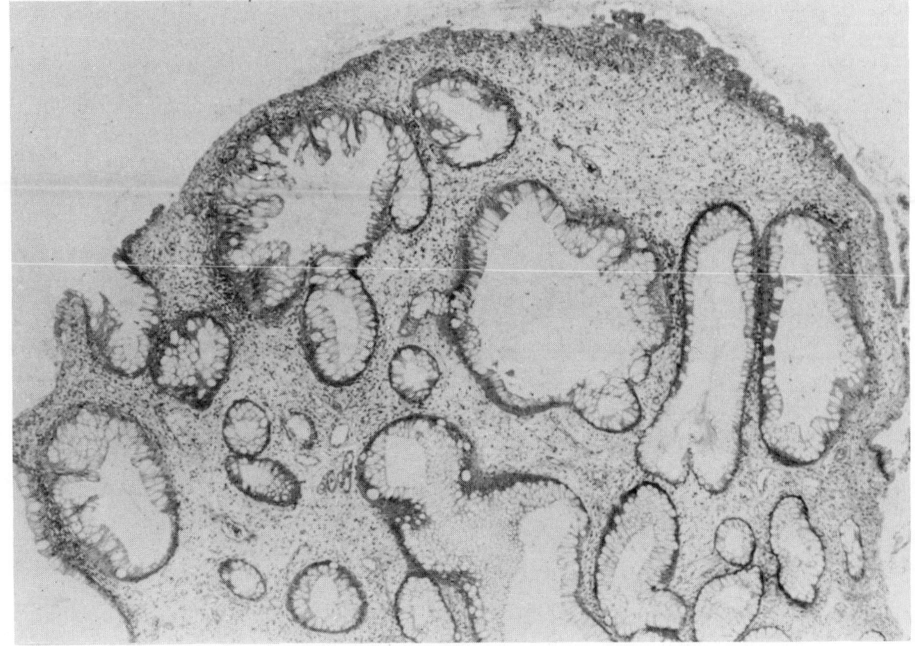

**12.** The lesion pictured in Figure 8–3:

A. Is a hamartoma
B. Occurs in long-standing inflammatory bowel disease
C. Is associated with orofacial melanotic pigmentation
D. Is associated with multiple osteomas
E. Has high potential for malignant transformation

**13.** All of the following statements about the lower esophageal sphincter are true EXCEPT:

A. It prevents reflux of gastric contents.
B. Its function is under neural control.
C. Its tone is unaffected by vagotomy.
D. It relaxes in response to swallowing.
E. It relaxes in response to gastrin.

**14.** All of the following statements about esophageal "webs" are true EXCEPT:

A. They are most often congenital.
B. They are composed of constricting bands of fibrous tissue.
C. They are morphologically identical to lower esophageal "rings."
D. They cause progressive dysphagia.
E. They sometimes are associated with anemia.

**15.** All of the following factors are causally related to the development of reflux esophagitis EXCEPT:

A. Increased gastric volume
B. Impaired clearance of refluxed gastric contents
C. Lower esophageal sphincter dysfunction
D. Increased acid production in the stomach
E. Sliding hiatal hernia

**16.** All of the following characteristics are associated with Barrett's esophagus EXCEPT:

A. Metaplastic goblet cells
B. Metaplastic parietal cells
C. Intranuclear inclusion bodies
D. Epithelial dysplasia
E. Adenocarcinoma of the esophagus

**17.** All of the following factors stimulate gastric acid secretion EXCEPT:

A. Gastric distention
B. Entry of sugars into the stomach
C. Entry of amino acids into the small bowel
D. Vagal stimulation
E. Histamine

**18.** Which of the statements listed below correctly describes angiodysplasia of the colon?

A. It is a frequent cause of lower gastrointestinal bleeding in the neonate.
B. The sigmoid colon is most frequently involved.
C. A congenital defect in the vascular media is present in colonic arterioles.
D. Multiple small arterial aneurysms are present in the submucosa.
E. Surgical resection is the only definitive therapy.

**19.** The "volcanic" lesion in the colon pictured in Figure 8–4 is characteristically produced by:

A. *Entamoeba histolytica*
B. *Clostridium difficile*
C. Enterohemorrhagic *Escherichia coli*
D. *Campylobacter jejuni*
E. *Yersinia enterocolitica*

**20.** In the acquired immunodeficiency syndrome, gastrointestinal disease is caused by all of the following EXCEPT:

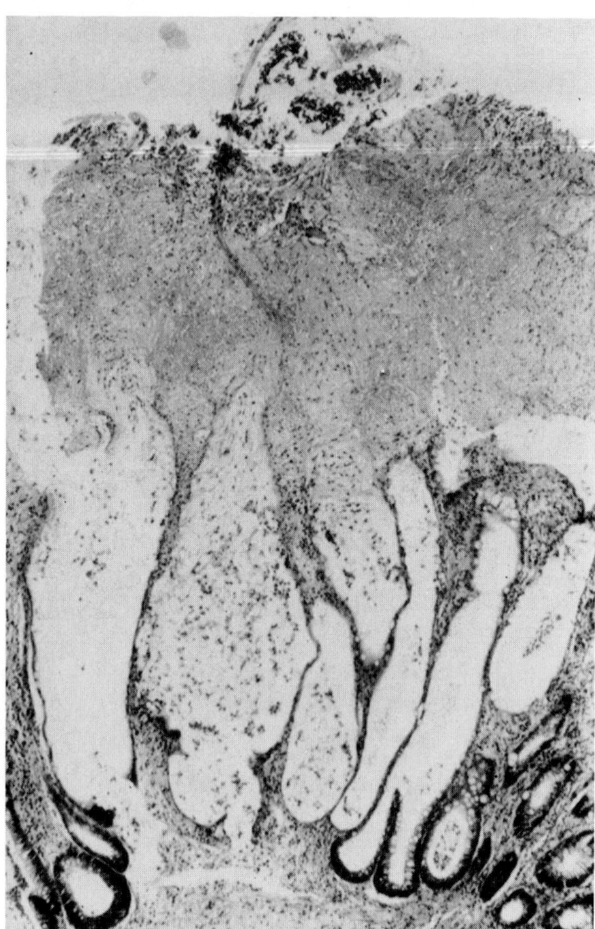

Figure 8–4

A. *Mycobacterium avium intracellulare*
B. *Cryptosporidium parvum*
C. Cytomegalovirus
D. Kaposi's sarcoma
E. *Pneumocystis carinii*

**21.** All of the following statements about acute appendicitis are true EXCEPT:

A. It is the most common acute abdominal condition treated surgically.
B. It is mainly a disease of adolescents.
C. Its clinical presentation resembles that of mesenteric lymphadenitis.
D. The diagnostic histologic feature is mucosal lymphoid hyperplasia.
E. It is accompanied by luminal obstruction in most cases.

**22.** Histologic changes commonly seen in reflux esophagitis include all of the following EXCEPT:

A. Intraepithelial eosinophils
B. Intraepithelial neutrophils
C. Hyperplasia of the mucosal basal zone
D. Elongated stromal papillae
E. Submucosal varices

**23.** All of the following statements about sporadic lymphomas of the gastrointestinal tract are true EXCEPT:

A. They most commonly involve the stomach.
B. The tumors are almost always of B-cell lineage.
C. They have a better prognosis than lymphomas arising in lymph nodes.
D. They usually arise in the lymph nodes of the associated mesentery.
E. It is possible to treat them effectively with surgical resection.

**24.** All of the following statements about acquired lactase deficiency are true EXCEPT:

A. It is the most common disaccharidase deficiency.
B. It is caused by a hypersensitivity immune response to milk (lactose).
C. It produces an osmotic diarrhea.
D. It produces no specific histopathologic changes of the mucosa on biopsy.
E. It is treated by dietary restriction.

**25.** All of the following descriptions apply to the disorder pictured in Figure 8–5 EXCEPT:

A. It occurs in an otherwise normal bowel.
B. It depends on peristalsis for development.
C. It causes intestinal obstruction.
D. It causes intestinal infarction.
E. It rarely occurs in children.

All of the following features are characteristic of the disorder pictured in Figure 8–6 EXCEPT:

A. Autosomal recessive transmission
B. Expression of disease early in life
C. Production of a malabsorption syndrome
D. Association with increased levels of very low density lipoproteins in the plasma
E. Association with acanthocytes ("burr cells") in the peripheral blood

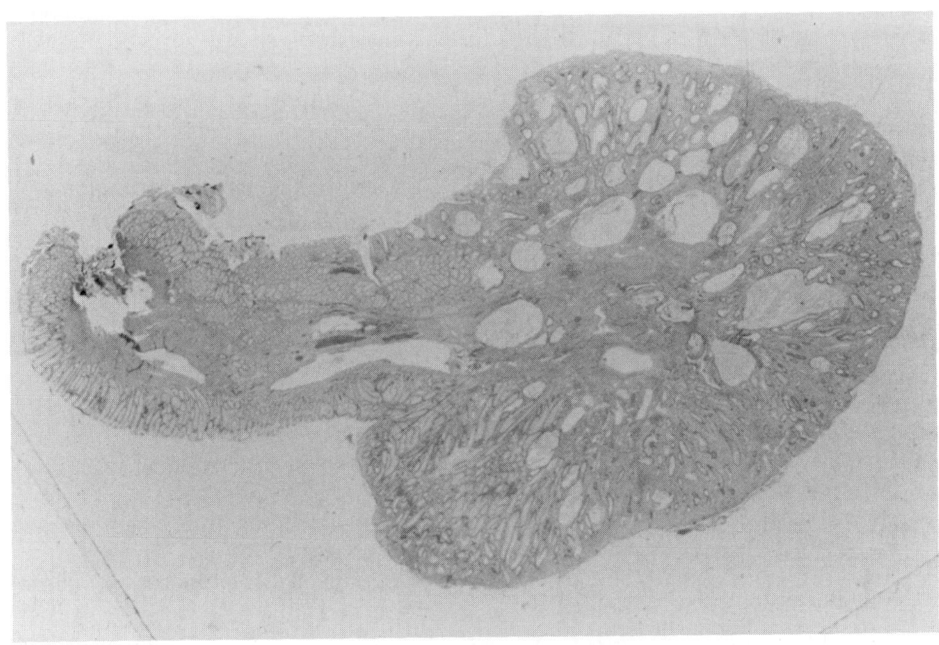

**Figure 8–5**

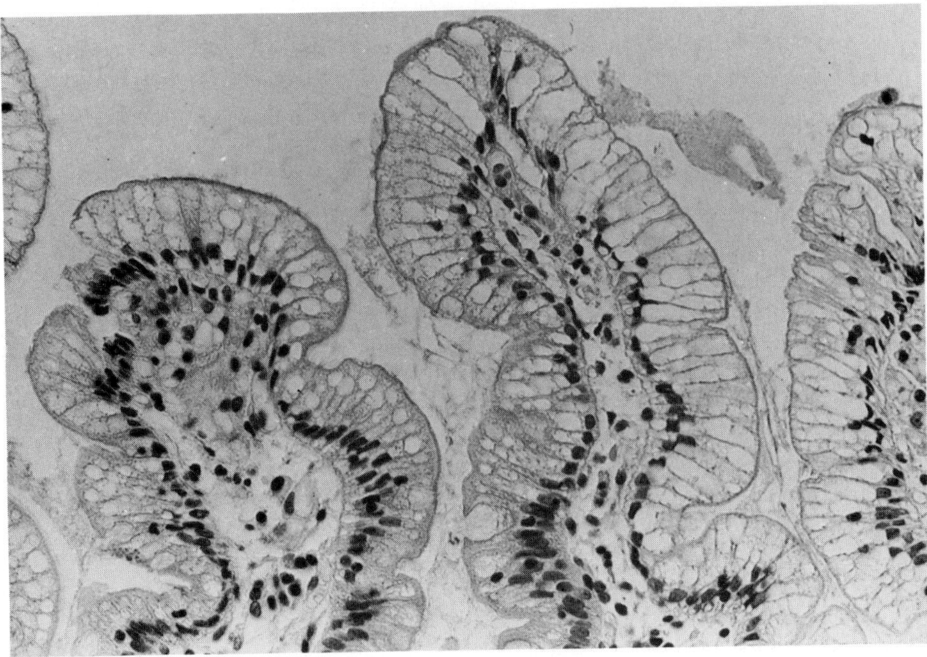

**Figure 8–6**

**DIRECTIONS:** For Questions 27 through 66, you are to decide whether EACH choice is TRUE or FALSE.

For each of the following statements about the normal esophagus, choose whether it is TRUE or FALSE.

**27.** The mucosa is composed of squamous epithelium that does not keratinize.
**28.** The serosal surface is lined by a single layer of mesothelial cells.
**29.** The wall of the upper third of the esophagus is composed of striated muscle.
**30.** Esophageal sphincters are composed of hypertrophied segments of muscularis mucosae.
**31.** The lumen narrows at the level of the bifurcation of the trachea.

For each of the following statements about esophageal varices, choose whether it is TRUE or FALSE.

**32.** They occur in the majority of patients with alcoholic cirrhosis.
**33.** They rarely are produced by biliary cirrhosis.
**34.** They are a common cause of epigastric pain in alcoholic patients.
**35.** Their rupture is associated with a high mortality rate.

For each of the following statements about peptic ulcer disease, choose whether it is TRUE or FALSE.

**36.** Peptic ulcers occur most commonly in the stomach.
**37.** Peptic ulcers occur most often as solitary lesions.
**38.** Peptic ulcers do not develop in individuals with achlorhydria.
**39.** Most patients with duodenal peptic ulcers secrete abnormally high levels of gastric acid.
**40.** Most patients with gastric peptic ulcers also have chronic gastritis.
**41.** Most patients with peptic ulcers are infected with *Helicobacter pylori*.
**42.** Most peptic ulcers eventually require surgical resection.
**43.** Most gastric carcinomas arise in gastric peptic ulcers.
**44.** Most duodenal carcinomas arise in duodenal peptic ulcers.

For each of the following statements about diverticular disease of the colon, choose whether it is TRUE or FALSE.

**45.** About half of Americans in the over-60 age group are affected by diverticular disease.
**46.** Multiple aneurysmal outpouchings of the colonic wall are characteristic of diverticula.
**47.** The cecum is the colonic region most frequently involved by the disease.
**48.** The muscularis propria between diverticula is characteristically hypertrophied.
**49.** Diverticulitis is initiated by diverticular perforation.
**50.** High-fiber diets have been shown to prevent development of the disease.
**51.** Surgical resection is required for most patients with acute diverticulitis.

For each of the following statements about carcinoma of the colon in the United States, choose whether it is TRUE or FALSE.

**52.** Colon carcinoma causes more deaths than any other form of cancer.
**53.** The high incidence of colon cancer is related to low dietary fiber.
**54.** Most colon cancers are detectable on digital rectal exam.
**55.** The vast majority of colon cancers arise from adenomatous polyps.
**56.** Stage is the most important prognostic factor in colon cancer.
**57.** Carcinoembryonic antigen is produced by most tumors.
**58.** Tumors that produce copious mucin have a better prognosis.
**59.** Stool testing for occult blood is a sensitive screening method for colon cancer.
**60.** Surgical resection of early lesions is usually curative.

For each of the following statements about carcinoid tumors, choose whether it is TRUE or FALSE.

**61.** They occur in the lung more often than in the gastrointestinal tract.
**62.** Their degree of histologic atypia (grade) usually correlates well with their metastatic potential.
**63.** They can be identified positively by their cytoplasmic secretory granules.
**64.** Those arising in the appendix rarely metastasize.
**65.** Small bowel carcinoid tumors do not produce the carcinoid syndrome in the absence of liver metastasis.
**66.** Gastrointestinal carcinoids are associated with an increased incidence of other malignant tumors of the gastrointestinal tract.

**DIRECTIONS:** For Questions 67 through 119, the set of lettered headings is followed by a list of numbered words or phrases. For each numbered word or phrase choose:

A—if the item is associated with (A) only
B—if the item is associated with (B) only
C—if the item is associated with *both* (A) and (B)
D—if the item is associated with *neither* (A) nor (B)

For each of the statements listed below, choose whether it describes esophageal carcinoma, gastric carcinoma, both, or neither.

A. Esophageal carcinoma
B. Gastric carcinoma
C. Both
D. Neither

**67.** Nearly all tumors are adenocarcinomas.
**68.** Blacks are affected more than whites.
**69.** Dietary factors are important in the pathogenesis.
**70.** Cigarette smoking is a significant risk factor.
**71.** Alcohol abuse is a significant risk factor.
**72.** Chronic inflammation is the most important predisposing factor.
**73.** Epigastric pain typically develops as an early symptom.
**74.** Krukenberg tumors of the ovary occur as a complication.

For each of the characteristics listed below, choose whether it describes acute gastritis, chronic gastritis, both, or neither.

A. Acute gastritis
B. Chronic gastritis
C. Both
D. Neither

**75.** Is associated with alcohol consumption
**76.** Is associated with cigarette smoking
**77.** Is causally related to autoantibodies against gastric mucosal cells
**78.** Is causally related to gastric mucosal hypoperfusion
**79.** Is associated with the use of aspirin
**80.** Is productive of gastrointestinal bleeding
**81.** Is associated with gastric peptic ulcers
**82.** Is associated with infection by *Helicobacter pylori*

For each of the features listed below, choose whether it describes Ménétrier's disease, the Zollinger-Ellison syndrome, both, or neither.

A. Ménétrier's disease
B. Zollinger-Ellison syndrome
C. Both
D. Neither

**83.** Marked enlargement of gastric rugal folds is characteristic.
**84.** Parietal and chief cell hyperplasia are common histologic features.
**85.** Excessive protein loss is an associated complication.
**86.** The risk of developing gastric lymphoma is increased.
**87.** The risk of developing gastric carcinoma is increased.
**88.** Pancreatic tumors are associated findings.
**89.** Pheochromocytoma and medullary carcinoma of the thyroid are associated disorders.

For each of the characteristics listed below, choose whether it describes hyperplastic gastric polyps, adenomatous gastric polyps, both, or neither.

A. Hyperplastic gastric polyps
B. Adenomatous gastric polyps
C. Both
D. Neither

**90.** Tend to be large (greater than 3.0 cm)
**91.** Usually occur in multiple numbers
**92.** Are commonly asymptomatic
**93.** Frequently undergo malignant transformation
**94.** Often are associated with carcinoma elsewhere in the stomach

For each of the features of inflammatory bowel disease listed below, choose whether it describes Crohn's disease, ulcerative colitis, both, or neither.

A. Crohn's disease
B. Ulcerative colitis
C. Both
D. Neither

**95.** Lesions occur at any level of the gastrointestinal tract.
**96.** Organ systems other than the gastrointestinal tract occasionally are involved.
**97.** The presence of granulomata is pathognomonic.
**98.** Viral particles usually are found in diseased bowel.
**99.** The disorder is associated with histocompatibility antigen HLA-B27.
**100.** Affected bowel usually becomes thickened and narrowed.
**101.** Toxic megacolon is an occasional complication.
**102.** Distribution of lesions is generally discontinuous.
**103.** Fissures and fistulas are characteristic.
**104.** Risk of amyloidosis is increased.
**105.** Incidence of gastrointestinal carcinoma is increased.

For each of the features listed below, choose whether it describes ischemic bowel disease producing transmural infarction, mucosal infarction, both, or neither.

A. Transmural bowel infarction
B. Mucosal bowel infarction
C. Both
D. Neither

**106.** Principally affects the small bowel
**107.** Results from venous thrombosis
**108.** Is produced by arterial occlusion
**109.** Is produced by atherosclerosis and hypotension
**110.** Is produced by hypotension alone
**111.** Grossly appears hemorrhagic
**112.** Is associated with a high mortality rate

For each of the characteristics listed below, choose whether it describes tropical sprue, Whipple's disease, both, or neither.

A. Tropical sprue
B. Whipple's disease
C. Both
D. Neither

**113.** The disease causes a malabsorption syndrome.
**114.** History of travel to an endemic area is essential to establishing the diagnosis.
**115.** Small bowel biopsy frequently shows flattened villi.
**116.** Antibiotic therapy is usually curative.
**117.** Systemic disease is present in addition to bowel involvement.
**118.** Macrophages laden with rod-shaped bacteria are found in the small bowel mucosa.
**119.** The disease is associated with an increased risk of small bowel lymphoma.

**DIRECTIONS:** Questions 120 through 151 are matching questions. For each numbered item, choose the most likely associated lettered item from those provided. Each numbered item has ONLY ONE answer. Within each group, each lettered item may be the answer to one, more than one, or none of the numbered items.

For each of the following statements about congenital gastrointestinal tract anomalies, choose whether it refers to the esophagus, stomach, small bowel, or large bowel.

A. Esophagus
B. Stomach
C. Small bowel
D. Large bowel

**120.** The most common location for congenital atresia
**121.** The most common location for a congenital stenosis
**122.** The most common location for congenital duplication
**123.** The most common location for congenital diverticula
**124.** The most common location for congenital absence of ganglion cells

For each of the characteristics listed below, choose whether it is characteristic of the gastric cardia, corpus (body), antrum, all of these regions, or none of these.

A. Cardia
B. Corpus (body)
C. Antrum
D. All of these
E. None of these

**125.** Gastrin production
**126.** Pepsin secretion
**127.** Intrinsic factor production
**128.** Location of endocrine (enterochromaffin) cells
**129.** Location of goblet cells
**130.** Location of Paneth's cells

For each of the features listed below, choose whether it is characteristic of the duodenum, jejunum, ileum, all of these segments of small bowel, or none of these.

A. Duodenum
B. Jejunum
C. Ileum
D. All of these
E. None of these

**131.** Paneth's cells
**132.** Peyer's patches
**133.** Brunner's glands
**134.** Serotonin-secreting endocrine cells
**135.** Vitamin $B_{12}$–intrinsic factor absorption
**136.** Meckel's diverticulum
**137.** Pancreatic rests

For each of the characteristics listed below, choose whether it describes *Salmonella* enterocolitis, *Shigella* enterocolitis, cholera, or none of these.

A. *Salmonella* enterocolitis
B. *Shigella* enterocolitis
C. Cholera
D. None of these

**138.** Shallow mucosal ulcers typically are produced.
**139.** Submucosal lymphoid hyperplasia is a characteristic feature.
**140.** Submucosal granulomas are a characteristic histologic feature.
**141.** The causative organism does not invade the mucosal epithelium.
**142.** The causative organism does not produce toxins.
**143.** The large bowel is involved preferentially.
**144.** The etiologic agent is a common cause of ulceroinflammatory proctitis in homosexual males.

For each of the features of colonic polyps listed below, choose whether it describes the hyperplastic polyp, tubular adenoma, villous adenoma, hamartomatous polyp, or none of these.

A. Hyperplastic polyp
B. Tubular adenoma
C. Villous adenoma
D. Hamartomatous polyp
E. None of these

**145.** Is the most common type of colonic polyp
**146.** Is the largest sized colonic polyp overall
**147.** Has the greatest likelihood of harboring cancer
**148.** Typically occurs in familial polyposis coli
**149.** Typically occurs in the Peutz-Jeghers syndrome
**150.** Occasionally causes a protein-losing enteropathy
**151.** Is characterized histologically by the presence of normal goblet cells

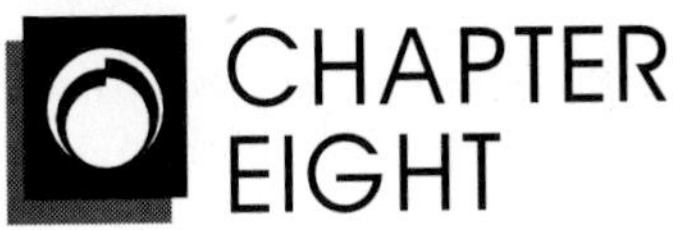

# The Gastrointestinal Tract

## ANSWERS

**1. (A)** Figure 8–1 illustrates the numerous (typically hundreds to thousands) adenomatous polyps of the colon that characterize the familial polyposis coli (FAP) or adenomatous polyposis coli (APC) syndrome. This is an autosomal dominant disorder now known to be associated with the mutation of a tumor suppressor gene (the APC gene) located on chromosome 5q21 and hereditary loss of one allele of this gene. The presence of the remaining mutated allele results in the development of innumerable colonic adenomas early in life. Whether a second event, such as the inactivation of the second allele, is required for malignant transformation is unclear. Nevertheless, malignant transformation of some of these adenomas virtually always occurs in the natural progression of the disease, and the risk of colon cancer in FAP is essentially 100%. The majority of sporadic colonic adenomas and carcinomas also contain a mutant APC gene and some (but not all) have homozygous loss of the APC gene.

In FAP, the colon appears normal at birth, and the benign tumors that are the precursors of carcinomas develop later in life, usually in the second or third decade. Progression to colon cancer occurs within 10 to 15 years after the onset of polyps. Thus, to prevent inevitable death from colon cancer, total colectomy is performed at the polyposis stage. Gardner's syndrome is a variation of FAP in which the polyposis occurs in association with multiple osteomas, epidermal cysts, and fibromatoses. The genetic alterations of the APC gene and the polyp-cancer progression sequence in Gardner's syndrome are identical to those of FAP. *(pp. 266; 813–815)*

**2. (E)** Achalasia is an uncommon disorder of esophageal motility whose pathogenesis is still poorly understood. The disease appears to represent a complex of functional abnormalities of the esophageal musculature. Primary among these defects is the failure of relaxation of the lower esophageal sphincter in advance of the propulsive peristaltic wave. In addition, diffuse esophageal spasm with aperistalsis and increased basal tone of the lower esophageal sphincter have also been noted. Although the etiology remains controversial, most studies show a loss of myenteric ganglion cells in the body of the esophagus. Muscular hypertrophy of the lower esophageal sphincter is not a feature of achalasia. The obstruction in achalasia is functional/neurologic in nature rather than stenotic/physical. *(pp. 757–758)*

**3. (A)** Esophagitis is a common problem among cancer patients and may result from a variety of factors. Cytotoxic chemotherapeutic drugs frequently cause esophageal injury and inflammation, as does therapeutic radiation. Furthermore, anticancer therapy produces immunologic deficiencies that predispose to viral and fungal infections of the esophagus. Antibiotics are used in the treatment of fungal esophagitis. They are not a cause of esophagitis. *(p. 761)*

**4. (D)** Esophageal disorders that lead to chronic regurgitation of ingested substances often are associated with pulmonary aspiration. Esophageal diverticula (e.g., Zenker's diverticulum of the upper esophagus) may become overdistended with food, leading directly to regurgitation and pulmonary aspiration. With the inability of ingested substances to pass through the tonically contracted lower esophageal sphincter in achalasia (see Question 2), nocturnal regurgitation and aspiration of undigested food often occur. In systemic sclerosis (scleroderma), fibrosis of the esophageal submucosa and muscular wall may occur. This produces a narrowed esophagus with markedly abnormal motor function, a consequence of which is chronic regurgitation. Esophageal carcinoma may lead to pulmonary aspiration through several mechanisms. Progressive physical obstruction may occur from intraluminal growth of fungating tumors, whereas infiltrating tumors may invade nerves and muscles and produce motor dysfunction. Furthermore, invasive esophageal carcinoma occasionally may produce a tracheoesophageal fistula through which ingested material can be aspirated directly into the bronchial tree.

Viral esophagitis, most commonly caused by herpes simplex virus or cytomegalovirus, produces superficial mucosal disease only (small discrete erosions or ulcerations). It does not produce obstruction or motor dysfunction of the esophagus and is not associated with aspiration pneumonia. *(pp. 210–213; 757; 759)*

**5. (C)** Focal acute gastric mucosal ulcerations are essentially a severe form of acute erosive gastritis and are known to occur in a number of well-defined, biologically stressful situations. Those that occur in association with conditions that raise intracranial pressure, such as brain tumors, head trauma, or intracranial surgery, are known as Cushing's ulcers, after the great neurosurgeon Harvey Cushing who first described them. Increased intracranial pressure is believed to stimulate vagal nuclei, causing hypersecretion of gastric acid, a phenomenon that has been documented only with Cushing's ulcers. In addition, neurogenic or catecholamine-induced vasoconstriction, with mucosal hypoperfusion and injury, contributes to their pathogenesis. Morphologically indistinguishable lesions are produced in other stressful conditions, such as extensive burns (Curling's ulcers), severe trauma, and severe sepsis. Toxic agents, including nonsteroidal anti-inflammatory drugs (particularly aspirin) as well as alcohol, cigarette smoke, chemotherapeutic drugs, and ingested acids or alkalis (e.g., suicide attempts) also may produce this pattern of injury.

Although the names may be confusing, Cushing's disease and Cushing's syndrome have nothing whatsoever to do with Cushing's ulcers. Cushing's syndrome (see Chapter 14, questions 23 through 25) is a metabolic disorder resulting from excess amounts of cortisol from any course. When the specific underlying problem producing Cushing's syndrome is an adrenocorticotrophic hormone–producing pituitary tumor driving excess cortisol production by the adrenals, the disorder is known as Cushing's disease. *(pp. 770; 777; 1151)*

**6. (E)** Mucosal ulceration in the affected bowel is characteristic of a number of infectious agents, including *Entamoeba histolytica*, *Campylobacter jejuni*, *Yersinia enterocolitica*, and *Salmonella* species. These organisms all have the ability to invade the bowel mucosa, causing ulcerative inflammation as well as diarrhea and abdominal pain. The stool typically contains pus and (often) blood originating from the mucosal lesions, and the diagnosis can be established by stool culture for enteric pathogens or by examination for ova and parasites (e.g., *E. histolytica*). Only when such specific causes of mucosal ulceration such as these have been ruled out can the diagnosis of idiopathic inflammatory disease (ulcerative colitis or Crohn's disease) be made with certainty.

Rotavirus is an important cause of viral gastroenteritis in infants and children. Although severe diarrhea may result, mucosal ulceration of the bowel usually is not observed. *(pp. 313; 328–334; 791–794)*

**7. (D)** Hirschsprung's disease is a congenital anomaly of the colon caused by failure of development of both Meissner's and Auerbach's plexuses. Neuroblasts from the neural crest fail to complete their distal migration, leaving a portion of distal colon devoid of ganglion cells. In over 80% of cases, only the rectum or rectosigmoid colon is involved. Involvement of the entire colon is extremely rare. Hirschsprung's disease may occur as an isolated lesion but often is associated with other congenital anomalies. Ten per cent of Hirschsprung's disease occurs in patients with Down's syndrome, and an additional 5% of cases are associated with serious neurologic abnormalities, suggesting generalized neural crest dysfunction. Hirschsprung's disease can be cured by surgical excision of the affected segment, which usually is not dilated. The dilated proximal bowel is usually normal. It becomes dilated with accumulated fecal material that cannot be moved through the aganglionic, aperistaltic segment and constitutes a functional down-stream obstruction to the passage of bowel contents. *(pp. 786–787)*

**8. (D)** The numerous granulomata within the bowel wall pictured in Figure 8–2 strongly suggest the diagnosis of gastrointestinal tuberculosis, although definitive diagnosis of this entity would require the identification of the characteristic acid-fast bacilli within the lesions by histochemical stain or by microbial culture. In the United States, involvement of the gastrointestinal tract by *Mycobacterium tuberculosis* is most commonly a secondary consequence of primary pulmonary tuberculosis. Organisms from a primary pulmonary focus are coughed up and swallowed, thereby gaining access to the gastrointestinal tract. Although any organ may be involved in systemic infection with *M. tuberculosis*, blood-borne spread to the gastrointestinal tract is much less common than direct infection from swallowed contaminated mucus originating from a pulmonary focus. With the elimination of *Mycobacterium bovus* infection from contaminated cows, primary bovine tuberculosis of the gastrointestinal tract has been virtually eliminated in the United States. *(pp. 324; 793–794)*

**9. (C)** Neoplasms of the small intestine, whether benign or malignant, are rare entities. Altogether they account for only 3 to 6% of all gastrointestinal tumors. Malignant tumors and benign tumors occur with nearly equal frequency, with benign tumors being only slightly more common. Of the benign mucosal tumors, adenomatous polyps are more common than hamartomas. As in the large bowel, adenomatous polyps are premalignant lesions that may undergo transformation to adenocarcinoma. However, among the benign tumors, both adenomas and hamartomas occur less frequently than leiomyomas. Among the malignant tumors of the small bowel, adenocarcinomas and carcinoid tumors occur with nearly equal frequency and are both more common than malignant lymphoma. Small bowel carcinomas often are discovered only in advanced stages, yet, compared to colorectal carcinoma, they have a better overall postresection 5-year survival rate (70% versus 52% [colorectal cancer statistics: American Cancer Society, 1991]). *(pp. 817–818)*

**10. (D)** Celiac sprue (gluten-sensitive enteropathy or nontropical sprue) is an immunologically mediated reaction to the gliadin constituent of dietary gluten (wheat protein) that causes small bowel mucosal injury and malabsorption. It is known to have a genetic predisposition and to be strongly linked to the HLA-DQw2 haplotype, which is present in 90 to 95% of cases. Histologically, the disorder is characterized by diffuse flattening of the villi of the small intestinal mucosa, although this feature is not pathognomonic for celiac sprue. Absorptive cell injury with loss of brush borders, increased numbers of intraepithelial lymphocytes, lymphoplasmacytic infiltration of the lamina propria, and reactive hyperplasia of the mucosal crypts are also characteristic. In many patients, antibodies to gliadin can be demonstrated in the serum. The pathologic changes in celiac sprue are typically more pronounced in the proximal small bowel, because the highest concentrations of gliadin are present there. The predominantly proximal distribution of the injury helps to differentiate celiac sprue from so-called tropical sprue, an infectious disease. Although tropical sprue may produce mucosal pathology indistinguishable from celiac disease, it often affects the distal small bowel almost exclusively and is cured with antibiotic treatment. Celiac sprue is treated effectively in most cases by simply avoiding the inciting antigen. This requires life-long adherence to a gluten-free diet. Once a gluten-free diet has been instituted, symptomatic disease rapidly disappears, and the small intestinal mucosal injury usually resolves completely. Immunosuppression rarely is needed to control the disease. Perhaps the most dire (although, happily, relatively uncommon) consequence of celiac sprue is an increased incidence of primary gastrointestinal tract lymphoma and carcinoma. In contrast to the great majority of MALTomas (lymphomas arising from *m*ucosal-*a*ssociated *l*ymphoid *t*issue) of the gastrointestinal tract, the lymphomas that occur in association with the celiac disease are mostly of T-cell lineage. *(pp. 876–877)*

**11. (C)** Endoscopic or radiologic diagnosis of benign gastric ulcers is based on distinguishing (virtually diagnostic) gross features that make it possible to differentiate them with great accuracy from ulcerating gastric cancers. Gastric peptic ulcers are characteristically small (i.e., usually less than 2 cm in diameter), round-to-oval, sharply demarcated ("punched-out") defects with straight walls. They most often are located on the lesser curvature at the interface between the gastric antrum and body. Although 40% of gastric cancers occur on the lesser curvature, they are often larger than benign lesions (i.e., usually greater than 4 cm in diameter) and have an irregular contour. The base of a benign tumor is composed of smooth scar tissue, cleaned of debris by peptic digestion. The base of a malignant ulcer is composed of bumpy tumor tissue. The edges of benign ulcers are slightly puffy from edema and inflammation but are not unevenly heaped-up and beaded like the edges of an expanding malignancy. Finally, contraction of the scar tissue at the base of a benign ulcer tends to draw the surrounding mucosa centripetally; consequently, the folds of the tethered mucosa fan out radially from the ulcer crater, a feature that produces a "sunburst" pattern on radiologic contrast studies of the stomach. This feature is characteristically lacking in malignant ulcers. *(pp. 774–775; 781–782)*

**12. (A)** The lesion pictured in Figure 8–3 is a juvenile polyp. These tumors are hamartomatous growths—that is, proliferations of cytologically normal colonic glands and lamina propria arranged in a haphazard, architecturally abnormal fashion. They are easily recognized by their relatively smooth surface and rounded contour; cystically dilated, mucin-filled glands; and abundant lamina propria. Most commonly, they occur as solitary sporadic lesions in the rectum of children less than 5 years of age and have no malignant potential. However, in the inherited juvenile polyposis syndrome, they are multiple, distributed throughout the gastrointestinal tract, and are associated with a slightly increased risk of colon cancer. Polyps that occur in long-standing inflammatory bowel disease are known as inflammatory polyps or pseudopolyps. They are neither neoplasms nor hamartomas but represent mucosal reparation and proliferation in response to chronic injury.

In the Peutz-Jeghers syndrome, hamartomatous polyps occur in association with orofacial melanotic pigmentation. However, Peutz-Jeghers polyps are histologically distinct from juvenile hamartomatous polyps. They are composed of tightly packed, highly arborized glands with little intervening lamina propria, and their mucosa typically is partitioned by bands of smooth muscle, a component juvenile polyps lack altogether.

Multiple hamartoma syndromes are to be contrasted with multiple adenoma syndromes such as familial polyposis coli (see Question 1) and its variant, Gardner's syndrome (multiple colonic adenomas plus multiple osteomas, epithelial cysts, and fibromatoses). In multiple adenoma syndromes, the risk of malignant transformation is extremely high (virtually 100%). Although tissue architectural abnormalities are seen in both hamartomas and adenomas, cytologic abnormalities are characteristic only of adenomas. They represent *de novo* proliferations of dysplastic epithelium and are comprised completely of atypical epithelium. Only in the rare hamartoma undergoing malignant transformation does adenomatous dysplasia arise within the epithelium of the preformed lesion. *(pp. 805; 810–811)*

**13. (E)** The function of the lower esophageal sphincter (LES) is to prevent reflux of gastric contents into the esophagus. It opens in response to swallowing to allow the passage of food and fluid from the esophagus to the stomach. The sphincter opens in anticipation of the peristaltic wave and closes again after the swallowing reflex. Control of LES function (maintenance of muscle tone with relaxation at the proper time) requires both active inhibition of the sphincter muscle by inhibitory neurons and cessation of tonic neural stimulation to the sphincter muscle. Although vagal innervation plays a role in maintaining LES function, vagotomy has virtually no effect on LES tone or relaxation.

Rather than relaxing the sphincter, gastrin acts to increase the sphincter tone, maintaining sphincter competence and preventing reflux of the ingested material that stimulated the hormone's release. *(p. 756)*

**14. (A)** Although they occur at different levels of the esophagus, esophageal "webs" (upper esophagus) and esophageal "rings" (lower esophagus) are morphologically identical lesions that consist of constricting bands of mural fibrosis, primarily involving the submucosa. Although they may occur as congenital lesions, they are much more often the result of esophageal injury secondary to factors such as gastric reflux, radiation, caustic chemicals, or underlying disease (e.g., scleroderma). Progressive dysphagia is the major symptom associated with these lesions. Webs occur most commonly in women and may be associated with anemia (the Paterson-Kelly or Plummer-Vinson syndrome). Like other disorders that predispose to esophageal stasis, webs (e.g., Plummer-Vinson syndrome) are associated with an increased risk of esophageal carcinoma. *(pp. 757; 764)*

**15. (D)** Reflux esophagitis is the most common inflammatory disorder of the esophagus. It is a multifactorial disorder and has been shown to be related to frequent and protracted reflux of gastric contents. Acid and pepsin, as well as bile and lysolecithin, in the refluxed fluid cause the esophageal mucosal injury and inflammation. Contributing causative factors include: (1) increased gastric volume (linked to increased volume of refluxate); (2) impaired clearance of refluxed material; (3) lower esophageal sphincter dysfunction with decreased efficacy of antireflux mechanisms; and (4) the presence of a sliding hiatal hernia. The common denominator among these factors is a failure to keep gastric contents away from the esophageal mucosa. Mechanisms related to gastric acid secretion itself do not appear to be involved, however. There is no evidence to suggest that the composition or acid concentration of gastric secretions in those with reflux esophagitis is fundamentally different from that in normal individuals. *(pp. 761–762)*

**16. (C)** Barrett's esophagus, a consequence of chronic gastrointestinal reflux, is characterized by metaplastic transformation of the stratified squamous epithelium of the normal esophageal mucosa into a columnar glandular epithelium. Three types of metaplastic secretory epithelium have been described: (1) intestinal type with goblet cells, absorptive cells, and Paneth's cells; (2) gastric antral type with mucin-producing epithelial surface cells resembling gastric surface cells, mucin-producing glands, and neuroendocrine cells; and (3) gastric fundic type with parietal cells and chief cells. Often these are admixed. Commonly, cells resembling gastric surface cells are admixed with goblet cells in the same epithelium. The most important consequence of these metaplastic structures is an increased risk of adenocarcinoma of the esophagus, an otherwise unusual entity. In the progression from metaplasia to carcinoma, the epithelium usually passes through various stages of increasing epithelial dysplasia. Thus, once individuals with Barrett's esophagitis are identified, biopsy surveillance may be carried out at regular intervals in order to monitor progression of disease. The goal of surveillance is early detection and treatment (surgical resection) of carcinoma or its immediate precursor, high-grade dysplasia.

Intranuclear inclusion bodies occur in viral esophagitis produced by herpes simplex virus or cytomegalovirus but do not occur with esophageal reflux. *(pp. 762–764)*

**17. (B)** Stimuli for the secretion of gastric acid are numerous and varied. Chemical, mechanical, neurologic, and hormonal factors are all known to be involved in the secretory process. Parasympathetic (vagal) stimulation of gastric parietal cells is the final common pathway for stimuli such as the sight, smell, and taste of food (the "cephalic phase" of stimulation). Gastric distention (the "gastric phase") stimulates mechanical and chemical receptors in the gastric wall. With the entry of digested proteins into the proximal small intestine (the "intestinal phase"), enteric mucosal hormones are released that promote gastrin output by antral G cells (the gastrin-producing neuroendocrine cells of the stomach). Gastrins are the most potent of all stimuli to gastric acid secretion. Histamine, a product of the neuroendocrine enterochromaffin-like cells (ECL cells) of the gastric body, is an important mediator in gastrin-stimulated acid secretion. In short, gastrin stimulates ECL cells to secrete histamine, which, in turn, stimulates the surrounding parietal cells to secrete acid. Thus, histamine is a potent acid secretagogue. In fact, blocking histamine receptors on parietal cells with chemical antagonists (e.g., cimetidine, ranitidine, etc.) effectively inhibits gastric acid secretion and is the basis of one form of current therapy for peptic ulcer disease.

In contrast to digested proteins in the intestinal phase of stimulation, other food substances, such as sugars and fats, have no effect on acid secretion. *(p. 768)*

**18. (E)** Angiodysplasia of the colon is one of the most frequent causes of lower gastrointestinal bleeding in elderly patients but rarely occurs before age 50. It is characterized by dilated, tortuous, submucosal capillaries, venules, and veins (not arteries or arterioles) that may rupture easily to produce bleeding. These pathologic changes almost always are limited to the right colon and most often are located within the cecum. Although it has been suggested that these lesions represent a congenital defect or even a neoplastic change, their pathogenesis now is believed to be related to bowel distention and increased intraluminal pressure from fecal impaction of the capacious cecum. These lesions are almost entirely intramucosal, so they usually cannot be detected by conventional radiologic imaging methods and can be difficult to diagnosis on endoscopy as well. Thus, selective mesenteric angiography may be required for clinical diagnosis. Even for pathologic diagnosis, injection of mesenteric vessels with colloidal contrast agents may be needed to localize lesions accurately in surgical resection specimens. Surgical resection of the colonic segment containing the abnormal vessels is the only definitive therapy. *(p. 789)*

**19. (B)** The so-called volcanic lesions pictured in the micrograph (Fig. 8–4) is considered pathognomonic of the acute phase of antibiotic-associated pseudomembranous colitis caused by *Clostridium difficile*. This organism is a normal denizen of the colon that may overgrow and cause disease when the microbial ecology of the gut is disturbed by antibiotic administration. The mucosal lesion pictured is characterized by the involvement of discrete groups of glands by highly destructive but superficial processes. Necrotic epithelial cells from the upper halves of the glands, inflammatory cells, and fibrin stream out of the mucosa in a fan-like array. These are the nascent pseudomembranes that eventually will become confluent over the mucosal surface as the process progresses. The injury is the result of toxin production by *Clostridium difficile* rather than invasion of the organism. Two toxins are elaborated: (1) toxin A, which is an enterotoxin and a potent chemoattractant for granulocytes; and (2) toxin B, which is cytopathic.

Among the other organisms mentioned (*Entamoeba histolytica*, enterohemmorhagic *Escherichia coli*, *Campylobacter jejuni*, *Yersinia enterocolitica*), only enterohemorrhagic *E. coli* may sometimes produce similar lesions. Most often, however, it causes a histologic picture of ischemia. *(pp. 339, 795)*

**20. (E)** *Mycobacterium avium intracellulare*, *Cryptosporidium parvum*, cytomegalovirus, and Kaposi's sarcoma are all common causes of gastrointestinal disease in acquired immunodeficiency syndrome (AIDS), but they are either highly uncommon (*Cryptosporidium parvum*) or not seen (e.g., Kaopsi's sarcoma) in immunocompetent individuals. *Pneumocystis carinii* is a ubiquitous fungus that does not infect normal individuals but is a common cause of disease in individuals with AIDS. It is the presenting feature in about 50% of AIDS cases. However, infection typically is limited to the lung and does not involve the gastrointestinal tract (although the liver rarely may be infected in systemic dissemination). *(pp. 228; 326–327; 352; 357)*

**21. (D)** Acute appendicitis occurs mainly in adolescents and young adults but may affect individuals of any age. It is characterized histologically by transmural neutrophilic infiltration and, in fulminant cases, mural necrosis. Lymphoid hyperplasia of the submucosa is not an indication of acute appendicitis. In fact, lymphoid hyperplasia is a finding of uncertain significance and even may be considered a variation of normal appendiceal morphology. Clinically, acute appendicitis most commonly is confused with acute mesenteric lymphadenitis caused by *Yersinia enterocolitica* or viral enterocolitis, which is often unrecognized prior to surgery. Although a false-positive diagnosis may be made in 20 to 25% of cases, the risks of appendiceal perforation (with a 2% mortality rate) necessitate prompt action on the part of the surgeon and more than justify the occasional "negative" laparotomy for suspected appendicitis. Luminal obstruction of the appendix predisposes to acute appendicitis, and fecaliths, calculi, tumors, or worms can be demonstrated in 50 to 80% of inflamed appendices. *(pp. 823–824)*

**22. (E)** Reflux esophagitis is the most common cause of esophageal pathology. To confirm the diagnosis, the distinctive features of reflux esophagitis may be sought on endoscopic biopsy. Characteristically, chronic reflux esophagitis produces reactive mucosal architectural changes such as expansion (hyperplasia) of the basal zone and elongation of the stromal papillae. However, the most sensitive and specific marker is the presence of intraepithelial eosinophils, with or without neutrophils. However, none of these changes is pathognomonic for reflux esophagitis, and clinical-pathologic correlation (e.g., detection of acid in the esophagus by pH probe analysis or visualization of reflux on radiologic barium swallow studies) may be required for diagnostic confirmation.

Submucosal varices are not a feature of any form of esophagitis. They are seen exclusively in diseases causing elevated pressures in the esophageal venous system, such as occurs in cirrhosis with portal hypertension. *(pp. 759–762)*

**23. (D)** The gastrointestinal (GI) tract is the most common site of primary extranodal lymphoma. Nevertheless, GI lymphoma is distinctly uncommon compared to other malignancies of the GI tract. The majority (55 to 60%) of sporadic GI lymphomas arise in the stomach, and almost all are B-cell tumors. They arise from the B cells of the mucosa-associated lymphoid tissue (MALT) which is the immunologic defense system of the GI tract. Overall, GI lymphomas have a better prognosis than either GI carcinomas or lymphomas arising in other extranodal sites. GI lymphomas are amenable to surgical resection and, in their early stages, may be curable with surgery alone. Gastric lymphoma is both the most common GI lymphoma and the one with the best prognosis. Gastric lymphoma, like gastric carcinoma, is now known to be etiologically related to *Helicobacter pylor* infection.

Primary GI lymphoma, by definition, arises directly from MALT and not from lymph nodes. Although primary nodal lymphomas may involve the GI tract in the course of their dissemination and GI lymphomas may involve lymph nodes secondarily, it is the site (tissue) of origin that classifies the tumor. The distinction is important because GI lymphomas differ biologically from nodal lymphomas. They are known to have different genotypic changes and to behave in a more indolent fashion (with a better prognosis). Furthermore, relapse of treated GI lymphoma curiously may be restricted to the GI tract. *(pp. 820–821)*

**24. (B)** Lactase deficiency is the most common disaccharidase deficiency of any kind, either acquried or congenital. Lactase is an enzyme associated with the apical brush border of the intestinal absorptive cell that breaks lactose into its component monosaccharides (glucose and galactose), a step requisite for absorption. Acquired lactase deficiency may occur as a result of intestinal mucosal injury (e.g., viral or bacterial enteritis) or may be unmasked by increased lactose intake. In either case, an underlying genetic predisposition (lactase deficiency has an unequal racial distribution) toward having a relative deficiency of the enzyme in the first place may be important. The osmotic gradient created by unabsorbed lactose causes watery diarrhea and malabsorption. The histopathologic changes in the small bowel mucosa are nonspecific. Thus, the diagnosis is usually made clinically. Individuals with acquired lactose intolerance can be treated only by dietary restriction (i.e., elimination of lactose-containing foods and substitution with "imitation" milk products). The ubiquitous presence of such products at the grocery store is an indication of the prevalence of this disorder. Disaccharidase deficiency with lactose intolerance is not a form of food allergy and is not immunologically mediated. It is a primary defect of the mucosal absorptive cell. *(pp. 791; 800)*

**25. (E)** The defect pictured in Figure 8–5 is an intussesception. This problem results when a segment of small bowel, while contracted in peristalsis, becomes telescoped into the lumen of the adjacent downstream segment and causes intestinal obstruction. As the intussusceptum is pushed by peristalsis deeper inside the enveloping segment, its mesentery gets pulled in after it, and the resultant vascular compromise leads to infarction. Intussusception is uncommon but occurs most often in an otherwise normal bowel in infants and children. In adults, intussusception may occur when an intraluminal mass (tumor or polyp) acts as a lead point for peristaltic propulsion into the distal bowel segment. Intussusception requires prompt surgical correction or resection. *(p. 809)*

**26. (D)** Figure 8–6 shows the pathognomonic changes of the small intestinal mucosal in abetalipoproteinemia, an autosomal recessive inborn error of the metabolism. The disorder is characterized by the inability to synthesize apoprotein B, the intracellular protein required for transepithelial transport of absorbed fat. Although the mucosal absorptive cells can absorb lipid, they cannot export it in the absence of apoprotein B, and lipid accumulates in their cytoplasm, giving it the characteristically bubbly appearance shown in the micrograph. The disease has dire consequences and usually expresses itself early in life as failure to thrive, with diarrhea and steatorrhea (malabsorption). Plasma levels of all lipoproteins containing apoprotein B, such as chylomicrons, very low-density lipoproteins, and low-density lipoproteins, are drastically reduced or absent. The systemic dearth of lipid, a major structural component of cell membranes, leads to cytologic abnormalities that in the red blood cell population typically are manifested by the appearance of acanthocytes ("burr cells").

**27. (True); 28. (False); 29. (True); 30. (False); 31. (True)**

**(27)** The esophagus is lined throughout its length by stratified squamous epithelium, which does not keratinize under normal conditions. **(28)** Its outer surface lacks a serosa and is covered instead by loose advential connective tissue. **(29)** The muscular wall of this hollow tube is composed of striated muscle in the upper third and smooth muscle in the lower two thirds. **(30)** Although functional studies have shown that sphincter function exists in both the upper and lower aspects of the esophagus, no anatomic counterpart for these functional sphincters has been discerned by morphologic studies. **(31)** The esophageal lumen narrows slightly at the level of the bifurcation of the trachea and at two other levels—the cricoid cartilage and the diaphragmatic haitus. *(pp. 755–756)*

**32. (True); 33. (True); 34. (False); 35. (True)**

Esophageal varices are dilated, tortuous, submucosal veins that are produced when flow through the hepatic portal system is compromised, increasing portal venous pressure and diverting flow through the coronary veins of the stomach into the esophageal plexus. Portal hypertension most commonly is caused by hepatic cirrhosis, yet the incidence of this complication varies markedly among the different forms of cirrhosis. **(32)** Portal hypertension and esophageal varices most commonly are found in association with alcoholic cirrhosis and occur in nearly two thirds of the patients with this disorder. **(33)** Curiously, however, they rarely occur in association with biliary cirrhosis or cardiac cirrhosis. **(34)** Whatever the etiology, esophageal varices are asymptomatic until they rupture. Thus, epigastric pain in alcoholic patients most likely would indicate acute gastritis or reflux esophagitis rather than the presence of esophageal varices, although they may well coexist. **(35)** Once rupture has occurred, the consequences are dire, and death occurs with the first episode of bleeding in about half of the cases. Even if the initial episode of bleeding can be controlled with medical or surgical measures, rebleeding is likely to occur. Overall, only operative procedures that reduce the pressure in the portal venous system by shunting the blood into the systemic system are capable of altering the course of this highly lethal consequence of advanced cirrhosis. *(pp. 759–761)*

**36. (False); 37. (True); 38. (True); 39. (False); 40. (True); 41. (True); 42. (False); 43. (False); 44. (False)**

Peptic ulcers are perhaps the most common chronic gastrointestinal disorder in industrialized nations. **(36)** Although they may occur at any level of the gastrointestinal tract exposed to gastric acid and pepsin, they occur most commonly in the first portion of the duodenum. The second most common site is the gastric antrum. **(37)** Peptic ulcers occur most commonly as solitary lesions. Occasionally, however, they may be multiple, especially in such disorders as the Zollinger-Ellison syndrome (see Question 84).

**(38)** Peptic ulcers result from mucosal damage caused by gastric acid and pepsin. In fact, without some level of acid-pepsin secretion, peptic ulcers do not develop and, therefore, are not seen in individuals with achlorhydria.

**(39)** Although some degree of gastric acid production is requisite to the genesis of peptic ulcers, abnormally high levels of gastric acid are not the major problem in peptic ulcer disease (PUD). With the exception of the Zollinger-Ellison syndrome, hyperacidity is found only in a small minority of cases of PUD. Thus, in most cases of PUD, the pathogenesis is more likely to be related to decreased mucosal defenses against acid-pepsin damage.

**(40 and 41)** Virtually all patients with PUD also have an associated chronic gastritis, usually caused by infection with *Helicobacter pylori*. In fact, *H. pylori* infection is present in 90 to 100% of patients with duodenal peptic ulcers and about 70% of patients with gastric peptic ulcers. Most cases of PUD not related to *H. pylori* infection are associated with chronic gastritis of other etiologies, such as alcohol or nonsteroidal anti-inflammatory drugs. This suggests that chronic gastritis may be the primary condition and that ulcer development is secondary. The etiologic link between *H. pylori* infection and PUD is very strong, although the exact pathogenetic mechanicsms are still imperfectly understood. The organism itself is found only in the stomach (it attaches only to gastric surface and foveolar cells), and never in the duodenum unless gastric metaplasia is present. Thus, in duodenal PUD, the ulcers appear to be the result of the pathophysiologic consequences of the gastritis rather than direct injury from the bacterium. In *H. pylori*–related PUD, definitive treatment of the ulcer disease, whether gastric or duodenal, requires eradication of the infection (which will lead to resolution of the gastritis) as well as pharmacologic blockade of acid output.

**(42)** With current medical therapies for PUD, including neutralization of gastric acid, pharmacologic blockade of gastric acid secretion (e.g., use of histamine receptor antagonists or inhibitors of parietal cell proton pumps), and antibiotic therapy for *H. pylori*, relatively few patients require surgery. Only ulcers refractory to aggressive medical treatment or those associated with complications such as perforation, bleeding, or gastric outlet obstruction require surgical intervention.

**(43 and 44)** Malignant transformation of peptic ulcers is exceedingly rare and has been reported only in gastric ulcers. Even in those cases, it is possible that the cancers did not derive from malignant transformation of a benign ulcer but rather represented unrecognized malignancies from the outset. Both PUD and gastric carcinoma are linked etiologically to chronic gastritis, usually caused by *H. pylori* infection, so it is likely that malignancy occurring in PUD is related primarily to the associated chronic gastritis rather than to the ulceration itself. *(pp. 770–777; 781)*

**45. (True); 46. (False); 47. (False); 48. (True); 49. (True); 50. (False); 51. (False)**

Diverticular disease is a disorder characterized by the development of saccular transmural outpouchings of the colonic mucosa that are prone to fecal impaction. **(45)** In industrialized Western countries, the disease is extremely common and currently is found in approximately 50% of individuals over the age of 60. The incidence of the disease increases with age and is rare in those under 30 years of age.

**(46)** Acquired colonic diverticula represent herniations of the colonic mucosa through "weak spots" in the muscularis propria where blood vessels penetrate the colonic wall. They are composed of mucosa and submucosa alone. An attenuated muscularis mucosa may or may not be present, but diverticula lack a muscularis propria entirely. **(47)** Although they may occur in any segment, 95% of colonic diverticula are located in the sigmoid colon. **(48)** Their development is believed to be related to increased intraluminal pressure from exaggerated peristaltic contractions. The common finding of hypertrophy of the muscularis propria in the affected segment supports this hypothesis.

**(49)** The delicacy of these thin-walled diverticular structures makes perforation an easily understood complication. Inflammatory changes usually are produced by perforation, with leakage of the contents into the adjacent pericolonic fat. The inflammatory response may be quite extensive, with pericolonic abscesses, sinus tracts, or even peritonitis. With chronic inflammation, pericolonic scarring with stricture formation may occur.

**(50)** Although clinical studies have failed to confirm that increased intraluminal pressure is essential in the pathogenesis of diverticular disease, they have shown that it correlates well with symptomatic disease. Thus, high-fiber diets that increase stool bulk and decrease peristaltic activity (hence intraluminal pressure) may not prevent the development of diverticular disease but are at least effective in reducing the symptomatology of this condition.

**(51)** The majority (about 80%) of individuals with diverticular disease are asymptomatic and never come to medical attention. When inflammation does occur, however, it most often resolves spontaneously. Only a small percentage of patients require surgical intervention for obstruction, free perforation, or inflammatory complications. *(pp. 806–808)*

**52. (False); 53. (True); 54. (False); 55. (True); 56. (True); 57. (True); 58. (False); 59. (False); 60. (True)**

**(52)** Adenocarcinoma of the colon is by far the most common malignant tumor of the gastrointestinal tract, but, overall, it ranks third among the leading causes of cancer deaths in the United States. In males, lung cancer and prostate cancer are the two leading causes of cancer death. In females, lung cancer and breast cancer are responsible for the most cancer deaths. **(53)** The high incidence of adenocarcinoma of the colon has been shown epidemiologically to be related to dietary factors such as low fiber content, high carbohydrate content, high fat content, and decreased protective micronutrients (e.g., vitamins A and C, which act as free radical scavengers).

**(54)** The distribution of cancers within the colon has been changing (moving proximally) over the last several decades. In the past, only about 10% of colon cancers occurred in the right colon, and, conversely, over 50% of cancers were readily detectable on digital or proctosigmoidoscopic examination. This is no longer true. Currently, about 25% of colonic carcinomas are found in the right colon, about 25% in the descending colon and proximal sigmoid, and about 25% in the rectum and distal sigmoid colon. Only those in the rectum and possibly distal sigmoid are palpable on digital rectal exam. **(55)** The vast majority of colon cancers have a similar origin and histologic appearance. Except for those that arise in inflammatory bowel disease, almost all colon cancers derive from malignant transformation of colonic adenomas (adenomatous polyps). Ninety-eight per cent of all colon cancers are adenocarcinomas, most being moderately to well differentiated. **(56)** Although stage is by far the most important indicator of outcome in colon cancer, certain histologic variations also may have prognostic significance. **(58)** For example, tumors of the rectosigmoid that produce copious amounts of mucin (known as mucinous or colloid carcinomas) tend to have a worse prognosis. It is believed that the elaboration of pools of extracellular mucin by the tumor aids in its ability to dissect through normal tissues and increase its potential for infiltration.

**(57)** Although by no means unique to colonic malignancies, most of these cancers produce the glycoprotein oncofetal antigen known as carcinoembryonic antigen (CEA). With removal of the primary tumor, the serum levels of CEA usually drop. Any subsequent rise in the serum CEA level may indicate recurrent or metastatic disease.

**(59 and 60)** Colon cancer is a surgical disease. Radiation therapy and chemotherapy largely are considered adjuvant treatment modalities for this disease. Although deadly in advanced stages, early-stage disease is curable with surgical resection. Resected tumors that are limited to the mucosa have a 5-year survival rate of virtually 100% and are almost always cured. Therefore, along with prevention, early detection is an important issue in this disease. Many tumors still occur within the reach of the palpating finger (thus the continued importance of rectal examination), but screening for more proximal malignancies most commonly is done by colorometric tests for occult blood in the stool. Unfortunately, these tests are both nonspecific (bleeding from any cause will yield a positive test) and insensitive (the intermittent pattern of bleeding from tumors produces many falsely negative tests). Colonoscopic examinations with direct visualization of the mucosa are both sensitive and specific, but they are labor intensive to perform and have significant procedure-associated risks (e.g., perforation). Thus, because stool examinations for occult blood are inexpensive and easily can be repeated to increase accuracy, they still are used commonly for screening purposes. Moreover, blood in the stool is always pathologic and should initiate investigation whether or not colon cancer is the underlying cause. *(pp. 253; 815–817)*

**61. (False); 62. (False); 63. (True); 64. (True); 65. (True); 66. (True)**

**(61)** Although they may occur in the lung as well as the breast, thymus, liver, gallbladder, ovary, or urethra, carcinoid tumors arise most often in the gastrointestinal tract. **(62)** No matter what their site of origin, carcinoid tumors tend to have the same histologic appearance. They are composed of a uniform population of round cells showing little cytologic atypia. The ability of these tumors to invade and metastasize cannot be predicted from their histologic appearance.

**(63)** Carcinoid tumor cells can be identified positively by their cytoplasmic content of neurosecretory granules, which have a characteristic affinity for soluble silver salts. These granules may contain a variety of amine and peptide products, including serotonin, adrenocorticotrophic hormone, pancreatic polypeptide, somatostatin, vasoactive intestinal polypeptide (VIP), insulin, gastrin, histamine, kallekrein, bradykinin, prostaglandins, and others. Most of these products can be identified in tissue sections of the tumor by immunohistochemistry. If production of a particular cell product predominates and causes a hormone-related clinical syndrome, the tumor usually is named for that secretory product (e.g., VIPoma).

**(64)** Although, in general, the biologic behavior of carcinoid tumors is somewhat unpredictable, carcinoids arising in the appendix (the most common site of gastrointestinal carcinoid tumors) are almost always indolent and rarely metastasize. Their behavior contrasts with that of extra-appendiceal carcinoid tumors, which tend to spread to local lymph nodes as well as the liver, lungs, and bone.

**(65)** The carcinoid syndrome results from the systemic effects of the secretory products of carcinoid tumors, especially serotonin and histamine. Because these substances are metabolized readily in the liver, the carcinoid syndrome is rarely produced by small intestinal carcinoid tumors in the absence of liver metastases. The secretory products of hepatic metastases enter the systemic circulation directly and bypass hepatic degradation.

**(66)** One of the most important and unfortunate features of gastrointestinal carcinoid tumors is their association with an increased incidence of other malignant tumors, both intestinal and extraintestinal. Concurrent malignant neoplasms are found in about 30% of patients with carcinoid tumors of the small intestine and in about 15% of those with appendiceal carcinoids. The majority of these concurrent cancers are found elsewhere in the gastrointestinal tract, and they are usually adenocarcinomas. *(pp. 818–820)*

**67. (B); 68. (C); 69. (C); 70. (A); 71. (A); 72. (C); 73. (D); 74. (B)**

**(67)** Gastric carcinomas are adenocarcinomas that arise from the glandular epithelium of the gastric mucosa. Most malignancies of the esophagus, however, are squamous cell carcinomas. Exceptions to this are represented by esophageal adenocarcinomas that arise from the metaplastic epithelium of a Barrett's esophagus or, rarely, from esophageal submucosal mucous glands.

**(68)** Although the reasons are completely unknown, epidemiologic studies have shown that, throughout the world, the incidence of esophageal carcinoma is significantly higher among blacks than whites. Racial predisposition also has been demonstrated for gastric carcinoma, and, in the United States, blacks, native Americans, and native Hawaiians are at increased risk compared to whites.

**(69)** Dietary factors are important in the pathogenesis of both esophageal and gastric malignancy. Diets rich in nitrites, nitrates, and nitrosamines have been linked causally to both esophageal and gastric carcinoma. Conversely, decreased dietary intake of foodstuffs rich in "antioxidant" nutrients such as vitamins A and C, which act as free radical scavengers, also has been implicated in these diseases.

**(70 and 71)** It has been shown by epidemiologic studies in the United States that esophageal carcinoma occurs six to seven times more frequently among smokers of cigarettes, cigars, or pipes than among nonsmokers. Alcohol abuse is also well known to represent a significant risk factor for esophageal cancer. However, neither cigarette smoking nor alcohol abuse has been demonstrated to influence the incidence of gastric carcinoma.

**(72)** Chronic inflammation is the important predisposing condition for both esophageal and gastric carcinoma. In fact, almost all epithelial malignancy in the upper gastrointestinal tract arises in a background of chronic inflammation. Chronic esophagitis of any cause and chronic gastritis, either autoimmune or related to *H. pylori* infection, are extremely important risk factors for the development of carcinoma. In these settings, cancers arise through progressive epithelial dysplasia, evolving to carcinoma *in situ* and, finally, invasive malignancy. This is to be contrasted with epithelial malignancy in the lower gastrointestinal tract, the vast majority of which arises in benign but premalignant tumors (adenomas).

**(73)** Unfortunately, both esophageal and gastric carcinoma tend to be diseases of insidious onset and rarely produce symptoms that bring the patient to early clinical attention. Both diseases are characteristically asymptomatic until late in their course, when pain may develop as a symptom. Alternatively, unexplained weight loss may be the first evidence of underlying malignancy.

**(74)** Bilateral metastatic adenocarcinomas in the ovaries are known as Krukenberg tumors. Although the primary tumor may originate from any abdominal viscus, it most frequently represents metastatic poorly differentiated ("signet ring") gastric carcinoma. Squamous carcinoma of the esophagus, by definition, never gives rise to Krukenberg tumors. Even adenocarcinoma of the esophagus, however, rarely produces this metastatic pattern. *(pp. 764–765; 779–783)*

**75. (A); 76. (A); 77. (B); 78. (A); 79. (A); 80. (A); 81. (B); 82. (B)**

Acute gastritis is an acute mucosal injury that may be accompanied by hemorrhage and/or erosion. It is usually symptomatic (sometimes dramatically so) but transient in nature. Acute gastritis commonly resolves completely following reversal of the etiologic condition or removal of the causative agent. Chronic gastritis, however, is defined histologically. It refers to a group of conditions that produce a continuum of increasing mucosal inflammation leading to atrophy of the gastric mucosa, which often is accompanied by metaplastic and/or dysplastic changes. Chronic gastritis is associated with an extended clinical course, but it commonly has ill-defined symptomatology or may even be asymptomatic. Two types generally are defined: (1) an autoimmune-mediated process targeted to the body/fundic mucosa, and (2) a nonimmune gastritis chiefly involving the antrum (by far the more common form). Chronic gastritis of either type is associated with an increased incidence of gastric carcinoma (see Question 72), particularly when intestinal metaplasia and/or dysplasia are present.

**(75, 76, and 79)** Acute gastritis may be produced by excessive alcohol consumption or heavy smoking. Alcohol, cigarette smoke, and nonsteroidal anti-inflammatory drugs (NSAIDs: e.g., aspirin, ibuprofen), the three most common causes of acute gastritis, are all agents known to produce direct damage to the gastric epithelium. They disrupt the tight junctions between mucosal cells and allow back-diffusion of gastric acids. Consequently, mucosal edema and inflammation and erosion of the gastric mucosal cells are produced. Although chronic gastritis possibly could develop from prolonged excessive exposure to these agents, only NSAIDs constitute a major etiologic association with chronic gastritis.

**(77)** The production of autoantibodies directed against gastric mucosal cells is a feature associated exclusively with chronic autoimmune fundal gastritis. In particular, patients with chronic fundal gastritis and pernicious anemia typically produce antibodies directed against gastric parietal cells and intrinsic factor. These antibodies may represent a secondary response to exposed antigens on gastric mucosal cells damaged by autoreactive T-cell responses.

**(78)** Adequate blood flow is primary among the factors necessary for normal function of the gastric mucosal cells and maintenance of the gastric mucosal barrier. Ischemia and shock (either hypovolemic or septic), with consequent hypoperfusion of the gastric mucosa, are major causes of acute gastritis. In contrast, hypoperfusion is not known to play an etiologic role in chronic gastritis.

**(80)** Only the acute form of gastritis, with its gastric epithelial cell damage, mucosal denudation, and exposure of delicate submucosal vessels is associated with gastrointestinal bleeding. Occasionally this can be massive, even fatal. In chronic forms of gastritis, mucosal atrophy is the rule, but the mucosa characteristically remains intact unless peptic ulcer disease supervenes (see Questions 36 through 44).

**(81 and 82)** Only the nonimmune form of chronic gastritis is commonly associated with concurrent gastric or duodenal peptic ulcers or with infection by *Helicobacter pylori*. *(pp. 607–608; 770–773)*

**83. (C); 84. (B); 85. (A); 86. (D); 87. (A); 88. (B); 89. (D)**

Ménétrier's disease and the Zollinger-Ellison syndrome are both considered forms of so-called hypertrophic gastropathy, although they are completely unique and unrelated disease processes. **(83)** Their only common feature is the diffuse hyperplasia of the gastric mucosa that they each produce. Thus, both Ménétrier's disease and the Zollinger-Ellison syndrome are characterized grossly by striking cerebriform enlargement of the gastric rugal folds.

**(84 and 88)** The Zollinger-Ellison syndrome typically is caused by a gastrin-secreting endocrine tumor, usually of pancreatic origin, producing hypergastrinemia. With continued excessive gastrin stimulation, hyperplasia of gastric glands occurs with increases of both parietal and chief cell numbers and individual cell volume. Hypersecretion of gastric acid by parietal cells is induced, leading to the production of numerous intractable peptic ulcers, the hallmark of the syndrome. In Ménétrier's disease, it is the surface mucous cells and foveolar cells of the gastric pits that undergo hyperplasia. In contrast to the Zollinger-Ellison syndrome, the specialized cells of the underlying glands usually undergo atrophy rather than hyperplasia. **(85)** The hypertrophic mucous cells secrete large amounts of mucoprotein and, in some patients, the protein loss is severe enough to produce hypoproteinemia. Thus, Ménétrier's disease sometimes constitutes a form of protein-losing gastroenteropathy.

**(86)** Although the heaped-up mucosal folds of Ménétrier's disease and the Zollinger-Ellison syndrome may bear a close resemblance to the mucosal thickening seen in gastric lymphoma and may be confused with lymphoma clinically on this basis, neither disorder actually is associated with lymphoma. **(87)** Ménétrier's disease, however, does impose a slightly increased risk of gastric carcinoma.

**(89)** The gastrin-producing pancreatic endocrine tumors of the Zollinger-Ellison syndrome may be part of a multiple endocrine neoplasia (MEN) syndrome. MEN syndromes can be divided into two major categories: those composed primarily of tumors of neural crest origin and those arising in endocrine organs that are not derived from the neural crest. The pancreatic adenomas of the Zollinger-Ellison syndrome belong to the latter group. They are associated with adenomas of the pituitary gland, the parathyroid, and the adrenal cortex. In contrast to this group of neoplasms, pheochromocytoma and medullary carcinoma of the thyroid are examples of tumors of neural crest origin and do not occur in association with pancreatic adenomas. Ménétrier's disease has no association with MEN syndromes. *(pp. 778; 1170)*

**90. (B); 91. (A); 92. (C); 93. (B); 94. (A)**

Although gastric polyps are in fact rare, they are among the most common benign neoplasms of the stomach. Histologically, gastric polyps are classified as either hyperplastic or adenomatous; the hyperplastic variety comprise 80 to 90% of all gastric polyps. **(90)** Adenomatous polyps, which are true neoplasms, tend to be large and may grow up to 3 to 4 cm in diameter. Hyperplastic polyps are seldom over 1 cm in diameter. **(91)** Hyperplastic polyps are usually multiple, whereas adenomatous polyps tend to occur singly. However, multiple adenomatous polyps may be present as part of an inherited polyposis syndrome such as familial polyposis coli. **(92)** All gastric polyps tend to be asymptomatic and are usually discovered incidentally. **(93)** The major significance of adenomatous gastric polyps is their tendency to undergo malignant transformation. Hyperplastic polyps represent regenerative non-neoplastic lesions and rarely undergo malignant transformation. **(94)** However, hyperplastic polyps may be associated with co-existent gastric carcinoma elsewhere in the stomach, because both are etiologically related to chronic gastritis. *(p. 779)*

**95. (A); 96. (C); 97. (D); 98. (D); 99. (D); 100. (A); 101. (B); 102. (A); 103. (A); 104. (C); 105. (C)**

Crohn's disease and ulcerative colitis are both idiopathic disorders with systemic manifestations that produce inflammatory disease of the bowel as their primary consequence. Although they have many overlapping features, leading to the hypothesis that the two diseases actually may represent opposite ends of the spectrum of host response to the same disease entity, in their classic forms the two processes can be distinguished on a number of bases.

**(95)** The distribution of the two diseases is usually quite distinctive. Crohn's disease involves the terminal ileum in the majority of cases (65 to 75%) and frequently affects the colon concurrently. The colon alone is involved in 20 to 30% of cases, but the lesions of Crohn's disease may be found at any level of the gastrointestinal tract, including the stomach. Ulcerative colitis is a process largely limited to the large intestine, although the terminal ileum is involved (so-called backwash ileitis) in 10% of cases.

**(96)** Extraintestinal involvement may occur in both conditions. The systemic complications are similar in both diseases and include: migratory polyarthritis, sacroiliitis, ankylosing spondylitis, uveitis, hepatobiliary involvement, and skin lesions.

**(97)** One of the primary pathologic features that distinguishes Crohn's disease from ulcerative colitis is the presence of granulomas. These appear in affected bowel segments in approximately 60% of the cases. However, the presence of granulomas is by no means pathognomonic. When granulomas are observed, specific causes of granulomatous enterocolitis, such as tuberculosis, must be considered, and special stains for organisms should be performed. In Crohn's disease, special stains for bacteria, fungi, parasites, or acid-fast bacilli fail to reveal microorganisms.

**(98)** The search for a specific etiologic microorganism in ulcerative colitis and Crohn's disease has proven unfruitful despite considerable effort expended in the investigation of a wide range of candidate pathogens.

**(99)** Crohn's disease and ulcerative colitis share many epidemiologic similarities, including age, race, and sex distribution, but no specific human lymphocyte antigen (HLA) profiles have been identified in association with these diseases. Although previous reports linked HLA-B27 to inflammatory bowel disease with ankylosing spondylitis, it is now clear that the antigen is associated only with the latter disorder with or without inflammatory bowel disease.

**(100)** In general, the gross appearance of the affected bowel in the two diseases differs in several specific respects. In Crohn's disease the inflammation is characteristically transmural and leads to marked fibrosis (scarring) of the submucosa and muscularis propria. The wall of the affected bowel becomes rigid, thickened, and narrowed. **(101)** In ulcerative colitis, the inflammatory process usually is limited to the mucosa, and the bowel wall is not significantly thickened. Occasionally, however, a severe acute attack of fulminant ulcerative colitis may produce sudden cessation of bowel function, dilation of the colon, and acute transmural inflammation with fraying and thinning of the muscularis propria (toxic megacolon). The danger of perforation in this situation is great, and the consequences may be lethal. Curiously, this drastic complication of ulcerative colitis is virtually never seen in Crohn's disease.

**(102)** The distribution of lesions in the involved bowel is another major distinguishing feature between ulcerative colitis and Crohn's disease. The lesions of Crohn's disease are typically discontinuous; affected areas are interrupted by uninvolved patches of normal-appearing bowel (known as "skip lesions"). This pattern contrasts with that of ulcerative colitis, in which the lesions are usually continuous: the ulceration characteristically begins in the rectum and progressively involves the proximal mucosa in a confluent manner. **(103)** The transmural nature of the inflammatory process in Crohn's disease leads to the formation of deep mural fissures and fistulous tracts, which are among the most important complications of this disease. Ulcerative colitis does not produce these deeply penetrating lesions; it is characterized instead by shallow superficial mucosal ulcerations.

**(104)** In long-standing inflammatory bowel disease of either type, reactive systemic amyloidosis may occur. This complication is a result of chronic stimulation of the liver by inflammatory cytokines (e.g., interleukins 1 and 6) to produce serum amyloid–associated protein (SAA). In susceptible individuals, SAA cannot be degraded completely and undergoes partial proteolysis to form amyloid deposits in tissue throughout the body. **(105)** One of the most important yet most unfortunate similarities between ulcerative colitis and Crohn's disease is the increased frequency of colonic carcinoma with which they are both associated. Although the overall risk of gastrointestinal carcinoma is much smaller in Crohn's disease than in ulcerative colitis, the risk increases with increasing duration of disease in both disorders. *(pp. 234–235; 800–806)*

**106. (A); 107. (A); 108. (A); 109. (C); 110. (B); 111. (C); 112. (A)**

Ischemic bowel disease is a broad term used to describe hypoxic injury to the gastrointestinal tract caused by any disorder that leads to enteric hypoperfusion. In general, the extent of the injury produced in the bowel is related directly to the severity of the reduction in blood flow. On the one hand, transmural infarction represents maximal injury to the bowel, producing ischemic necrosis of all layers of the bowel wall. Mucosal infarction, on the other hand, is the result of minimal ischemic damage, involving only the layer that is most remote in the end-arterial system (i.e., the mucosa). Thus, in mucosal infarction, the muscularis and the serosa are spared.

**(106)** Mucosal infarction may occur at any level of the bowel, from stomach to anus, without particular predilection for any specific region. Transmural infarction, however, most commonly affects the small bowel. Unlike the colon, which throughout most of its length receives collateral circulation from the posterior abdominal wall to which it is attached, the small bowel is entirely dependent on the mesenteric vascular supply.

**(107 and 108)** Although transmural infarction most often is produced by arterial occlusion with total or near-total reduction in blood flow, it occurs as a result of venous thrombosis in a minority of cases. In contrast to total arterial or venous occlusion, which completely halts the flow of blood, conditions that reduce but do not arrest the flow of blood may produce mucosal injury but rarely lead to transmural infarction. **(109)** The combination of atherosclerosis and hypotension may, according to the severity of these elements, produce any degree of ischemic injury, from mucosal to mural to transmural infarction. **(110)** In the absence of significant atherosclerosis, hypotension alone virtually never produces transmural infarction. Conversely, low-flow states (shock) with reflex splanchnic vasoconstriction are the major causes of mucosal infarction.

**(111)** Ischemic bowel disease, no matter what the level of injury, commonly appears grossly hemorrhagic. In mucosal infarction, the hemorrhage is limited to the superficial layers of the gut, but in transmural infarction hemorrhage may be seen throughout the deeper levels as well. **(112)** Because the hemorrhagic necrosis of mucosal infarction is of a limited and superficial nature, it rarely has grave consequences. Transmural infarction, in contrast, is a highly lethal disorder that is associated with a mortality rate of 50 to 75%. It requires prompt diagnosis and surgical intervention before perforation of the dead bowel and abdominal catastrophe ensue. *(pp. 787–789)*

**113. (C); 114. (A); 115. (A); 116. (C); 117. (B); 118. (B); 119. (D)**

**(113)** Tropical sprue and Whipple's disease are two uncommon infectious causes of malabsorption. In Whipple's disease, the causative agent is *Tropheryma whippelii*, a periodic acid–Schiff (PAS)-positive bacillus that cannot be cultivated *in vitro*. In tropical sprue, no specific causative agent has been identified, but bacterial overgrowth by enterotoxigenic organisms such as *Escherichia coli* and *Haemophilus* has been implicated in the pathogenesis. **(114)** Only tropical sprue is associated with travel to an endemic area (the Caribbean, for example). The pathologic changes in the small bowel are not pathognomonic, so a history of travel to an endemic area is essential to its diagnosis. **(115)** Small bowel biopsy in tropical sprue usually shows flattening of villi, as in celiac sprue, whereas villi in Whipple's disease are usually distended with macrophages, giving the mucosa a shaggy appearance.

**(116)** Not surprisingly, both tropical sprue and Whipple's disease can be cured by antibiotic therapy. Even before the identification of the associated pathogenic agents, the dramatic response of these diseases to antibiotics strongly suggested that they were indeed of bacterial origin. **(117)** Although Whipple's disease once was thought to be a disease limited to the small bowel, it is now clear that it is systemic in distribution. The skin, central nervous system, joints, heart, blood vessels, kidney, lungs, serosal membranes, lymph nodes, spleen, and liver may all be involved. With systemic dissemination, Whipple's disease can be fatal if undiagnosed, yet completely curable with antibiotics. Tropical sprue, in contrast, produces disease only in the small intestine. **(118)** One of the primary pathologic features of Whipple's disease is the presence of PAS-positive, glycoprotein-laden macrophages in the small bowel mucosa that contain the characteristic rod-shaped bacilli. Electron microscopic identification of the bacilli may be required to confirm the diagnosis. **(119)** Neither disease is associated with an increased risk of gastrointestinal lymphoma or carcinoma. *(pp. 798–799)*

**120. (C); 121. (B); 122. (C); 123. (C); 124. (D)**

Congenital anomalies may occur at any level of the gastrointestinal tract and lead to bowel obstruction and other serious gastrointestinal problems in the neonate. Many of these developmental defects are life-threatening, so they must be recognized early and surgically corrected before disastrous consequences occur. Thus, knowledge of the most prevalent lesions and their most common sites of occurrence is critical.

**(120)** Congenital atresia (failure of a bowel segment to develop, leaving behind a solid, cord-like remnant) occurs most often in the small intestine. **(121)** Intestinal stenosis refers to luminal narrowing from any cause. The most frequent developmental abnormality producing intestinal stenosis is hypertrophy of the gastric pylorus. Hypertrophic pyloric stenosis is unique among the congenital stenoses, because most of the others are caused by hypoplastic, rather than hyperplastic, segments of bowel wall or luminal strictures. Hypertrophic pyloric stenosis is easily cured by pylorotomy.

**(122)** Congenital duplication occurs as a consequence of a defect in transformation from the solid to the hollow luminal phase of bowel development early in gestation. Although rare, this anomaly occurs most frequently in the small intestine.

**(123)** Congenital diverticula, which represent herniations or outpouchings of the entire intestinal wall (complete with muscularis propria), are uncommon lesions and are often asymptomatic. The most common congenital diverticulum, known as Meckel's diverticulum, is located in the small intestine and represents a remnant of the vitelline duct. Other congenital diverticula represent primary defects in the bowel wall and are unrelated to antecedent embryologic structures.

**(124)** Ganglion cells, which are critical to the transmission of the parasympathetic stimulus to peristalsis, migrate into the gut from the neural crest. Most commonly, they fail to reach the most distal bowel segment, the rectosigmoid region of the large bowel. The aganglionic segment cannot propagate a peristaltic wave and acts as a functional bowel obstruction (see Question 8). *(pp. 757; 759; 769; 786–787)*

**125. (C); 126. (B); 127. (B); 128. (D); 129. (E); 130 (E)**

**(125)** Gastrin, a peptide hormone that stimulates hydrochloric acid production by gastric parietal cells, is produced primarily in the gastric antrum, which itself is devoid of parietal cells. **(126)** Pepsin is produced by the zymogenic chief cells of the gastric glands in the body and fundus. **(127)** It is also in the specialized glands of the corpus that parietal cells are located. In addition to the production of hydrochloric acid, parietal cells elaborate intrinsic factor—a glycoprotein that plays an essential role in the absorption of vitamin $B_{12}$. **(128)** Gastric endocrine cells are scattered throughout the glands of all the gastric regions and indeed throughout the entire gut, making the gastrointestinal tract the largest endocrine organ in the body. **(129)** The goblet cell is a cell type characteristically found in the small and large intestine but not in the normal stomach. Although gastric surface cells and neck cells as well as glandular cells in the cardia and antrum all secrete mucus, they contain finely dispersed mucigen granules in their cytoplasm rather than the single, large, apical vacuoles containing intestinal-type mucins that characterize goblet cells. **(130)** Similarly, in the normal gastrointestinal tract, Paneth's cells are found only in the small intestine. Therefore, the appearance of Paneth's cells or goblet cells in the gastric mucosa always indicates a pathologic metaplastic change and usually occurs in association with chronic gastritis. *(pp. 767–768; 772; 783–785)*

**131. (D); 132. (C); 133. (A); 134. (D); 135. (C); 136. (C); 137. (D)**

**(131)** Two microscopic features that are unique to the normal small intestine allow for its ready histologic identification. On a cytologic level, the easily recognizable, intensely eosinophilic Paneth's cells, which occur almost exclusively in the small bowel, can be identified in the mucosal crypts of all small bowel segments. The second singular feature of the small bowel is the unique architectural arrangement of the surface mucosal epithelium into projections known as villi. **(132)** Peyer's patches are prominent lymphoid nodules (germinal centers) that characterize the ileal segment of small bowel, whereas **(133)** Brunner's glands, elaborately branched submucosal mucus glands, are found only in the duodenal segment.

**(134)** Endocrine cells (argentaffin or enterochromaffin cells), which produce a panoply of peptide hormones, are found in the mucosal crypts throughout the length of the small intestine. Although histologically identical, endocrine cells represent a family of unique cell types, each capable of elaborating a particular hormone. Besides serotonin, these cells are known to produce gastrin, somatostatin, substance P, vasoactive intestinal peptide, bombesin, and other hormones. However, serotonin-producing endocrine cells do not appear to be anatomically segregated from endocrine cells producing any of these other intestinal hormones, and are found scattered among other argentaffin cells in all small bowel segments.

**(135)** Like the intestinal endocrine cells, mucosal absorption cells in the small bowel are histologically identical but, at least in some aspects, functionally unique. The best studied example of such functional uniqueness is that of vitamin $B_{12}$–intrinsic factor absorption by the surface absorptive cells of the ileum. These cells produce a specific receptor protein for intrinsic factor–vitamin $B_{12}$ complex, which they display on the luminal surface of their cell membrane. The receptor protein is not produced by absorptive cells elsewhere in the small intestine; thus, vitamin $B_{12}$ deficiency is a common consequence of ileal resection or severe mucosal disease involving the ileum.

**(136)** Meckel's diverticulum is a remnant of the omphalomesenteric duct, an embryologic structure that connects the primitive gut with the yolk sac. Although it may vary slightly in position, it is always located in the ileal segment of small bowel, usually within 12 inches of the ileocecal valve. **(137)** Pancreatic rests, in contrast, may occur anywhere in the small bowel. They occur as small foci of ectopic, yet normal, pancreatic tissue that are considered to be congenital anomalies but, unlike Meckel's diverticula, have no normal embryologic counterpart. *(pp. 783–786)*

**138. (B); 139. (A); 140. (D); 141. (C); 142. (D); 143. (B); 144. (D)**

The pathologic characteristics of bacterial enterocolitides vary according to three basic properties of the infecting agent; (1) invasive potential, (2) toxin production, and (3) antigenic potential (ability to elicit immune responses in the host). The infectious enterocolitides produced by *Salmonella, Shigella,* and *Vibrio cholerae* organisms are major causes of infectious gastrointestinal disease that represent classic examples of these three pathogenetic features. **(138)** The *Shigella* bacillus is the cause of the clinical syndrome known as bacillary dysentery. This organism directly penetrates the bowel mucosa through the epithelial cells and replicates within the lamina propria. Here the organism liberates an endotoxin that is cytodestructive and leads to shallow mucosal ulcerations, the characteristic feature of Shigella enterocolitis. **(139)** Although *Salmonella* organisms are capable of mucosal penetration and liberation of endotoxins, mucosal ulceration is not a prominent feature. Instead, *Salmonella* enterocolitis is characterized by an intense immune response producing massive hypertrophy of submucosal lymphoid follicles. In the prototypic *Salmonella* gastroenteritis, typhoid fever, *S. typhi* organisms tend to localize within the Peyer's patches of the ileum, which become greatly hypertrophied and are seen grossly as plaque-like mucosal elevations. The mucosa overlying these hypertrophied follicles undergoes secondary necrosis, presumably as a result of pressure-induced ischemia but not as a direct consequence of bacterial toxicity.

**(140)** Granulomatous inflammation is not characteristically produced by any of these three organisms. The presence of granulomata would suggest infection with mycobacteria (tuberculosis), fungi, or strains of bacteria, such as *Yersinia enterocolitica,* that induce granulomatous inflammation.

**(141)** Enterocolitis produced by *Vibrio cholerae* causes few anatomic changes in the affected bowel. Because the organism does not invade the bowel mucosa, no mucosal ulcerations are produced. The profuse watery diarrhea that is the hallmark of this infection is caused by an enterotoxin elaborated by the bacillus. The enterotoxin activates membrane-bound adenyl cyclase, causing increased intracellular levels of cyclic adenosine monophosphate (cAMP). Thus, salt and water absorption are inhibited, and active secretion of water, chloride, and bicarbonate by mucosal crypt cells is stimulated.

**(142)** As indicated, all three of these organisms are capable of toxin production. In *Shigella* enterocolitis and cholera, toxin production by the causative organism is the principal pathogenetic factor.

**(143)** Among these three forms of enterocolitis, only shigellosis preferentially involves the large bowel. The tissue damage in *Shigella* enterocolitis is limited almost entirely to the mucosa of the colon, although the ileum is sometimes involved. *Salmonella* enterocolitis classically involves both small and large intestine, whereas cholera is primarily a disease of the small bowel.

**(144)** Although ulceroinflammatory proctitis of infectious etiology may be seen among homosexual males, it is not particularly associated with any of the above forms of bacterial enterocolitis. The most common causative agents are *Treponema pallidum, Neisseria gonorrhoeae* (gonococci), *Chlamydia,* and herpes simplex virus. *(pp. 328–333; 791–794)*

**145. (A); 146. (C); 147. (C); 148. (B); 149. (D); 150. (C); 151. (D)**

Any benign proliferation of colonic mucosal elements that has an exophytic growth pattern and protrudes above the level of the surrounding mucosa is called a colonic polyp. The term, however, refers only to the gross morphology of the lesion. Microscopically, most colonic polyps can be divided into two major categories: non-neoplastic lesions (hyperplastic polyps and hamartomas) and neoplastic epithelial lesions (adenomas). Among the adenomas, several different morphologic types may be distinguished that correspond to differing tendencies to undergo neoplastic transformation.

**(145)** The hyperplastic polyp is the most common type of colonic polyp, comprising 90% of all colonic epithelial polyps at autopsy. Clinically, they are usually discovered only incidentally on endoscopy because they are virtually always asymptomatic. Hyperplastic polyps are not considered to be true neoplasms but rather reactive proliferations of mature, well-differentiated, non-neoplastic epithelial cells separated by connective tissue resembling the lamina propria.

**(146)** Although the definitive identification of any colonic polyp depends on its histologic appearance, the gross size and configuration of the polyp often provide clues to the recognition of specific types. Overall, villous adenomas are the largest in size. They are slow-growing, velvety lesions that, unlike other types of adenomatous polyps, are rarely pedunculated. In general, hyperplastic polyps are the smallest lesions. Tubular adenomas and hamartomatous polyps tend to be intermediate in size between hyperplastic polyps and villous adenomas.

**(147)** In true adenomatous polyps (tubular adenomas, villous adenomas, and tubulovillous adenomas, a histologic composite of these two types), there is a positive correlation between the size of the lesion and the probability of neoplastic transformation. Thus, villous adenomas, the largest of the adenomatous polyps, have the highest likelihood of containing carcinoma. Nonadenomatous polyps (hyperplastic polyps and hamartomatous polyps) seldom undergo neoplastic transformation.

**(148)** Familial polyposis coli is a hereditary autosomal dominant disorder characterized by the formation of extremely large numbers of adenomatous polyps in the colon (see Question 1) and occasionally in the small bowel and stomach as well. Typically, the entire colonic mucosa is covered by closely packed polyps, giving the surface a shaggy appearance. The vast majority of the polyps are small tubular adenomas, although an occasional villous adenoma may occur. Eventual malignant transformation of one or more of these polyps is virtually inevitable in this disease; therefore, it commonly is treated with total colectomy at an early age.

**(149)** The Peutz-Jeghers syndrome is also an autosomal dominant disorder characterized by diffuse intestinal polyposis. In contrast to familial polyposis coli, however, the polyps of Peutz-Jeghers syndrome occur mainly in the small intestine and are of the hamartomatous variety.

**(150)** Villous adenomas in general tend to be symptomatic more often than other adenomatous polyps and often cause rectal bleeding. Occasionally, villous adenomas may be associated with copious mucin production, causing a protein-losing enteropathy, a complication not usually associated with other types of colonic polyps.

**(151)** Although the hamartomatous polyps of the Peutz-Jeghers syndrome resemble tubular adenomas grossly, they are easily differentiated from the latter by histologic examination. Instead of the closely aggregated neoplastic glands of the tubular adenomas, hamartomatous polyps are composed of tightly packed, highly arborized glands that are lined primarily by normal-appearing goblet cells. The glands often are separated by strands of smooth muscle. As the name implies, hamartomatous polyps are composed of proliferations of the three normal elements of the colonic mucosa: mucosal epithelial cells, loose connective tissue (lamina propria), and smooth muscle (muscularis mucosae). *(pp. 810–815)*

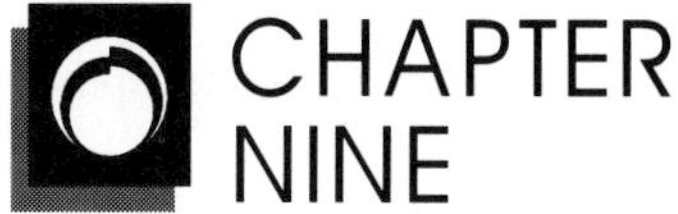

CHAPTER NINE

# The Liver, Biliary Tree, and Pancreas

**DIRECTIONS:** For Questions 1 through 22, choose the ONE BEST answer to each question.

**1.** Conditions that predispose to the disorder pictured in Figure 9–1 include all of the following EXCEPT:

A. Pregnancy
B. Crohn's disease
C. Hyperlipidemia
D. Obesity
E. Ulcerative colitis

**2.** All of the following characteristically cause fatty change in the liver EXCEPT:

A. Reye's syndrome
B. Diabetes mellitus
C. Total parenteral nutrition
D. Tetracycline toxicity
E. Acute viral hepatitis B

**3.** Which of the following histologic features of hepatocellular injury is prognostically LEAST favorable?

A. Councilman body formation
B. Bile lake formation
C. Collagen formation
D. Ballooning of hepatocytes
E. Lobular inflammatory cell infiltrates

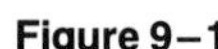
**Figure 9–1**

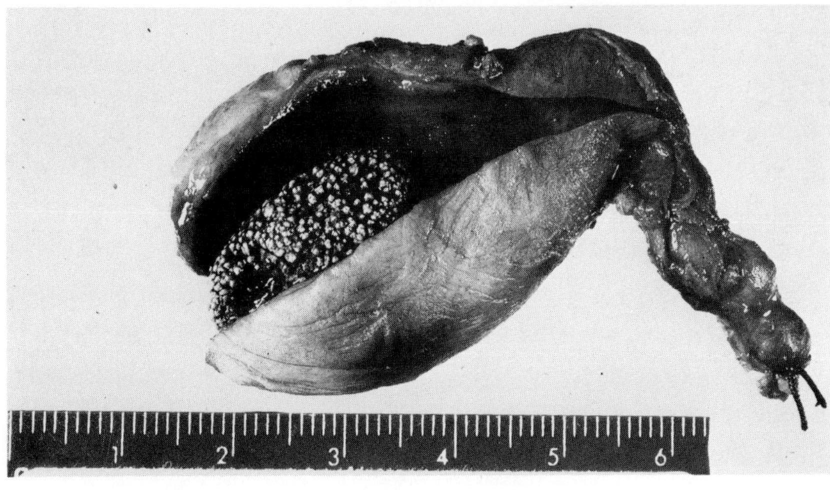

**4.** The hepatorenal syndrome refers to which of the following?

A. Functional failure of a morphologically normal kidney associated with severe liver disease
B. Simultaneous toxic damage to the liver and kidneys with functional failure of both
C. Immune complex glomerulopathy from chronic antigenemia associated with chronic viral hepatitis
D. Acute tubular necrosis from hypotension following a gastrointestinal bleed in the cirrhotic patient
E. All of these

**5.** Which one of the following statements about centrilobular hemorrhagic necrosis of the liver is TRUE?

A. Pressure necrosis from distended central veins and sinusoids is the major causal factor.
B. Congestive heart failure is the most common cause.
C. Its gross appearance is identical to that of nutmeg toxicity ("nutmeg liver").
D. In chronic cases, it frequently produces micronodular cirrhosis.
E. It is frequently a consequence of portal vein thrombosis.

**6.** All of the following statements about fulminant viral hepatitis are true EXCEPT:

A. It is more common than fulminant hepatitis caused by drugs.
B. Its severity is proportional to the immune response to the virus.
C. Death usually occurs within 24 hours of the onset of symptoms.
D. Histologically, it is commonly indistinguishable from drug-induced fulminant hepatitis.
E. Survivors usually have lifelong immunity to recurrent infection.

**7.** The liver condition pictured in Figure 9–2 predisposes to all of the following disorders EXCEPT:

A. Hemorrhoids
B. Cholesterol gallstones
C. Hyperaldosteronism
D. Splenomegaly
E. Hepatocellular carcinoma

**8.** Causes of hepatitis in the neonate include all of the following EXCEPT:

A. Wilson's disease
B. $\alpha_1$-Antitrypsin deficiency
C. Toxoplasmosis
D. Extrahepatic biliary atresia
E. Galactosemia

**9.** All of the following statements about Wilson's disease are true EXCEPT:

A. It is caused by increased copper absorption.
B. Kayser-Fleischer rings in the eyes are diagnostic.
C. Excess copper in the liver is rarely visible on liver biopsy.
D. Cirrhosis eventually develops in virtually all patients.
E. Serum ceruloplasmin levels are characteristically low.

**10.** All of the following features are characteristic of hepatocellular carcinoma EXCEPT:

A. Bile production
B. $\alpha$-Fetoprotein production
C. Mucin production
D. Tumor embolization to the lung
E. Intraperitoneal hemorrhage

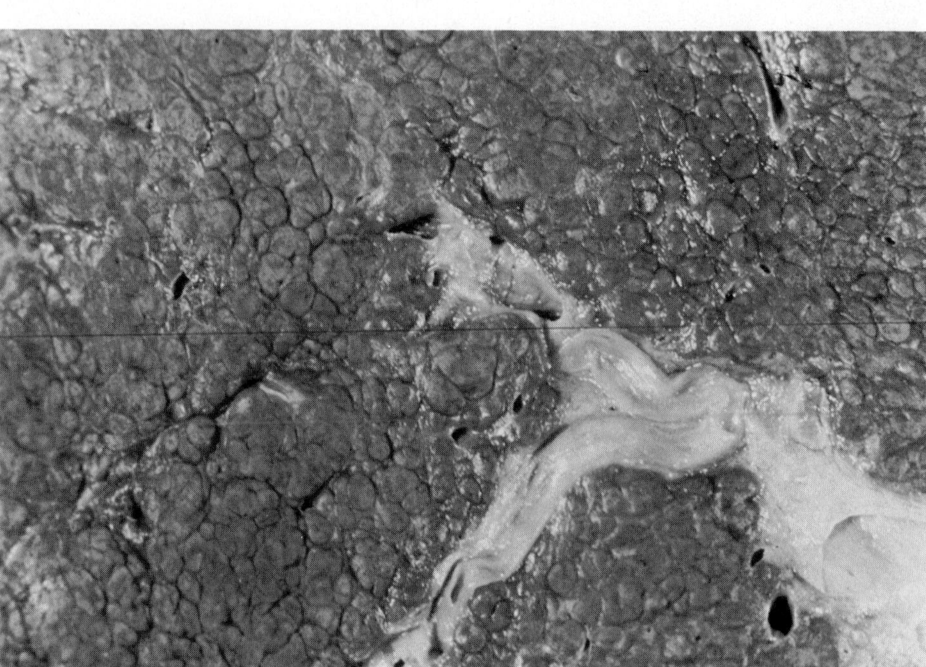

**Figure 9–2**

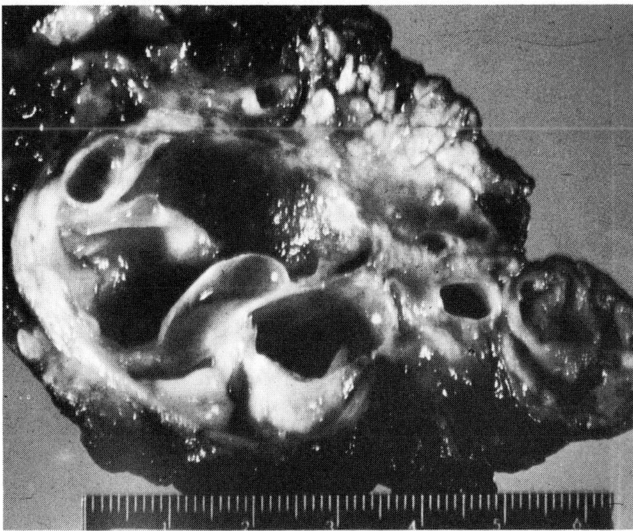

Figure 9–3

**11.** Hepatic complications associated with liver allograft transplantation include all of the following EXCEPT:

A. Drug toxicity
B. Nonfunction resulting from hypoxic preservation injury
C. Acute rejection
D. Recurrence of the original disease
E. Graft-versus-host disease

**12.** The solitary lesion pictured in Figure 9–3 was removed from the head of the pancreas and was lined by benign epithelial cells making mucin. This lesion is associated with:

A. Angiomas of the retina and cerebellum
B. Pancreatitis
C. Mucin-producing adenocarcinoma
D. Cystic fibrosis
E. Cysts in the liver and kidney

**13.** In which of the following conditions is the unconjugated (indirect) fraction of bilirubin increased more than the conjugated (direct) fraction?

A. Primary biliary cirrhosis
B. Recurrent jaundice of pregnancy
C. Rotor syndrome
D. Thalassemia
E. Obstruction of the common bile duct by gallstones

**14.** Metabolic effects of alcohol that contribute to fatty change in the liver include all of the following EXCEPT:

A. Increased lipid absorption from the small bowel
B. Increased lipid mobilization from adipose tissue
C. Increased triglyceride formation in hepatocytes
D. Decreased fatty acid of oxidation
E. Decreased lipoprotein formation

**15.** In which of the following conditions is the intracellular material pictured in Figure 9–4 found within hepatocytes?

A. Carbon tetrachloride toxicity
B. $\alpha_1$-Antitrypsin deficiency
C. Viral hepatitis A
D. Alcoholic liver disease
E. Hemochromatosis

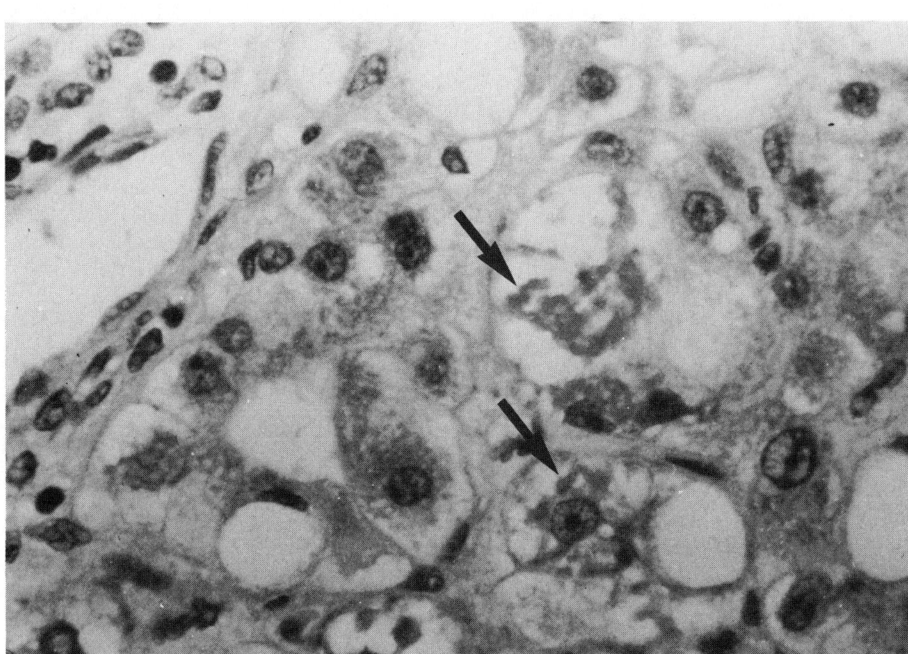

Figure 9–4

**16.** All of the following features are characteristic of hepatic encephalopathy EXCEPT:

A. Occurs with cirrhotic portal hypertension
B. Characteristically causes asterixis
C. Frequently responds to antibiotic treatment
D. Frequently is associated with generalized cerebral edema
E. Does not occur when serum ammonia levels are normal

**17.** A hereditary hyperbilirubinemia that is incompatible with survival to adulthood is:

A. Crigler-Najjar syndrome type I
B. Crigler-Najjar syndrome type II
C. Dubin-Johnson syndrome
D. Gilbert's disease
E. Rotor's syndrome

**18.** All of the following statements about hepatitis A virus infection are true EXCEPT:

A. Acute infection is often asymptomatic.
B. Ingestion of contaminated food or water is the most common mode of transmission.
C. Chronic hepatitis sometimes results.
D. Fatal fulminant hepatitis sometimes results.
E. No carrier state exists.

**19.** Causes of chronic active hepatitis include all of the following EXCEPT:

A. Wilson's disease
B. Methyldopa
C. $\alpha_1$-Antitrypsin deficiency
D. Alcohol
E. Hemochromatosis

**20.** Prescription drugs may cause any of the following types of hepatic disease EXCEPT:

A. Bile stasis
B. Liver abscesses
C. Massive hepatic necrosis
D. Chronic active hepatitis
E. Liver cell adenoma

**21.** All of the following statements about primary idiopathic hemochromatosis are true EXCEPT:

A. Increased intestinal uptake of iron occurs.
B. Cirrhosis is a common consequence.
C. The HLA-A3 genotype is present in most cases.
D. The risk of hepatocellular carcinoma is increased greatly.
E. Diabetic patients are at increased risk of developing the disease.

**22.** Carcinoma of the pancreas:

A. Arises from pancreatic acinar cells
B. Is decreasing in incidence in the United States
C. Occurs most often in the tail of the pancreas
D. Is associated with spontaneous venous thrombosis
E. Is usually cured by total pancreatectomy

**DIRECTIONS:** For Questions 23 through 41, you are to decide whether EACH choice is TRUE or FALSE.

For each of the following statements about hepatitis B virus (HBV) infection, choose whether it is TRUE or FALSE.

**23.** The virus causes cytotoxic damage to the liver cells.
**24.** Antibody production to the HBV surface antigen is defective in HBV carriers.
**25.** Antibody production to the HBV core antigen confers lifelong immunity.
**26.** The presence of HBV e-antigen in serum indicates infectivity.
**27.** HBV is the only hepatotrophic virus associated with an asymptomatic carrier state.
**28.** The histologic finding of ground-glass cytoplasm in liver cells is diagnostic of hepatitis B.
**29.** HBV is the most common cause of virally induced chronic active hepatitis.
**30.** Infection with hepatitis D virus (HDV) occurs only in HBV-infected individuals.
**31.** Co-infection with HDV protects against chronic complications of HBV disease.

For each of the following statements about extrahepatic biliary obstruction, choose whether it is TRUE or FALSE.

**32.** The increased serum levels of alkaline phosphatase help to differentiate it from primary biliary cirrhosis.
**33.** The increased serum levels of conjugated bilirubin cause pruritus.
**34.** The associated bleeding diathesis is a result of platelet dysfunction.
**35.** The associated darkening of the urine differentiates it from hemolytic causes of jaundice.
**36.** The most common cause is impaction of a gallstone in the cystic duct.

For each of the following statements about acute cholecystitis, choose whether it is TRUE or FALSE.

**37.** Virtually all patients with gallstones eventually develop acute cholecystitis.
**38.** Bacterial infection is the initiating factor in acute cholecystitis in the majority of cases.
**39.** Chronic cholecystitis usually is preceded by repeat episodes of acute cholecystitis.
**40.** Right upper quadrant pain is the most common presentation of acute cholecystitis.
**41.** Surgical removal of the gallbladder is the treatment of choice.

**DIRECTIONS:** For Questions 42 through 67, the set of lettered headings is followed by a list of numbered words or phrases. For each numbered word or phrase choose:

A—if the item is associated with (A) only
B—if the item is associated with (B) only
C—if the item is associated with *both* (A) and (B)
D—if the item is associated with *neither* (A) nor (B)

For each of the following characteristics, choose whether it describes hepatic vein thrombosis, portal vein thrombosis, both, or neither.

A. Hepatic vein thrombosis
B. Portal vein thrombosis
C. Both
D. Neither

**42.** The mortality rate is high.
**43.** The disorder is known as the Budd-Chiari syndrome.
**44.** An enlarged and tender liver is characteristic.
**45.** Intra-abdominal tumor is a common cause.
**46.** Pregnancy is a risk factor.
**47.** Peritoneal sepsis is a risk factor.
**48.** Cirrhosis is a predisposing factor.

For each of the statements listed below, choose whether it describes acute cholangitis, primary sclerosing cholangitis, both, or neither.

A. Acute cholangitis
B. Primary sclerosing cholangitis
C. Both
D. Neither

**49.** It is characterized by a neutrophilic inflammatory infiltrate.
**50.** It is associated with cholelithiasis (gallstones).
**51.** It is associated with inflammatory bowel disease.
**52.** It produces an elevated serum alkaline phosphatase.
**53.** It usually is accompanied by bile stasis.
**54.** It responds to antibiotic therapy.
**55.** It predisposes to cholangiocarcinoma.

For each of the characteristics listed below, choose whether it describes primary biliary cirrhosis, hepatic sarcoidosis, both, or neither.

A. Primary biliary cirrhosis
B. Hepatic sarcoidosis
C. Both
D. Neither

**56.** Produces granulomas in the liver
**57.** Is associated with Sjögren's syndrome
**58.** Is associated with a hyperglobulinemia
**59.** Is associated with cutaneous anergy
**60.** Is associated with anti-mitochondrial antibody

For each of the characteristics listed below, choose whether it describes acute cholecystitis, acute pancreatitis, both, or neither.

A. Acute cholecystitis
B. Acute pancreatitis
C. Both
D. Neither

**61.** Strongly resembles perforated peptic ulcer on clinical presentation
**62.** Is associated with gallstones
**63.** Is associated with hyperlipidemia
**64.** Is associated with hypercalcemia
**65.** Is associated with alcoholism
**66.** Causes markedly elevated serum amylase levels
**67.** Causes adult respiratory distress syndrome

**DIRECTIONS:** Questions 68 through 81 are matching questions. For each numbered item, choose the most likely associated lettered item from those provided. Each numbered item has ONLY ONE answer. Within each group, each lettered item may be the answer to one, more than one, or none of the numbered items.

For each of the characteristics listed below, choose whether it describes liver cell adenoma, hepatocellular carcinoma, hepatic cholangiocarcinoma, gallbladder carcinoma, or none of these.

A. Liver cell adenoma
B. Hepatocellular carcinoma
C. Hepatic cholangiocarcinoma
D. Gallbladder carcinoma
E. None of these

**68.** Is associated with cirrhosis
**69.** Is associated with cholelithiasis
**70.** Usually produces elevated serum levels of $\alpha$-fetoprotein
**71.** Is associated with Thorotrast exposure
**72.** Is associated with oral contraceptive use
**73.** Occasionally causes the Budd-Chiari syndrome
**74.** Usually produces elevated serum levels of human chorionic gonadotropin

For each of the following causes of hepatic injury, choose the histologic feature with which it commonly is associated:

A. Fatty change
B. Cholestasis
C. Councilman bodies
D. Granulomas
E. None of these

**75.** Hepatic duct obstruction
**76.** Sulfa drugs (sulfonamides)
**77.** Tetracycline
**78.** Anabolic steroids
**79.** Yellow fever
**80.** Acute viral hepatitis
**81.** Cardiogenic shock

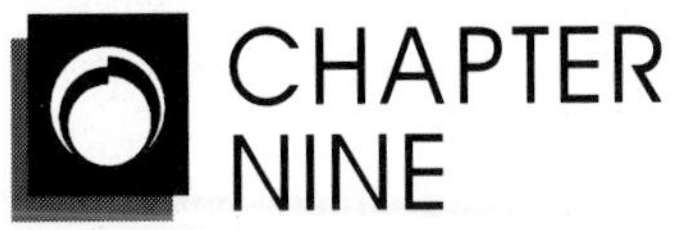

# The Liver, Biliary, Tree, and Pancreas

## ANSWERS

**1. (E)** The gallbladder pictured in Figure 9–1 contains a large, crystalline, yellow-flecked cholesterol gallstone. Most gallstones (approximately 80%) are composed largely of cholesterol, a steroid molecule that is largely insoluble in water. In bile, cholesterol's solubility is dependent on its combination with bile salts and lecithins. These molecules increase the solubility of cholesterol several million-fold. In normal bile the concentraiton ratio of bile salts and lecithins to cholesterol usually exceeds 13:1. When this equilibrium is disturbed by either increasing the cholesterol or decreasing the bile salts or lecithin, cholesterol may precipitate out and form stones. Estrogens inhibit bile acid synthesis and increase cholesterol secretion as well. Thus, females are affected twice as often by gallstones as males, and factors that alter estrogen levels in females, such as pregnancy or oral contraceptive steroid use, further increase the risk of gallstone formation. Obesity is associated with increased hepatic cholesterol secretion and, thus, is a risk factor for gallstones. Some forms of hyperlipidemia are characterized by increased cholesterol synthesis and predispose to gallstones (as well as cardiovascular disease).

Of the two types of inflammatory bowel disease, only Crohn's disease predisposes to cholelithiasis. The ulceroinflammatory process of Crohn's disease mainly involves the terminal ileum—the site of bile salt resorption—and leads to bile salt depletion, with the loss of bile salts from the enterohepatic circulation. In contrast, ulcerative colitis produces disease largely limited to the colon and does not interfere with the enterohepatic circulation of bile salts. *(pp. 482; 804; 884–888)*

**2. (E)** The accumulation of fat within liver cells is one of the most common patterns of hepatic injury. Although the pathogenesis is not fully understood in some diseases, such as Reye's syndrome, most conditions that cause fatty liver are believed to involve one or more of the following metabolic/biochemical abnormalities in hepatocyte lipid metabolism: (1) excessive entry of free fatty acids into the liver; (2) interference with conversion of fatty acids to phospholipids; (3) increased esterification of fatty acids to triglycerides; (4) decreased synthesis of lipid acceptor proteins (apoproteins) to which triglycerides must be coupled in order to be exported from the liver cell; (5) impaired coupling of lipid to lipid acceptor proteins; or (6) impaired lippoprotein secretion from the liver.

Among the systemic diseases causing hepatocellular fatty change, diabetes mellitus is one of the most common. Diabetes causes excessive breakdown of fat stores and an increased presentation of fatty acids to the liver. Total parenteral nutrition is associated with fatty change because the lipid content of the solutions presents an increased free fatty acid load to the liver. Many drugs cause fatty change in the liver, and tetracycline is thought to do so by reducing apoprotein synthesis.

Fatty change is not a feature typical of acute viral hepatitis, however. The hepatotrophic viruses cause lymphocyte-mediated immune attack on infected liver cells, producing diffuse liver cell injury and patchy necrosis. Although hepatitis C may cause mild fatty change in the affected liver, hepatitis with significant lipid accumulation usually suggests an alcoholic or drug-related etiology. *(pp. 25–26; 857; 865–866)*

**3. (C)** The liver is an organ with impressive regenerative capacity and may recover fully from disorders that cause liver cell death. However, the severity, duration, and type of injury are counterbalancing factors in the recovery process. Chronic or profound injuries frequently lead to scar (collagen) formation in the damaged liver. Although fibrosis is reversible to a variable extent during the early stages of chronic injury if the source of the injury is removed, removal of the injurious agent is frequently difficult (alcoholism) or impossible (some cases of chronic active viral hepatitis or primary biliary cirrhosis). Thus, collagen formation often heralds the development of cirrhosis and is prognostically the least favorable histologic feature of hepatic injury.

Councilman body formation and ballooning degeneration of hepatocytes are the histologic manifestations of apoptosis and cellular swelling, respectively. They are hallmarks of liver cell injury and death. A bile lake refers to an area of confluent necrosis of groups of hepatocytes from chemical (bile) injury. The liver, through regeneration, may recover fully from any of these events.

Lobular inflammatory infiltrates may be the cause of or the result of hepatocyte necrosis and are a variable feature of hepatocyte injury. They may resolve completely or contribute to the formation of fibrosis. Thus, their prognostic significance is more variable than fibrosis itself. *(pp. 14–21; 79–82; 833–835; 839)*

**4. (A)** The hepatorenal syndrome is defined as functional renal failure in the absence of morphologically overt renal damage occurring in patients with severe liver disease (most often advanced cirrhosis). Although the pathogenesis of the hepatorenal syndrome has not been elucidated fully, there is evidence that it may be related to generalized renal vasoconstriction, which is more marked in the cortex than in the medulla. Reduction of renal cortical blood flow leads to decreased glomerular filtration and marked sodium retention. Although hepatic and renal failure may occur simultaneously in various toxic or immune complex disorders, these specific cases are defined by their underlying etiology and are not included in the concept of the hepatorenal syndrome. Likewise, acute tubular necrosis from hypotension following a gastrointestinal bleed in a patient with cirrhosis would be excluded according to the above definition. *(p. 842)*

**5. (B)** Centrilobular hemorrhagic necrosis of the liver is a severe form of chronic passive centrilobular congestion and hypoperfusion and most commonly is caused by congestive heart failure. Necrosis of hepatocytes in the centrilobular zone is primarily the result of hypoxia secondary to arteriolar hypoperfusion. However, pressure necrosis from retrograde congestion may play a secondary role in the injury. Grossly, the cut surface of the liver has a mottled pattern of deep red, blood-filled centrilobular zones rimmed by pale tan zones of necrotic hepatocytes in a background of normal red-brown parenchyma. Oddly, the resultant pattern resembles the cut surface of a nutmeg and thus has become known as "nutmeg" liver. (Eggnog drinkers note: Nutmeg is not a hepatotoxin and is not the cause of nutmeg liver.) In cases of chronic hypoperfusion and passive congestion, delicate centrilobular scarring may result, but true cirrhosis rarely develops. Thrombosis of the portal vein produces an obstruction to hepatic inflow (not outflow) and would not be associated with passive congestion of the central veins. This is to be contrasted with hepatic vein thrombosis (Budd-Chiari syndrome), which creates a profound obstruction to hepatic vascular outflow and severe centrilobular congestion and necrosis. *(pp. 97; 523; 872–874)*

**6. (C)** Fulminant hepatitis refers to an uncommon but often lethal form of hepatocellular disease characterized by submassive to massive necrosis of liver cells and precipitous hepatic failure. Most cases (about 50 to 65%) are caused by viral hepatitis, but 25 to 30% of cases are related to drugs and chemicals. In contrast to the drug-induced forms of fulminant hepatitis, in which the damage may be caused either by a hypersensitivity reaction to the drug or by direct toxic damage from a metabolite of the offending compound, fulminant viral hepatitis is most often an immunologically mediated phenomenon. In viral hepatitis, liver injury is produced mainly, if not exclusively, by immune responses to the virally infected, antigenically altered hepatocytes, and the severity of the injury is proportional to the strength of the immune response. If there is no immune response, there is no liver injury, as in the healthy carrier state of viral hepatitis B or C.

Histologically, all forms of fulminant hepatitis tend to look alike. Massive necrosis of the liver cells occurs, leaving behind only the intact portal structures and the collapsed reticulin framework of the cords. The severity and distribution of the necrosis tend to be variable. Although the mortality rate in fulminant viral hepatitis is high, those who do survive almost never become carriers but, rather, acquire lifelong immunity to recurrent infection. Fulminant hepatitis causes rapidly progressive hepatic insufficiency, resulting in death from 2 to 3 weeks after the onset of symptoms. Although rapidly fatal, fulminant liver failure does not produce "sudden death" (within 24 hours after onset). *(pp. 843–855)*

**7. (B)** Figure 9–2 shows the cut surface of a liver with micronodular cirrhosis, the form of cirrhosis most commonly caused by alcohol abuse. The fibrous scarring and regenerative nodules of the sclerotic liver greatly increase resistance to flow through the portal venous system, and the hydrostatic pressure in the portal vein increases. With the rising portal pressure, flow is diverted into the systemic venous system through common portosystemic collateral channels. The principal sites of these portosystemic shunts are the veins around the rectum (hemorrhoids), gastroesophageal junction (esophageal varices), retroperitoneum, and the falciform ligament of the liver (periumbilical or abdominal wall varices). Blood flow also is diverted preferentially into the splenic vein, which is a major tributary of the portal vein, and congestive splenomegaly results.

Secondary hyperaldosteronism and sodium retention also occur in association with cirrhosis. This is thought to be due to sequestration of blood within the splanchnic bed, decreasing the circulating blood volume. Renal perfusion is decreased, and renin is released from the juxtaglomerular cells, causing increased aldosterone secretion.

In addition, impaired hepatic metabolism and excretion of the hormone contribute to the hyperaldosteronism.

Cirrhosis predisposes to the development of hepatocellular carcinoma. In the United States, about 85 to 90% of liver cell carcinomas arise in cirrhotic livers. The risk of developing hepatocellular carcinoma varies with different etiologic types of cirrhosis (high risk in pigment cirrhosis; low risk in alcoholic cirrhosis), but all forms impose some risk.

Cholesterol gallstones may be associated with cirrhosis (secondary biliary cirrhosis) because they can cause the condition through chronic duct obstruction, but gallstones do not occur as a consequence of having cirrhosis. Cholesterol gallstones result from hepatic production of bile with abnormal proportions of cholesterol and bile salts, and cirrhosis does not usually predispose to this problem. *(pp. 834–837; 867–868; 879)*

**8. (A)** A wide variety of infections, hereditary metabolic defects, congenital anomalies, and drug-related toxic disorders can produce severe liver injury in the neonate. Some of the causes of neonatal hepatitis may even lead to cirrhosis in infancy or early chldhood. Although no specific etiology can be found in most cases of neonatal hepatitis (which are then classified as "idiopathic neonatal hepatitis"), the most commonly occurring specific causes of the condition are extrahepatic biliary atresia (EHBA) and $\alpha_1$-antitrypsin deficiency. EHBA is a congenital condition characterized by defective development of the extrahepatic biliary tree and is incompatible with life unless the problem is corrected surgically (if possible) or the patient receives a liver transplant. Galactosemia and tryosinemia are two errors of metabolism that produce severe liver disease and even cirrhosis in infancy if survival is sustained long enough.

A long list of infectious agents can cause neonatal hepatitis. Some of the most common offending agents are transmitted transplacentally from the mother and are known as the "TORCH" infections. These include toxoplasmosis ("T"), rubella ("R"), cytomegalovirus ("C"), herpes viruses ("H"), and other ("O") bacterial and viral agents. It is important to identify infectious forms of neonatal hepatitis and to differentiate them from structural or metabolic forms so that specific therapy can be instituted as quickly as possible.

Wilson's disease, in contrast, is an autosomal recessive disorder of copper metabolism that rarely becomes symptomatic before 5 to 10 years of age and in half of the patients remains asymptomatic until adolescence (see Question 9). It is not a cause of neonatal hepatitis. *(pp. 443; 450–451; 863–867; 890)*

**9. (A)** Wilson's disease (hepatolenticular degeneration) is a hereditary defect of copper metabolism with an impairment of excretion of copper by the liver. Copper accumulates in the parenchyma of various organs, most importantly the liver and brain. However, the process of accumulation is usually slow and is compatible with prolonged survival even when untreated. Wilson's disease usually remains asymptomatic until adolescence, when liver damage (hepatitis or cirrhosis) becomes manifest, and the degenerative changes in the brain generally develop during adulthood. Deposition of copper granules in Descemet's membrane close to the limbus of the cornea produces one of the most characteristic and diagnostic features of Wilson's disease, Kayser-Fleischer rings. Although toxic accumulations of copper in the liver first may produce active hepatitis, the disease inevitably results in cirrhosis. However, with early diagnosis and chelating drug (e.g., penicillamine) therapy, the buildup of copper in the liver, brain, and other organs is prevented, and life expectancy is normal.

Ironically, however, copper may be difficult to identify on liver biopsy in Wilson's disease. Copper is rarely visible in routine histologic preparations and may or may not be demonstrable with special histochemical techniques. A more easily identified abnormality consistently present in all patients with Wilson's disease, however, is a reduction of the serum ceruloplasmin level. Ceruloplasmin is an $\alpha_2$-globulin produced by the liver to which absorbed copper is bound before release into the circulation, and accounts for 90 to 95% of the total plasma copper. Normally, the ceruloplasmin-bound copper then is recycled to the liver for excretion through the bile. In Wilson's disease, the hepatic accumulations of copper cause cellular injury and suppression of ceruloplasmin production. Thus, serum ceruloplasmin levels consistently are reduced. Nevertheless, total serum copper remains relatively normal, because "free" copper loosely bound to albumin is proportionately increased. Free copper is the toxic culprit that causes all the extrahepatic tissue damage in Wilson's disease and is the target of chelating drug therapy. *(pp. 863–864)*

**10. (C)** Hepatocellular carcinoma (HCC or hepatoma) often displays some of the distinctive features reminiscent of its cell of origin, the liver cell. Among normal cells, bile production is a feature unique to hepatocytes. Likewise, bile production by malignant cells identifies them as hepatocellular in origin. The production of $\alpha$-fetoprotein (AFP) by HCC is also highly characteristic but not diagnostic because other tumor types, such as germ cell tumors, also may manufacture this protein. The production of AFP by HCC recapitulates the characteristic production of this protein by the embryonic liver.

Another distinctive feature of HCC is its striking propensity for venous invasion. It commonly invades the hepatic vein and may extend into the inferior vena cava. Fragments of intravascular tumor then may break off and embolize to the lung, a phenomenon associated with only a few other tumors, including renal cell carcinoma, choriocarcinoma, and gastric or breast carcinoma metastatic to the liver. Another common pattern of growth that HCC exhibits is direct extension through the liver capsule with penetration of surrounding structures. Capsular penetration may give rise to severe intraperitoneal bleeding, which is occasionally the presenting feature of the disease.

It is important to recognize, however, that HCC is not a mucin-secreting adenocarcinoma. Primary hepatic mucin-secreting adenocarcinomas originate from the bile duct epithelium and are known as cholangiocarcinomas.

Rarely, HCC and cholangiocarcinoma may exist simultaneously in a so-called mixed pattern, but the two elements may be differentiated on the basis of bile production and mucin production, respectively. A bigger problem in differential diagnosis is distinguishing cholangiocarcinoma from the far more common metastatic adenocarcinomas of the liver. There are usually no distinctive features for either one, and they cannot be differentiated from one another on histopathologic grounds alone. *(pp. 300; 879–882)*

**11. (E)** The increasing use of allograft transplantation for chronic liver disease necessitates recognition of the somewhat unique set of pathologic processes that may complicate this therapy. As with any surgery, technical problems may occur, and in this situation problems with vascular and bile duct anastomoses may be considerable. Hepatotoxicity from drugs used for immunosuppression or infection also may occur. The liver may fail to function altogether after transplantation as a result of hypoxic injury incurred during the process of allograft preservation and transport. Not surprisingly, acute immunologic rejection is a common cause of hepatic injury in the early post-transplantation period (after 2 months). Recurrence of the disease that necessitated transplantation in the first place (e.g., primary biliary cirrhosis, primary sclerosing cholangitis, viral hepatitis) may complicate the late post-transplantation period.

Liver injury caused by graft-versus-host (GVH) disease is seen only with bone marrow transplantation, not liver transplantation. In GVH disease, an immunologic attack on the recipient's native liver is mounted by the allogeneic immunocompetent cells and their precursors in the bone marrow, which have been transferred to a host immunosuppressed by native disease and/or iatrogenic immunosuppression (e.g., radiation, chemotherapy). Although GVH disease rarely is associated with hepatic allograft transplantation, the allograft itself would be the only tissue spared if it did occur (the immune cell mounting the response and the liver would be homogeneic). *(pp. 194; 876–878)*

**12. (C)** The lesion pictured in Figure 9–3 is a multiloculated neoplastic pancreatic neoplasm known as a mucinous cystic tumor (MCT). These lesions are uncommon but are important to recognize because of their premalignant potential. The lining of a MCT is composed of mucin-secreting cells that may be admixed with serous cells. Extensive histologic examination of these tumors is required to rule out the presence of a mucin-producing adenocarcinoma in some portion of the wall. These lesions must be differentiated clinically from pseudocysts, by far the most common cystic lesion of the pancreas, and from congenital cysts or retention cysts. Only pseudocysts are invariably associated with pancreatitis. They are caused by severe inflammation with focal necrosis and fluid accumulation that subsequently is walled off by fibrosis. This results in a cystic lesion without a true epithelial lining (therefore a "pseudocyst" rather than a true cyst). Congenital cysts of the pancreas are believed to develop from anomalous pancreatic ducts and may occur singly or multiply. They sometimes are associated with cysts in the liver and kidney as well. Rarely, pancreatic cysts occur as part of a syndrome known as von Hippel-Lindau disease, in which they are associated with angiomas in the retina, cerebellum, or brain stem and cysts of the liver and kidney. Retention cysts refer to dilated pancreatic ducts that develop from ductal obstruction. For example, they occur in cystic fibrosis secondary to ductal obstruction by inspissated secretions. Pseudocysts, congenital cysts, and retention cysts all tend to be unilocular lesions. The presence of a multilocular cyst, such as the one pictured, suggests a neoplastic lesion: namely, a MCT. Benign MCTs are known as cystadenomas, and malignant MCTs as cystadenocarcinomas. However, given the difficulty in definitively excluding malignancy in an otherwise benign-appearing MCT, the term cystadenoma (implying benignity) has been largely abandoned. *(pp. 904–905)*

**13. (D)** Bilirubin is a catabolic product of heme metabolism that is delivered to the liver bound to albumin, taken up by the hepatocytes, conjugated with glucuronide, and excreted in bile. Disorders that cause defects in the excretion of bile from the hepatocyte or block its flow through the biliary tree cause an increase in serum levels of conjugated bilirubin (direct fraction). Unconjugated bilirubin (indirect fraction) is elevated in disorders that increase the amount of bilirubin delivered to the liver, impair hepatic uptake of unconjugated bilirubin, or impair the conjugation process within the liver cells. In thalassemia, for example, bilirubin production is increased greatly as a result of hemolysis, the conjugation capacity of the liver is overwhelmed, and the indirect fraction of bilirubin in the serum rises.

Primary biliary cirrhosis, large duct obstruction by gallstones, recurrent jaundice of pregnancy, and the Rotor syndrome all cause increases in the direct fraction of bilirubin. They are examples of underexcretion rather than overproduction of bilirubin. The capacity of the liver cell to conjugate bilirubin is unimpaired in these conditions. In primary biliary cirrhosis, intrahepatic bile ducts are injured, and flow through the injured duct is consequently impaired. In obstructive cholelithiasis, it is usually the large extrahepatic ducts that are obstructed, preventing bile outflow from large drainage areas or even the entire liver. In the Rotor syndrome and recurrent jaundice of pregnancy, secretion of bile into the bile canaliculus is impaired. Consequently, bilirubin conjugated in the hepatocytes cannot be eliminated and backs up into the serum. *(pp. 838–841; 868–869)*

**14. (A)** Intake of alcohol is the most common cause of fatty change in the liver. The abnormal accumulation of neutral fat in the hepatocytes is the result of a combination of pathogenetic mechanisms. Alcohol causes increased mobilization of lipid from adipose tissue stores, leading to excessive entry of free fatty acids into the liver. Concomitantly, alcohol increases the esterification of fatty acids to triglycerides while reducing fatty acid oxidation. In addition, the formation of lipoproteins and their release from the hepatic cells also are impaired by alcohol. Alcohol has no known effect on lipid absorption from the small bowel, however. *(pp. 25–26; 857–861)*

**15. (D)** Figure 9–4 is a micrograph of hepatocytes containing Mallory's hyaline. This eosinophilic material is found in the liver cell cytoplasm in certain forms of hepatocellular injury and is considered to be highly characteristic of alcoholic injury. However, it also occurs in less common disorders such as Wilson's disease, primary biliary cirrhosis, chronic cholestatic syndromes, Indian childhood cirrhosis, focal nodular hyperplasia, and hepatocellular carcinoma. Mallory's hyaline is composed primarily of aggregates of prekeratin intermediate filaments. These aggregates result from alcohol-induced depolymerization of tubulin and defective assembly of microtubules required for intracytoplasmic transport of proteins. Overall, this type of injury occurs in relatively few hepatocellular disorders. It is not seen in either carbon tetrachloride toxicity, viral hepatitis, $\alpha_1$-antitrypsin deficiency, or hemochromatosis. *(pp. 24; 858)*

**16. (E)** Hepatic encephalopathy occurs as a complication of liver failure, usually with cirrhosis and portal-systemic shunting. It is a metabolic disorder of the central nervous system characterized by alteration in consciousness, neurologic signs, and electroencephalographic changes. It produces a characteristic flapping tremor of the upper extremities known as asterixis. Although the pathogenesis of these manifestations is uncertain, it is believed to be related to the production of a toxin in the intestine derived from protein metabolism by intestinal bacteria. With cirrhosis and portal hypertension, toxic substances absorbed from the bowel would be shunted into the inferior vena cava from the portal system through intra- or extrahepatic anastomoses, bypassing liver cells and escaping detoxification. Support for this concept is derived from the observations that high protein intake exacerbates the encephalopathy, whereas low protein intake and/or antibiotics administered to reduce the intestinal flora are effective treatments. Although ammonia has been implicated as the toxic agent, hepatic encephalopathy may occur in the absence of hyperammonemia. Pathologic findings in the brain are variable in hepatic encephalopathy but usually include generalized cerebral edema as well as alterations in neurons and laminar necrosis. The changes are reversible if hepatic function is restored. *(pp. 842; 1340)*

**17. (A)** The Crigler-Najjar syndrome type I is characterized by the near-complete impairment of glucuronyltransferase (more precisely known as uridine diphosphate glucuronosyltransferase, or UGT), the enzyme responsible for bilirubin conjugation in the liver. Death inevitably occurs in infancy from extensive brain damage caused by severe unconjugated hyperbilirubinemia. In contrast, the type II Crigler-Najjar syndrome is generally mild. In this form of the disease, UGT activity is somewhat decreased but responds to medical therapy with phenobarbital. Gilbert's disease is a completely benign hereditary disorder producing mild defects in hepatocyte uptake of unconjugated bilirubin, mild deficiencies in UGT, and in 50% of the cases a mildly increased hemolysis. There are no pathologic alterations in the liver and the disease is usually asymptomatic, at most producing a mild jaundice (see Question 9). *(pp. 840–841)*

**18. (C)** In the vast majority of cases, hepatitis A virus infection is a mild or asymptomatic transient disease from which lifelong immunity is acquired. In about 25% of cases, the infection is contracted by the fecal-oral route from infected humans, the natural reservoir of the virus during the stage of fecal viral shedding. More often, the infection is contracted from contaminated food, water, milk, or shellfish. The hepatitis A virus produces neither a carrier state nor a chronic disease process. Therefore, it is never associated with the dire complications of chronic hepatotrophic viral infection (i.e., cirrhosis or hepatocellular carcinoma). Nevertheless, it can be lethal because infection occasionally produces fulminant hepatitis and massive hepatic necrosis. Fortunately, this is rare, making the mortality rate for this disease less than 0.1%. Overall, hepatitis A virus is responsible for about 2 to 4% of cases of fulminant hepatitis of viral origin and less than 1% of all fulminant hepatitis cases. *(pp. 843–844)*

**19. (E)** Chronic active hepatitis is a serious disorder of varied etiology that is characterized by chronic destructive inflammation and fibrosis in the liver. It is a progressive disorder that often ends in cirrhosis and death. Although well known to occur in 5 to 10% of cases of hepatitis B and in more than 50% of cases of hepatitis C, chronic active hepatitis also may occur in association with Wilson's disease, drug toxicity or hypersensitivity, $\alpha_1$-antitrypsin deficiency, autoimmune (lupoid) hepatitis, and alcoholic liver disease. The most common drugs known to cause chronic active hepatitis are methyldopa, oxyphenacetin, isoniazid, and acetaminophen. In hemochromatosis, the accumulation of parenchymal iron produces chronic hepatocellular injury and leads to cirrhosis. Nevertheless, the process is not inflammatory in nature and does not produce chronic active hepatitis. *(pp. 856–865)*

**20. (B)** The liver is the major site of metabolic breakdown of most drugs (both prescription and nonprescription drugs). Thus, the liver is more susceptible to drug-related injury than any other organ in the body. For all physicians, awareness of the potential adverse effects of the drugs that they prescribe is essential in order to recognize hepatic complications and intervene in a timely manner. Even though the offending drug may be part of a therapeutic regimen, it sometimes may be necessary to withdraw the drug or replace it with other therapies in order to prevent significant morbidity or even mortality from hepatic damage. Drugs can produce a wide variety of hepatic injuries, many of which mimic hepatic disease of other specific etiologies. The pathogenesis of individual drug injuries is also varied and may include direct toxic effects as well as immune-mediated injury, with the drug acting as the antigen or hapten. Often, the mechanism of injury is unknown. It is important to be familiar with some of the more common causes of drug-related hepatic injury and the patterns of injury that they typically produce. Only a few are discussed here.

Bile stasis in the absence of bile duct obstruction may occur as a result of the impact of a drug on bile secretory mechanisms. It sometimes is seen in association with anabolic steroids, chlorpromazine, oral contraceptive steroids, or erythromycin, to name a few common examples. Massive hepatic necrosis is a dire (but fortunately uncommon) consequence of drug-mediated hepatic injury and has been linked to halothane, α-methyldopa, isoniazid, and acetaminophen (a widely used over-the-counter drug). α-Methyldopa and isoniazid also may cause chronic active hepatitis, as may nitrofurantoin, phenytoin, oxyphenacetin, and others. Drugs may even (although uncommonly) cause hepatic tumors. One example, hepatocellular adenoma caused by oral contraceptive steroids, is of particular interest because this neoplasm very rarely occurs in the absence of exposure to "the pill."

Liver abscesses are never caused by drugs. They are almost always the result of infection, either parasitic or bacterial. *(pp. 856–857)*

**21. (E)** Primary idiopathic hemochromatosis or hereditary hemochromatosis (HHC) is an inherited disorder of iron metabolism transmitted as an autosomal recessive trait and closely linked with the HLA-A3 genotype. In this disorder, iron uptake from the gastrointestinal tract is increased greatly (it is normally quite limited), and severe systemic iron overload is produced. Profound parenchymal damage from iron toxicity occurs in liver, pancreas, myocardium, pituitary, adrenal, thyroid and parathyroid, joints, and skin. Micronodular "pigment" cirrhosis results from damage to the liver, characteristically the most severely affected organ. Pigment cirrhosis poses a considerable risk (200-fold above the general population) of subsequent development of hepatocellular carcinoma, the leading causes of death from established hemochromatosis. Although early diagnosis and therapeutic intervention with regular, lifelong iron depletion (phlebotomy) may prevent the development of pigment cirrhosis, they do not completely eliminate the risk of hepatoma.

In HHC, iron is deposited both in the exocrine and the endocrine cells of the pancreas, and the injury leads to atrophy and fibrosis. Loss of pancreatic islets produces a secondary type of diabetes late in the course of the disease. This is to be distinguished from primary diabetes mellitus, neither form of which (i.e., insulin dependent or non–insulin dependent) is related to HHC. In short, diabetes commonly occurs in primary hemochromatosis, but hemochromatosis does not commonly occur in diabetic patients. *(pp. 861–863)*

**22. (D)** Carcinoma of the pancreas refers to neoplastic transformation of the pancreatic ductal elements. Pancreatic acini may give rise to malignant tumors but do so rarely and make up less than 1% of all pancreatic malignancies. Pancreatic endocrine ("islet cell") tumors are separately categorized neoplasms that are pathogenetically distinctive, not always malignant, and not generally included under the term "pancreatic carcinoma." The pathogenesis of pancreatic carcinoma is still obscure, but the three-fold rise in incidence of this malignancy over the past 60 years is thought to be related to smoking, diet, and chemical carcinogen exposure. Most tumors (60%) arise in the head of the pancreas and may cause early obstructive symptoms. Although only 5% arise in the tail and 15 to 20% in the pancreatic body, these tumors are particularly insidious because they often grow silently for long periods of time and are usually metastatic by the time the patient comes to clinical attention. In the remainder of cases, the disease is so diffuse when discovered that it is difficult to pinpoint the site of origin within the organ. Overall, fewer than 15% of pancreatic carcinomas are surgically resectable at the time of diagnosis, and only 20% of patients survive for a year (only 3% survive 5 years).

One of the most characteristic paraneoplastic syndromes associated with pancreatic carcinoma is that of spontaneous venous thrombosis, also referred to as migratory thrombophlebitis and known clinically as Trousseau's sign. The pathogenesis of this condition is thought to be related to platelet-activating and procoagulant factors produced by the malignancy, leading to a hypercoagulable state. *(pp. 905–907)*

**23. (False); 24. (True); 25. (False); 26. (True); 27. (False); 28. (True); 29. (False); 30. (True); 31. (False)**

**(23)** Hepatitis B virus (HBV) is one of a group of hepatotropic viruses that are themselves not cytotoxic for liver cells (with the possible exception of the hepatitis C virus). Damage to the liver is produced by the host immune responses mounted against the virally infected liver cells. **(24)** Individuals who fail to respond immunologically (i.e., have a defective response) to HBV harbor the virus indefinitely but fail to sustain liver disease. Such individuals are known as "healthy" carriers. **(25)** Antibody to the HBV core antigen usually is produced early in the course of the disease in normally responding individuals, but it serves only as a marker of current or recent infection. It does not confer immunity to the virus. Only antibody to the HBV surface antigen is capable of eradicating the HBV infection and conferring lifelong immunity. **(26)** HBV "e" antigen is associated with the DNA-containing viral core but is immunologically distinct from both HBV core antigen and surface antigens. The e antigen is detectable in the serum early in the course of acute infection when the disease is most transmissible and disappears before the onset of recovery. It is a marker of active viral replication and infectivity.

**(27)** Although HBV is associated with an asymptomatic carrier state as outlined, it is not the only hepatotropic virus to produce such a condition. Hepatitis C virus (HCV) and hepatitis D virus (HDV) also are known occasionally to produce chronic carrier states. With rare exceptions, no known chronic carrier state is produced with hepatitis A virus (HAV) or hepatitis E virus.

**(28)** Overall, the histologic findings in acute viral hepatitis are similar whether produced by HAV, HBV, or

HCV. The histologic findings are so nonspecific and overlapping in these three disease states that the best way to distinguish them is through serologic studies. Occasionally, however, hepatocytes infected with HBV may show an amorphous eosinophilic area within their cytoplasm known as ground-glass cytoplasm. This finding represents focal collections of virions and is pathognomonic for HBV infection. Unfortunately, it usually is seen only in chronic carrier states and only infrequently is present in acute hepatitis B.

**(29)** Chronic active hepatitis, a progressive fibrosing inflammatory disorder, follows only about 5% of cases of acute HBV in adults, but about 50% of HCV goes on to chronic active disease. HAV does not produce chronic hepatitis (or only extremely rarely does so).

**(30 and 31)** Hepatitis D virus is a very small, defective RNA virus that can replicate or cause infection only when it is encapsulated by HBV surface antigen. Thus, it can infect only HBV carriers or those with HBV hepatitis. Basically, it makes any form of HBV infection worse. Healthy HBV carriers develop acute hepatitis; those with mild HBV hepatitis progress to fulminant disease; and the incidence of chronic progressive hepatitis and subsequent cirrhosis increases. *(pp. 843–856)*

**32. (False); 33. (False); 34. (False); 35. (True); 36. (False)**

Extrahepatic biliary obstruction causes hepatic cholestasis, secondary hepatocellular dysfunction, and malabsorption from the absence of bile acids in the gut. It is characterized by hyperlipidemia with increased plasma levels of cholesterol and phospholipids. **(32)** Increased serum levels of alkaline phosphatase originating from damaged ductal epithelial cells occur in extrahepatic duct obstruction but do not help to differentiate this disorder from other causes of cholestasis. Indeed, in primary biliary cirrhosis, significant elevations of alkaline phosphatase result from the widespread destruction of bile ducts, the hallmark of this disease. **(33)** One of the most characteristic clinical features of extrahepatic cholestasis is the development of pruritus, believed to be caused by the accumulation of bile acids in the serum. The elevated serum levels of conjugated bilirubin occurring in extrahepatic cholestasis cause jaundice, not pruritus.

**(34)** The absence of bile salts from the intestine seriously affects the absorption of fat and fat-soluble vitamins, including vitamin K. The synthesis of prothrombin and other vitamin K–dependent coagulation factors may become seriously impaired in extrahepatic cholestasis and may cause a bleeding diathesis. Platelet function is not known to be altered, however.

**(35)** In hemolytic causes of jaundice, excessive production of bilirubin results in an unconjugated hyperbilirubinemia. Unconjugated bilirubin is water insoluble and is bound to albumin in the serum; thus it is not filtered across the glomerulus into the urine. In extrahepatic biliary obstruction, however, jaundice is produced by conjugated hyperbilirubinemia. Conjugated bilirubin is water soluble, so it appears in the glomerular filtrate and produces a characteristically dark-colored urine (choluric jaundice).

**(36)** By far the most common cause of obstruction of the extrahepatic biliary tree is gallstones. In order to cause cholestasis in the liver, however, the stone must lodge in either the hepatic duct or the common bile duct. If lodged in the cystic duct, it may give rise to acute cholecystitis, but because hepatic biliary drainage is unimpaired, extrahepatic cholestasis will not occur. *(pp. 837–839; 868–869)*

**37. (False); 38. (False); 39. (False); 40. (True); 41. (True)**

**(37)** Although the great majority (about 90%) of cases of acute cholecystitis are associated with gallstones, the converse is not true. In fact, most individuals with cholelithiasis (70 to 80%) remain asymptomatic throughout their lifetime.

**(38)** Bacterial infection may be a contributing factor to acute cholecystitis in 5 to 10% of cases; however, the major etiologic factor is direct chemical irritation and inflammation of the gallbladder wall by concentrated bile in the setting of bile outflow obstruction. This occurs in the absence of infection and only later in the course of the disease, once the mucosal injury has occurred, is the process sometimes complicated by superimposed infection.

**(39)** Although repeat attacks of acute cholecystitis may result in chronic changes with fibrosis of the gallbladder wall, most cases of chronic cholecystitis are not preceded by repeated bouts of acute disease. Most commonly, chronic cholecystitis is an insidious disorder producing vague complaints. As in acute cholecystitis, most cases are associated with gallstones. In contrast to acute calculus cholecystitis, however, duct obstruction by stones is not requisite to its pathogenesis.

**(40)** Chronic cholecystitis usually is characterized by intolerance to fatty foods, belching, and distress, whereas acute cholecystitis usually manifests itself as an acute abdominal emergency. It commonly produces progressive right upper quadrant or epigastric pain, often referred to the right shoulder, which may be accompanied by fever, anorexia, tachycardia, diaphoresis, and/or nausea and vomiting.

**(41)** The treatment of choice in acute cholecystitis is surgical removal of the gallbladder to prevent catastrophic complications such as perforation with pericholecystic abscess formation, generalized peritonitis, ascending cholangitis, liver abscess formation, subdiaphragmatic abscesses, or septicemia. *(pp. 888–890)*

**42. (A); 43. (A); 44. (A); 45. (C); 46. (A); 47. (B); 48. (B)**

**(42, 43, 44)** The Budd-Chiari syndrome is a rare but catastrophic event caused by thrombosis of the hepatic veins. Because the liver has a dual blood supply from the hepatic artery and the portal vein but a single venous outflow, occlusion of the hepatic veins has more serious consequences than any other major form of hepatic vascular occlusion. It is associated with a high mortality rate, with some patients dying within days of its onset and most dying within months. The liver is enlarged and tender, and intractable ascites is produced. In contrast, portal vein thrombosis is much better tolerated. The liver is neither enlarged nor tender, and the outlook for survival is good when the problem is corrected surgically with a splenorenal shunt.

**(45)** One of the most common causes of thrombosis of either the portal or hepatic vein is vascular invasion by tumor. Hepatic vein thrombosis frequently is caused by tumors with a propensity for invasion of the vena cava, such as hepatocellular, renal cell, or adrenal carcinoma, whereas portal vein thrombosis is caused most often by tumors arising within the abdominal cavity.

**(46)** About half the cases of hepatic vein thrombosis are associated with conditions that produce thrombotic tendencies, such as polycythemia vera, pregnancy and the postpartum state, oral contraceptive use, paroxysmal nocturnal hemoglobinuria, and intra-abdominal malignancies (in order of frequency). Vascular invasion from intra-abdominal malignancy is also a common cause of portal vein thrombosis, but it is the only major risk factor shared with hepatic vein thrombosis.

**(47)** Intrahepatic rather than peritoneal infections are common causes of hepatic vein thrombosis. In contrast, portal vein thrombosis is associated with intraperitoneal sepsis and secondary portal phlebitis. Furthermore, because the portal vein is anatomically continuous with the splenic vein, disorders that initiate thrombosis in the splenic vein, such as pancreatitis or pancreatic carcinoma, may produce portal vein thrombosis through retrograde propagation of the thrombus. Pancreatitis, however, does not cause thrombosis of the hepatic veins. **(48)** Cirrhosis is the most common intrahepatic cause of portal vein thrombosis, but it does not predispose to hepatic vein thrombosis. *(pp. 871–872; 874)*

**49. (A); 50. (A); 51. (B); 52. (C); 53. (A); 54. (A); 55. (D)**

**(49)** Cholangitis refers to suppurative inflammation of the intrahepatic or extrahepatic bile ducts and is characterized histologically by neutrophilic inflammatory infiltrates within the walls or lumens of affected ducts. **(50)** Acute cholangitis is almost always produced by extrahepatic duct obstruction, which most commonly is caused by impaction of a gallstone in the common bile duct.

**(51)** Primary sclerosing cholangitis (PSC) is an inflammatory process of the intra- and extrahepatic bile ducts that leads to scarring and stricture formation. The strictures produce a characteristic "bleeding" pattern on radiologic contrast studies of the biliary tree. PSC is believed (but not fully proven) to be an autoimmune process. It is strongly associated with inflammatory bowel disease.

**(52)** Both acute cholangitis and PSC produce elevated serum alkaline phosphatase levels. Compared with cholangitis, however, the degree of alkaline phosphatase elevation occurring with PSC is usually modest.

**(53)** Acute cholangitis is almost always caused by extrahepatic duct obstruction; therefore, it is almost invariably accompanied by bile stasis. In PSC, bile stasis may occur but is predictably seen only in advanced disease.

**(54)** Antibiotic therapy is usually effective in cholangitis, a process caused by direct bacterial infection of the bile duct. Although there may be a rationale for immunosuppressive chemotherapy in PSC (or a need for liver transplantation in end-stage disease), PSC does not respond to antibiotic administration. **(55)** Neither cholangitis nor PSC is associated with subsequent neoplastic transformation of bile ducts. *(pp. 195; 869–870; 888–889)*

**56. (C); 57. (A); 58. (C); 59. (C); 60. (A)**

**(56)** Primary biliary cirrhosis (PBC) and sarcoidosis are both diseases that are associated with abnormal immunologic findings and may produce granulomas in the liver. **(57)** PBC is thought to be an autoimmune disease whose primary target is the intrahepatic biliary tree. The disease is associated with other autoimmune diseases such as rheumatoid arthritis, Hashimoto's thyroiditis, and Sjögren's syndrome. Sarcoidosis is characterized by hyperreactive cellular and humoral immunity but is not believed to be autoimmune in nature. **(58)** Both diseases are associated with a hyperglobulinemia. In sarcoidosis, abnormally high levels of antibodies to commonly encountered antigens typically occur. In PBC, the hyperglobulinemia is usually of the immunoglobulin M class.

**(59)** Abnormal cellular immunity also is observed in both diseases, and impaired T-cell reactivity with cutaneous anergy is characteristic. **(60)** PBC usually can be distinguished, however, on the basis of its histopathology (lymphohistiocytic inflammatory infiltration of the portal tracts and bile ducts with biliary epithelial injury) and by the presence of anti-mitochondrial antibodies in the serum. These are found in more than 90% of patients with PBC. Antibodies to mitochondrial pyruvate dehydrogenase (so-called M2 antibodies) are particularly characteristic of PBC. *(pp. 712–714; 868–869)*

**61. (C); 62. (C); 63. (C); 64. (B); 65. (B); 66. (B); 67. (B)**

**(61)** Acute cholcystitis and acute pancreatitis are diseases that may closely resemble one another at presentation, because the onset of both diseases is usually marked by the sudden development of acute abdominal pain, a situation known as an "acute abdomen." Thus, they must be differentiated not only from one another but from other common causes of acute abdomen, such as perforated peptic ulcer or bowel infarction. **(62)** The two diseases share some etiologic conditions as well. Gallstones are implicated in the pathogenesis of almost all (90%) cholecystitis and, in the United States, are second only to alcohol intake as the most common cause of acute pancreatitis. However, only a small percentage of patients with gallstones develop either of these conditions. Direct damage to the organ caused by bile salts and lecithin is believed to be a major etiologic factor in both disorders.

**(63)** Both acute cholecystitis and pancreatitis are also more common among individuals with hyperlipidemia. Type IV hyperlipidemia predisposes to biliary calculus formation, which, as mentioned, is strongly related to the pathogenesis of acute cholecystitis. Types I and V hyperlipidemia are more closely associated with acute pancreatitis. In contrast to acute cholecystitis, acute pancreatitis associated with hyperlipidemia is believed to develop from activation of pancreatic lipase with local production of free fatty acids that are toxic to acinar cells and blood vessels. **(64)** Similarly, direct activation by calcium of another pancreatic enzyme, trypsinogen, is believed to be the underlying cause of acute pancreatitis associated with hypercalcemia. Trypsin, in turn, is able to activate the majority of proenzymes in the pancreas, such as proelastase and prophospholipase, initiating a catastrophic process of autodigestion in the pancreas. Very rarely, calcium may be the major constituent of gallstones (calcium carbonate gallstones), which conceivably could cause duct obstruction and acute cholecystitis. However, the formation of these calculi is poorly understood and does not appear to be related to hypercalcemia.

**(65)** One of the conditions most strongly associated with acute pancreatitis (or, more precisely, acute exacerbations of chronic pancreatitis) is alcoholism. Alcohol is known to stimulate output of protein-rich pancreatic secretions that may become inspissated within small ducts, causing obstruction. Alcohol also has been postulated to have direct toxic effects on acinar cells. Furthermore, it causes deranged intracellular transport of pancreatic enzymes, leading to intracellular activation by lysosomal enzymes and consequent cellular injury. Alcohol does not appear to be related to the pathogenesis of acute cholecystitis, however.

**(66)** Amylase is one of many pancreatic enzymes released into the serum during an attack of acute pancreatitis. Elevation of serum amylase usually occurs within the first 24 hours of an acute attack and serves as an early marker for the disease. Although amylase is somewhat less specific for pancreatic disease than other pancreatic enzymes, assay methods for amylase are simple and widely used. Serum amylase remains elevated during the active phase of the disease and falls to basal levels 2 to 5 days after the acute attack. Amylase is not an enzyme produced by the gallbladder and is not associated with cholecystitis.

**(67)** The adult respiratory distress syndrome (diffuse alveolar damage in the lungs) is an ominous complication of acute pancreatitis. The pathogenesis is thought to be related to enzymatic destruction of pulmonary surfactants by circulating pancreatic phospholipase released into the serum during an acute attack of pancreatitis. *(pp. 888–889; 899–902)*

**68. (B); 69. (D); 70. (B); 71. (C); 72. (A); 73. (B); 74. (E)**

**(68)** Chronic infection with hepatitis B virus (HBV) is the most common condition associated with hepatocellular carcinoma on a worldwide basis. However, in countries such as the United States, where HBV is not endemic, cirrhosis is the most common predisposing condition and is present in 85 to 90% of cases of hepatoma. The risk of developing hepatocellular carcinoma (HCC) varies among the specific forms of cirrhosis. Hepatoma occurs with high frequency in hereditary tyrosinemia (40% of patients develop HCC) and in pigment cirrhosis (hemochromatosis). Chronic infection with hepatitis C virus also may be a significant cause. Although alcoholic cirrhosis is the most common form of cirrhosis in the United States, HCC is relatively rare in this disease, perhaps because the natural course of the disease is usually relatively short.

**(69)** Gallstones are present in the great majority of cases (75 to 90%) of carcinoma of the gallbladder. It is postulated that chronic inflammation of the gallbladder associated with gallstones may be an important factor in the pathogenesis of gallbladder carcinoma. Furthermore, metabolic derivatives of cholic acid, a bile component, are known to be potent carcinogens and also may contribute to the origin of this malignancy.

**(70)** High serum levels of $\alpha$-fetoprotein (AFP) are present in up to 75% of patients with hepatocellular carcinoma. Although mildly elevated serum levels of AFP may occur in nonmalignant liver disease, very high levels (greater than 1000 ng/mL) strongly suggest the presence of either HCC or yolk sac tumors of germ cell origin, two malignant tumors known to produce large quantities of this protein.

**(71)** Hepatic cholangiocarcinoma (carcinoma of the intrahepatic bile ducts) occurs with increased frequency in individuals exposed to Thorotrast, a contrast agent formerly used in radiography of the biliary tree. Thorotrast exposure also is associated with the otherwise rare angiosarcoma of the liver but does increase the risk of other hepatobiliary malignancies.

**(72)** Liver cell adenoma used to be a very rare tumor. Although still uncommon, it now appears more frequently in women between 20 and 40 years of age who have used oral contraceptives.

**(73)** Hepatocellular carcinoma has a propensity for hepatic vein invasion and may even extend into the inferior vena cava and right side of the heart. With extensive hepatic vein invasion, venous outflow from the liver is blocked and the Budd-Chiari syndrome is produced.

**(74)** With rare exceptions, the only malignancies that produce elevated levels of human chorionic gonadotropin are those that originate from germ cells and have trophoblastic differentiation. The primary hepatic and biliary neoplasms discussed do not produce this hormone. *(pp. 300–301; 857; 878–882; 1074)*

**75. (B); 76. (D); 77. (A); 78. (B); 79. (C); 80. (C); 81. (E)**

**(75)** Very few histologic patterns of liver injury are pathognomonic for a given disease process. However, many causes of liver injury do predictably produce patterns that suggest the diagnosis. Hepatic duct obstruction, for example, characteristically produces cholestasis in the liver. Cholestasis is first seen in centrilobular zones, and, if the obstruction persists, progressively involves the peripheral zones of the lobule and portal bile ducts. Although cholestasis may occur in other forms of liver disease, extrahepatic bile duct obstruction occasionally produces an additional unique feature called bile lakes or bile "infarcts." These are produced by leakage of bile from small portal bile ducts with necrosis of surrounding liver cells. Bile lakes are diagnostic of extrahepatic duct obstruction but occur in only 20% of cases.

**(76)** Drug-induced hepatic injuries fall into two basic categories: toxic injury and hypersensitivity reactions. In general, toxic injuries produce predictable pathologic changes. Hypersensitivity reactions are much less consistent in the pattern of injury they produce. They may result in cholestasis, nonspecific eosinophilic inflammation, granuloma formation, or injury resembling viral hepatitis ranging in severity from focal to massive hepatocellular necrosis. A few drugs tend to be more predictably associated with a specific type of hypersensitivity response than others. Reactions to sulfonamides, for example, most frequently produce a granulomatous hepatitis. **(77 and 78)** Tetracycline and anabolic steroids are examples of agents that produce toxic liver injury. They commonly produce fatty change and cholestasis, respectively.

**(79)** Yellow fever is an acute viral disease that classically produces focal coagulative necrosis (apoptosis) of liver cells. The dead hepatocytes become small, rounded, eosinophilic masses that are called Councilman bodies, after the renowned pathologist who first described them. Councilman bodies are not specific for yellow fever, however. They occur in numerous other types of liver disease as well. **(80)** Acute viral hepatitis caused by any of the hepatotrophic viruses, for example, produces focal random necrosis of liver cells (Councilman body formation). **(81)** Cardiogenic shock typically produces marked centrilobular congestion in the liver and may result in centrilobular zonal necrosis. However, it is not characteristically associated with fatty change, cholestasis, Councilman body formation, or granulomas. *(pp. 843; 850–851; 857; 868; 872–873)*

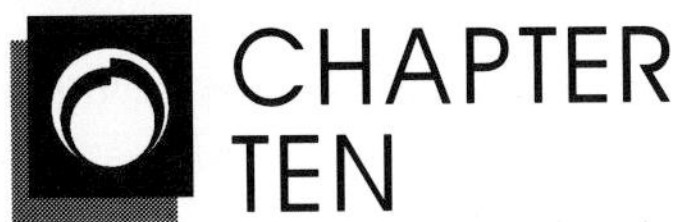

CHAPTER TEN

# The Kidney and Urinary Tract

**DIRECTIONS:** For Questions 1 through 21, choose the ONE BEST answer to each question.

**1.** All of the following substances are components of the glomerular basement membrane EXCEPT:

A. Fibronectin
B. Heparin sulfate
C. Laminin
D. Type IV collagen
E. Fibrin

**2.** Most forms of chronic renal failure produce increased serum levels of all of the following substances EXCEPT:

A. Calcium
B. Aldosterone
C. Phosphate
D. Parathormone
E. Renin

**3.** Uremia is associated with all of the following abnormalities EXCEPT:

A. Peripheral neuropathy
B. Gastritis
C. Polycythemia
D. Pericarditis
E. Diffuse alveolar damage

**4.** Glomerular injury caused by circulating complexes occurs with all of the following disorders EXCEPT:

A. Syphilis
B. Goodpasture's syndrome
C. Hepatitis B
D. Systemic lupus erythematosus
E. Lung cancer

**5.** Diabetes mellitus is associated with all of the following renal disorders EXCEPT:

A. Diffuse glomerulosclerosis
B. Nodular glomerulosclerosis (Kimmelstiel-Wilson disease)
C. Benign nephrosclerosis
D. Urate nephropathy
E. Acute pyelonephritis

**6.** Clinical manifestations associated with the kidney tumor pictured in Figure 10–1 include all of the following EXCEPT:

A. Hyperlipidemia
B. Cushing's syndrome
C. Polycythemia
D. Hypercalcemia
E. Feminization

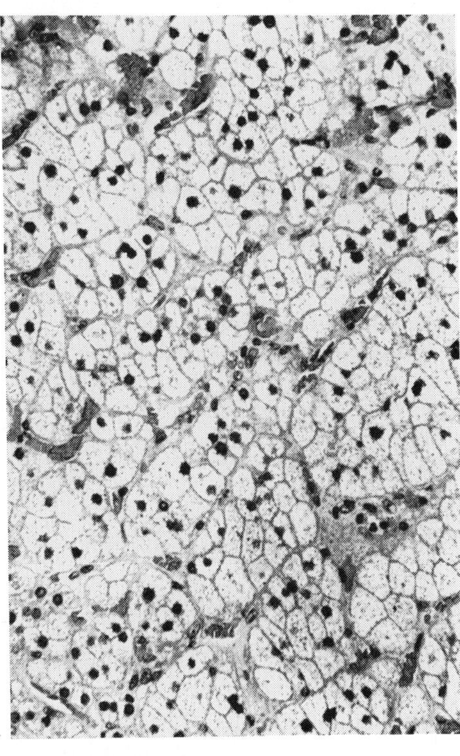

**Figure 10–1**

**7.** All of the following conditions predispose to urolithiasis EXCEPT:

A. Sickle cell nephropathy
B. Hyperparathyroidism
C. Gout
D. *Proteus* pyelonephritis
E. Enteric hyperoxaluria

**8.** Of the factors listed below, the one LEAST likely to cause acute pyelonephritis is:

A. Pregnancy
B. Nephrolithiasis
C. Catheterization of the bladder
D. Prostatic hypertrophy
E. Septicemia

**9.** Mesangial cells are associated with all of the following properties EXCEPT:

A. Ingestion of macromolecules
B. Connection with Lacis cells
C. Ability to contract
D. Production of renin
E. Production of basement membrane proteins

**10.** In immunologically mediated glomerulonephritis, all of the following cells contribute to the glomerular injury EXCEPT:

A. Mast cells
B. Macrophages
C. Platelets
D. Neutrophils
E. Mesangial cells

**11.** Systemic lupus erythematosus gives rise to all of the following patterns of glomerular injury EXCEPT:

A. Focal proliferative glomerulonephritis
B. Diffuse membranous glomerulonephritis
C. Diffuse proliferative glomerulonephritis
D. Lipoid nephrosis
E. Mesangial proliferative glomerulonephritis

**12.** Renal papillary necrosis usually occurs in the ABSENCE of infection in:

A. Urinary tract obstruction
B. Analgesic abuse nephropathy
C. Diabetes mellitus
D. Urate nephropathy
E. Multiple myeloma

**13.** All of the following statements correctly describe chronic pyelonephritis EXCEPT:

A. It causes asymmetrically scarred kidneys.
B. It is associated with vesicoureteral reflux in most cases.
C. It characteristically spares the calyces and pelvis.
D. It typically produces thyroidization of tubules.
E. It is an important cause of end-stage renal disease.

**14.** All of the following statements correctly describe analgesic abuse nephropathy EXCEPT:

A. It is associated with ingestion of about a kilogram of analgesic per year.
B. It is caused most commonly by analgesic compounds containing phenacetin.
C. It causes an inability to concentrate urine.
D. It often improves with drug withdrawal.
E. It predisposes to the development of renal cell carcinoma.

**15.** The substance produced by the kidney that raises systemic blood pressure is:

A. Platelet-activating factor
B. Kininogen
C. Prostaglandin
D. Renin
E. Aldosterone

**16.** Renal diseases producing systemic hypertension include all of the following EXCEPT:

A. Acute glomerulonephritis
B. Acute pyelonephritis
C. Chronic glomerulonephritis
D. Chronic pyelonephritis
E. Renal vasculitis

**17.** Histologic features of malignant nephrosclerosis include all of the following EXCEPT:

A. Fibrinoid necrosis of arterioles
B. Medial thickening of arterioles
C. Fibromuscular dysplasia of the renal artery
D. Necrotizing glomerulitis
E. Focal renal parenchymal infarction

**18.** All of the following statements correctly describe renal artery stenosis EXCEPT:

A. It is an uncommon form of hypertension.
B. It is the most common curable form of hypertension.
C. It is usually caused by atherosclerotic plaque.
D. It produces high renin levels in the venous blood of the ischemic kidney.
E. It is treated by surgical removal of the ischemic kidney.

**19.** Obstetrically related renal disease includes all of the following disorders EXCEPT:

A. Nephrocalcinosis
B. Diffuse cortical necrosis
C. Adult hemolytic uremic syndrome
D. Eclampsia
E. Hydronephrosis

**20.** Hematuria is a characteristic clinical feature of all of the following diseases EXCEPT:

A. Glomerulonephritis
B. Malakoplakia
C. Nephrolithiasis
D. Renal cell carcinoma
E. Bladder papilloma

**21.** The tumor pictured in Figure 10–2 is associated with all of the following predisposing factors EXCEPT:

A. Exposure to azo dyes
B. *Schistosoma haematobium* infection
C. Cigarette smoking
D. Von Hippel-Lindau disease
E. Exposure to cyclophosphamide

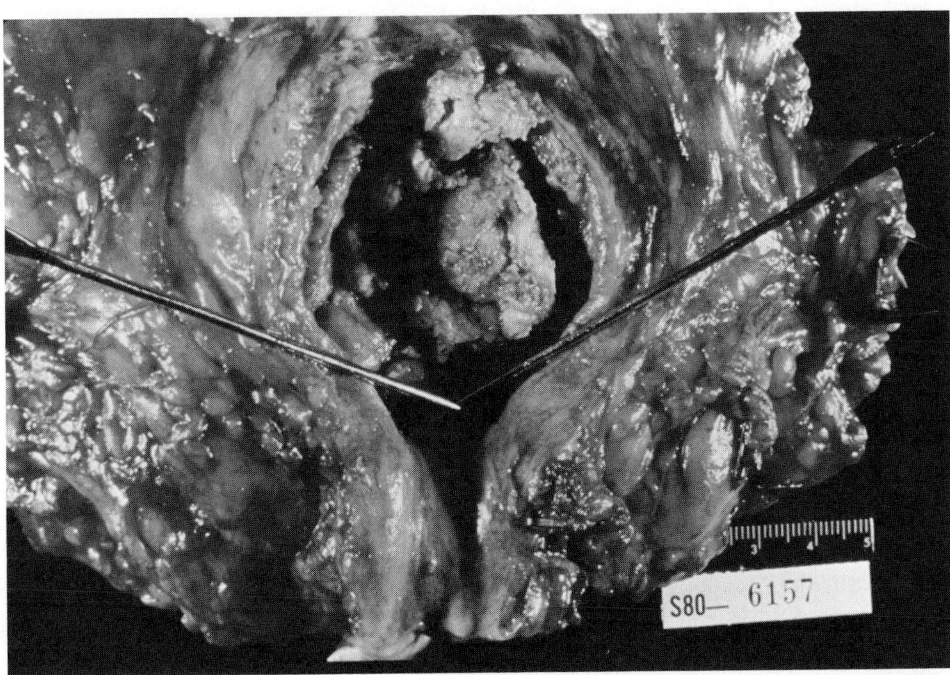


**Figure 10–2**

**DIRECTIONS:** For Questions 22 through 26, you are to decide whether EACH choice is TRUE or FALSE.

For each of the following statements about acute tubular necrosis (ATN), choose whether it is TRUE or FALSE.

**22.** ATN is the most common cause of acute renal failure.
**23.** ATN occurs as a result of isolated ischemic damage to tubules.
**24.** ATN occurs as a result of isolated toxic damage to tubules.
**25.** Oliguria is the sine qua non of the diagnosis of ATN.
**26.** Recovery from ATN depends on compensatory hypertrophy of uninjured tubules.

**DIRECTIONS:** For Questions 27 through 33, the set of lettered headings is followed by a list of numbered words or phrases. For each numbered word or phrase choose:

A—if the item is associated with (A) only
B—if the item is associated with (B) only
C—if the item is associated with *both* (A) and (B)
D—if the item is associated with *neither* (A) nor (B)

For each of the conditions associated with kidney disease listed below, choose whether it is a cause of rapidly progressive glomerulonephritis, the nephrotic syndrome, both, or neither.

A. Rapidly progressive glomerulonephritis
B. Nephrotic syndrome
C. Both
D. Neither

**27.** Streptococcal infection
**28.** Immunoglobulin A nephropathy (Berger's disease)
**29.** Penicillamine therapy
**30.** Synthetic penicillin (e.g., methicillin) therapy
**31.** Wegener's granulomatosis
**32.** Goodpasture's syndrome
**33.** Systemic lupus erythematosus

**DIRECTIONS:** Questions 34 through 50 are matching questions. For each numbered item, choose the most likely associated lettered item from those provided. Each numbered item has ONLY ONE answer. Within each group, each lettered item may be the answer to one, more than one, or none of the numbered items.

For each of the following statements about cystic disease of the kidney, choose whether it describes childhood polycystic kidney disease, adult polycystic kidney disease, medullary sponge kidney, all of these, or none of these.

A. Childhood polycystic kidney disease
B. Adult polycystic kidney disease
C. Medullary sponge kidney
D. All of these
E. None of these

**34.** The disease is inherited as an autosomal dominant trait.
**35.** Renal function is usually normal.
**36.** Berry aneurysms are associated anomalies.
**37.** Cysts arising from collecting ducts are present in the medulla.
**38.** Cysts arising from proximal tubules are present in the cortex.

For each of the statements about primary glomerular disease listed below, choose whether it describes lipoid nephrosis, membranous glomerulonephritis, membranoproliferative glomerulonephritis, immunoglobulin A (IgA) nephropathy, or none of these.

A. Lipoid nephrosis
B. Membranous glomerulonephritis
C. Membranoproliferative glomerulonephritis
D. IgA nephropathy
E. None of these

**39.** It is the most common cause of the nephrotic syndrome in children.
**40.** It is the most common cause of the nephrotic syndrome in adults.
**41.** Glomeruli appear normal by light microscopy.
**42.** Basement membrane splitting is seen in glomeruli by light microscopy.
**43.** Cellular "crescents" are typically seen in glomeruli by light microscopy.
**44.** Subendothelial dense deposits are seen in glomeruli by electron microscopy.
**45.** Mesangial dense deposits are seen in glomeruli by electron microscopy.
**46.** It occurs in association with malignant epithelial tumors.
**47.** It occurs in association with prophylactic immunizations.
**48.** It occurs in association with thyroiditis.
**49.** It involves primary activation of the alternate complement pathway.
**50.** It has a very good long-range prognosis.

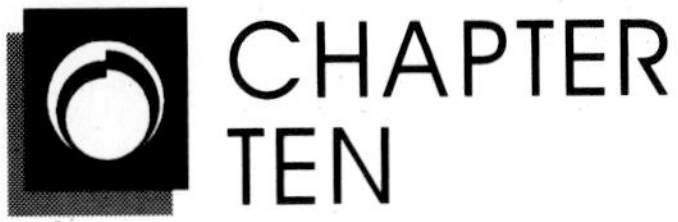

CHAPTER
TEN

# The Kidney and Urinary Tract

## ANSWERS

**1. (E)** The glomerular basement membrane is the structure that is primarily responsible for the molecular size–dependent permeability barrier in the glomerulus. Its normal biochemical components include fibronectin, heparan sulfate (the most important of the polyanionic proteoglycans responsible for the charge-dependent glomerular filtration barrier), entactin, laminin, and type IV collagen, which gives structural support to the capillary wall. Fibrin is not a normal component of the glomerular basement membrane. Its presence would indicate a pathologic alteration of glomerular permeability with leakage of fibrinogen such as occurs in glomerulonephritis (GN). Fibrinogen is a protein of high molecular weight that does not normally filter thorugh the glomerulus. With glomerular injury, fibrinogen may leak into Bowman's space, where it may itself serve as a mediator of further glomerular damage. Fibrin deposition then may occur as a result of macrophage procoagulant activity. Fibrinogen and fibrin stimulate cell proliferation in the glomerulus (e.g., crescent formation in rapidly progressive GN), and, in some experimental models of GN, pretreatment with anticoagulants prevents proliferative glomerular lesions. The rationale for using anticoagulant therapy in the treatment of human GN is based on this observation. *(pp. 929–930; 943)*

**2. (A)** Chronic renal disease of any etiology ultimately produces the same major physiologic abnormalities and clinical manifestations. Hyperaldosteronism is produced as a consequence of increased renin production. It compounds the problem of salt and water retention that results from impaired glomerular filtration. Phosphate begins to be retained as soon as the glomerular filtration rate drops below 25% of normal and overt uremia develops. Increased serum phosphate leads to increased entry of calcium into bone and a fall in serum calcium levels. The failing kidney further contributes to hypocalcemia by its inability to synthesize 1,25-dihydroxy–vitamin $D_3$, the active metabolite of vitamin D, which increases calcium absorption from the gut (see Chapter 3, Question 4). Hypocalcemia, in turn, stimulates the production of parathormone by the parathyroid glands, producing secondary hyperparathyroidism and renal osteodystrophy. *(pp. 415–416; 486–487; 932–933)*

**3. (C)** Uremia is a clinical syndrome resulting from chronic renal failure. It refers to a state of azotemia (elevated blood urea nitrogen and creatinine) in association with a constellation of metabolic and endocrine abnormalities that result from biochemical derangements in end-stage chronic renal disease. The severity of the clinical signs and symptoms of uremia correlates only roughly with the degree of azotemia.

Uremia produces clinical abnormalities in nearly every major organ system as well as systemic derangements of fluid, electrolyte, and acid-base balance. Neurologic manifestations include peripheral neuropathy, myopathy, and encephalopathy. In the gastrointestinal tract, nausea and vomiting, bleeding, gastritis, esophagitis, and colitis occur. Cardiopulmonary abnormalities commonly include uremic pericarditis and, less commonly, diffuse alveolar damage with hyaline membrane formation (uremic pneumonitis).

Uremia is associated with an increase in one of the two major endocrine functions of the kidney: renin production. The other major renal endocrine function, erythropoietin production, is diminished. Therefore, anemia (not polycythemia) is the major hematologic manifestation of uremia. *(pp. 932–933)*

**4. (B)** A nephritis initiated by circulating antigen-antibody complexes occurs as a secondary consequence in a variety of diseases. In nephritis of this type, the antibodies have no immunologic specificity for glomerular constituents.

The complexes are simply trapped in the glomerular basement membrane (GBM) as a result of their intrinsic physicochemical properties and of the hemodynamic forces within the glomerulus. Once the immune complexes have localized in the GBM, injury is mediated by a variety of mechanisms, including complement activation, neutrophil and monocyte infiltration, platelet activation, and fibrin deposition (see Question 10).

The underlying immune response in circulating immune complex nephritis may be directed against either exogenous or endogenous antigens. Diseases in which the inciting antigen is microbial in origin include syphilis, hepatitis B or C, malaria, and certain streptococcal infections. Diseases associated with immune complex nephritis in which the antibodies are directed against endogenous antigens include systemic lupus erythematosus and cancer (the antibody targets being native DNA and tumor-specific or tumor-associated antigen, respectively).

The glomerular injury in Goodpasture's syndrome is not the result of circulating immune complexes. On the contrary, autoantibodies against intrinsic components of the GBM (specifically, the α3 chain of type IV collagen) form immune complexes *in situ* as they are filtered through the glomerulus. Goodpasture syndrome is the archetypal example of anti-GBM nephritis. *(pp. 1024–1025; 1027–1028)*

**5. (D)** Diabetes mellitus (DM) is a major cause of renal morbidity and mortality. Among the organs affected in DM, the kidney typically sustains the greatest amount of injury. Pathologically, DM produces a wider variety of renal lesions than any other single disease. The spectrum of diabetic nephropathy includes glomerular, vascular, and tubulointerstitial disease. Diabetic glomerulosclerosis may be either diffuse or nodular, the latter being known as Kimmelstiel-Wilson disease. Diabetic glomerulosclerosis results from both a metabolic defect leading to nonenzymatic glycosylation of proteins ("advanced glycosylation end-products") and an increase in mesangial matrix production (mechanism unknown). The microangiopathy associated with DM is often more pronounced in the kidney than in other organs and typically produces both arteriolosclerosis and benign nephrosclerosis. Acute pyelonephritis also occurs more frequently in diabetics than nondiabetics and, in severe cases, may be further associated with necrotizing papillitis (see Question 12), a consequence of the coincidence of acute bacterial infection (to which diabetics are predisposed) and impaired papillary circulation.

Urate nephropathy is caused by precipitation of uric acid crystals in the kidneys of individuals with hyperuricemia. Urate crystals may precipitate in the tubules (causing obstruction of nephrons), deposit in the medullary interstitium, or form stones in the collecting system. Hyperuricemia and urate nephropathy are principally associated with either primary or secondary gout (e.g., chemotherapeutic treatment of leukemias and lymphomas with increased cell destruction and urate formation) (see Chapter 15, Questions 26 through 32). However, urate nephropathy is not associated with DM. *(pp. 920–921; 961–963; 974)*

**6. (A)** The photomicrograph in Figure 10–1 illustrates the typical "clear cell" appearance of renal cell carcinoma. This tumor, which arises from tubular epithelium, is the most common renal cancer in adults. It is also one of the great "mimics" in medicine, because it is capable of manufacturing a wide variety of hormones that produce a number of diverse systemic syndromes. For example, Cushing's syndrome may result from the secretion of glucocorticoids by the tumor. Polycythemia may result from the production of erythropoietin. Secretion of a parathyroid-like hormone leads to hypercalcemia. Feminization or masculinization may occur if gonadotropins are elaborated by the tumor. Although renal cell carcinomas are known to contain a large amount of lipid and glycogen, giving them a clear cell appearance on histologic section, they do not secrete lipid and are not associated with hyperlipidemia. *(pp. 986–987)*

**7. (A)** Urolithiasis (kidney stones) is a common clinical problem, affecting 5 to 10% of the American population. Some stones may be asymptomatic or may produce only painless hematuria. However, stones that result in ureteral obstruction cause one of the most severe forms of pain in all of clinical medicine (ureteral colic—an unforgettable experience for most of the afflicted). Although stones may be formed at any level in the urinary tract, most uroliths originate in the kidney itself (nephroliths). The majority of urinary stones (about 75%) are composed of calcium salts (calcium oxylate or calcium oxylate/calcium phosphate) and occur in association with conditions producing hypercalcemia and/or hypercalciuria, such as hyperparathyroidism. Five per cent of calcium-containing stones are associated with hyperoxaluria, either primary (hereditary) or acquired by increased intestinal absorption of oxalates ("enteric hyperoxaluria"). No matter what their composition, all stones are the result of supersaturation of the urine with the stone-forming substance, a situation favored by overproduction combined with low urine volume.

Primary and secondary gout increase serum urate levels and lead to the formation of urate stones. Infections by urea-splitting bacteria (such as *Proteus mirabilis*), which convert urea to ammonia and create an alkaline urine, lead to the precipitation of magnesium ammonium phosphate salts in the urine. The result is the formation of very large urinary stones, frequently assuming the outline of the renal pelvis and calyces ("staghorn" calculi).

Sickle cell nephropathy causes a spectrum of renal changes, including hematuria, decreased concentrating ability, proteinuria, and even papillary necrosis, but, unlike the previous disorders, is not associated with stone formation. *(pp. 981; 984–985)*

**8. (E)** Acute pyelonephritis (APN) is suppurative inflammation of the renal pelvis, tubules, and interstitium caused by bacterial infection. Ascending infection from the lower urinary tract (usually caused by gram-negative enteric organisms such as *Escherichia coli*) associated with vesicoureteral reflux is by far the most common cause. Thus, conditions that predispose to lower urinary tract obstruction and/or infection increase the risk of acquiring APN. Such conditions include pregnancy, nephrolithiasis, prostatic hypertrophy (see Chapter 11, Question 7), and tumors. Instrumentation of the urinary tract (e.g., catheterization of the bladder) also predisposes to APN in the absence of obstruction or pre-existing renal lesions.

Hematogenous infection of the kidney is much less common than ascending infection. It usually occurs only in debilitated or immunosuppressed patients, in the presence of an underlying renal abnormality such as ureteral obstruction or previous renal injury, or with nonenteric organisms such as staphylococci and certain fungi. Septicemia alone seldom causes APN because the kidney is remarkably resistant to blood-borne organisms. *(pp. 967–971)*

**9. (D)** In addition to forming a branching cellular framework that supports the glomerular capillary tufts, mesangial cells have a number of other important functions. They ingest macromolcules that have leaked across the glomerulus. They are also contractile and thereby may serve to regulate intraglomerular blood flow. They are capable of laying down both basement membrane–like mesangial matrix and collagen. They can be stimulated to elaborate a number of biologically active mediators, such as cytokines, growth factors, eicosanoids, and endothelin. They are connected with the Lacis (mesangial-like) cells of the juxtaglomerular apparatus, which is the organelle that senses changes in afferent arteriolar pressure and is the principal source of renin production. Mesangial cells themselves, however, do not elaborate renin. *(pp. 930–931; 943)*

**10. (A)** Most glomerulonephritis is caused by antibody- and cell-mediated mechanisms of immunologic damage. Once immune complexes (either circulating and passively trapped [see Question 4] or formed *in situ*) become localized in the glomerulus, glomerular injury is produced by a combination of secondary mechanisms. Activation of complement produces neutrophil chemotactic agents (mainly C5a). Neutrophils, in turn, release proteases and oxygen-derived free radicals that cause cellular and basement membrane damage. Macrophages and monocytes also infiltrate the glomerulus and release a large number of biologically active molecules, free radicals, and proteases that contribute to glomerular damage. Platelets, which aggregate in the glomerulus during immune-mediated injury, release arachidonic acid metabolites (eicosanoids) and growth factors. These platelet products are believed to act as mediators of glomerular injury and reduced glomerular filtration rates. Resident mesangial cells are also believed to play an active role in the process. Mesangial cells can be stimulated to produce inflammatory mediators (such as free radicals, cytokines, and eicosanoids) that are capable of mediating glomerular inflammation and injury.

It is important to recognize that all immunologically mediated glomerular diseases involve mechanisms related only to hypersensitivity responses of types II (antibody mediated), III (immune complex mediated), and IV (cytotoxic T-cell mediated), never type I (immunoglobulin E and mast cell mediated). This may be because there are no mast cells in the normal glomerulus. *(pp. 77; 943)*

**11. (D)** Systemic lupus erythematosus (SLE) gives rise to a number of different patterns of glomerular injury, including focal proliferative glomerulonephritis, diffuse proliferative glomerulonephritis, diffuse membranous glomerulonephritis, and a mesangial proliferative pattern (increased number of mesangial cells plus increased amounts of mesangial matrix) that is rather unique to SLE. Thus, renal lesions may result that are indistinguishable from idiopathic membranous glomerulonephritis, membranoproliferative glomerulonephritis, or typical crescentic glomerulonephritis (see Question 27). However, the pattern of lipoid nephrosis (normal glomerular histology but fusion of epithelial foot processes seen electron microscopically) is not produced by SLE. *(pp. 204–205; 959–960)*

**12. (B)** Renal papillary necrosis (necrotizing papillitis) is a distinctive, dramatic form of tubulointerstitial disease resulting in necrosis and sloughing of renal papillae. It occurs only in well-defined sets of circumstances. Papillary necrosis may occur as a complication of suppurative urinary tract infection in severe cases of acute pyelonephritis but, in this setting, is seen most often diabetics and in those with urinary tract obstruction. Papillary necrosis rarely is produced in the absence of infection, but notable exceptions include both analgesic abuse nephropathy and sickle cell anemia. In these conditions, the necrosis is a direct result of toxic or anoxic damage, respectively.

Gout and multiple myeloma are both causes of tubulointerstitial disease. However, they are not typically associated with papillary necrosis unless both infection and urinary tract obstruction are produced in the course of the disease. In the urate nephropathy of gout, monosodium urate crystals deposit in the interstitium and tubular lumens. Papillary necrosis might rarely occur as a complication in this disease only if infection were to occur in the setting of urinary tract obstruction by urate stones. Multiple myeloma is associated with renal amyloidosis as well as urinary tract obstruction with secondary infection. With the latter, as with any cause of obstruction plus infection, papillary necrosis may occur as a complication. *(pp. 971; 973–975)*

**13. (C)** Chronic pyelonephritis (CPN) refers to chronic tubulointerstitial inflammation and scarring in association with pathologic involvement of the calyces and pelvis. The distinction is important because all causes of tubulointerstitial disease of the kidney typically spare the calyces except for analgesic nephropathy (see Question 14) and CPN with chronic bacterial infection (usually associated with either vesicoureteral reflux [VUR] or urinary obstruction). Between the two forms of CPN, that occurring with VUR is more common than that associated with obstruction.

CPN typically causes asymmetrical, irregular renal scarring, in contrast to the symmetrically scarred kidneys of chronic glomerular disease. On microscopic examination, varying amounts of interstitial inflammation and fibrosis are seen, as well as varying degrees of tubular atrophy and reactive hypertrophy. Tubules may be strikingly dilated and filled with colloid casts, a pathologic change known as "thyroidization" because of the resemblance of the involved tubules to thyroid follicles. An important cause of end-stage kidney disease, CPN accounts for about 11 to 20% of patients requiring chronic hemodialysis or renal transplant for renal failure. The majority of renal failure (about 50%) is caused by chronic glomerulonephritis. *(p. 971)*

**14. (E)** Analgesic abuse nephropathy is a form of chronic tubulointerstitial nephritis with renal papillary necrosis caused by excessive intake of analgesics (typically mixed compounds containing phenacetin). Intriguingly, the disease is almost always caused by drug mixtures and is rarely produced by single agents alone. The offending mixtures commonly contain aspirin, acetaminophen (a phenacetin metabolite), or codeine in addition to phenacetin. Most individuals who develop this disease ingest between 2 and 3 kilograms of a phenacetin-containing analgesics over a period of 3 years. The injury is largely targeted to the renal papillae, ultimately producing papillary necrosis (see Question 12), so early findings include the inability to concentrate urine. Pyuria is also an early clinical manifestation and occurs in virtually every patient. Although the pyuria is often sterile, bacterial infection complicates about 50% of cases. If the drug abuse is continued, renal failure often ensues. If drug use is discontinued and infectious complications are treated properly, renal function will stabilize or even improve in most cases. Unfortunately, even with discontinued drug use, neoplastic complications may develop. Specifically, transitional papillary carcinoma of the renal pelvis has been found to occur with increased frequency in long-term survivors of this disorder. Increased risk of development of renal cell carcinoma, however, has not been noted. *(pp. 973–974)*

**15. (D)** In addition to its central role in the regulation of fluids and electrolytes that maintain extracellular fluid and blood volume, the kidney further participates in the control of blood pressure by secreting substances that have pressor effects as well as substances that lower blood pressure. Renin secretion (in response to decreased pressure in afferent arterioles, decreased sodium or chloride load delivered to the macula densa, or adrenergic stimulation), is the major renal mechanism for increasing blood pressure. Renin raises blood pressure in two ways: (1) it catalyzes the first step in the enzymatic conversion of angiotensinogen to angiotensin II (a potent vasoconstrictor and the major effector molecule of the renin-angiotensin system); and (2) it stimulates aldosterone secretion by the adrenal cortex, thereby producing sodium retention. The kidney itself, however, does not produce aldosterone.

Vasodepressor (antihypertensive) substances secreted by the kidney include platelet-activating factor, kininogen (the basis of the urinary kallikrein-kinin system), prostaglandins, and nitric oxide. The vasodepressor substances are believed to counterbalance the vasopressor effects of angiotensin II. *(pp. 485–486)*

**16. (B)** Systemic hypertension is a common complication of renal diseases involving stimulation of renin secretion by the juxtaglomerular apparatus. Renin is the precursor of angiotensin II, both a potent vasoconstricting (pressor) agent and a stimulator of aldosterone secretion (see Question 15 above). Aldosterone, in turn, causes sodium retention that increases blood volume. Thus, renal diseases producing systemic hypertension include all forms of acute disease that target the arteries, arterioles, or glomeruli and all chronic renal disease, whether glomerular or tubulointerstitial in type. Specifically, these would include renal vasculitis, all forms of acute glomerulonephritis, chronic glomerulonephritis, and chronic pyelonephritis; all are causes of secondary (i.e., not "essential" or primary) hypertension that is renal in origin. In chronic tubulointerstitial disease, the glomeruli eventually are affected as well. Destruction of a tubule (the outflow tract for the glomerular filtrate) produces secondary injury to its associated glomerulus, and ultimately, the entire nephron degenerates. In the acute form of pyelonephritis, however, the glomeruli are not involved in the process and the juxtaglomerular apparatus is not activated. Pain, fever and malaise are produced, but hypertension is not part of the clinical picture. *(486–487; 970; 977t)*

**17. (C)** Malignant nephrosclerosis refers to the renal disease associated with the malignant or accelerated phase of hypertension. It may develop in previously normotensive individuals but more commonly is superimposed on pre-existing essential hypertension or chronic renal disease. The characteristic histologic finding in malignant nephrosclerosis is fibrinoid necrosis of arterioles. Often, the involved arterioles also show mural inflammation (necrotizing arteriolitis). Medial smooth muscle proliferation and concentric intermyenteric fibrosis are seen in the interlobular arteries and arterioles (hyperplastic arteriolitis, also known as "onion skinning"). Glomerular thrombosis and necrosis (necrotizing glomerulitis) often are present as well. Distal to the abnormal vessels, ischemic atrophy and infarction may be present.

Fibromuscular dysplasia of the renal artery is a cause of nephrogenic hypertension rather than an effect of accelerated systemic hypertension. It refers to a heterogeneous group of lesions of unknown etiology characterized by fibrous or fibromuscular thickening of the renal artery leading to stenosis (see Question 18). *(pp. 977–979)*

**18. (E)** Although it is a relatively rare problem overall, renal artery stenosis is the most common curable form of hypertension. It is most frequently caused by an atheromatous plaque at the origin of the renal artery but also may result from fibromuscular dysplasia of the renal artery (see Question 17). The resultant reduction in blood flow to the kidney stimulates the renin-angiotensin system, which in turn elevates blood pressure. Elevated renin levels in the plasma and/or in renal vein blood from the stenotic side are typical, and a fall in blood pressure in response to administration of angiotensin antagonists can be demonstrated in nearly all patients. About 80% of patients with fibromuscular dysplasia and about 60 to 75% of those with atherosclerotic renal artery senosis are cured following removal of the kidney on the *nonstenotic* side and surgical correction of the stenosis. Ironically, the kidney on the stenotic side is protected from the arteriolosclerotic effects of the hypertension it induces because the increased arterial pressure is not transmitted through the narrowed renal artery. However, the contralateral nonstenotic kidney typically is devastated by the effects of the hypertension and must be removed surgically. *(pp. 978–979)*

**19. (A)** A number of serious renal diseases may occur in association with pregnancy or childbirth. Both diffuse cortical necrosis and the adult hemolytic uremic syndrome (HUS) are life-threatening delivery-associated renal disorders that have a high mortality rate. Diffuse cortical necrosis is a complication of disseminated intravascular coagulation (DIC) (see Chapter 7, Question 5) but is a more severe form of injury in which DIC occurs in association with vasoconstriction. It produces a histologic picture of acute ischemic infarction, sharply limited to the renal cortex, with variable degrees of vascular thrombosis and necrosis. As an obstetric complication, DIC may be initiated either by release of tissue factor and activation of the extrinsic coagulation pathway (e.g., retained dead fetus or placenta) or by widespread injury to endothelial cells and activation of the intrinsic pathway (e.g., septic absorption, amniotic fluid embolism, toxemia). Diffuse cortical necrosis most often occurs following obstetrical emergencies such as abruptio placenta (premature placental separation from the uterine wall), septic shock, or extensive surgery. When bilateral, it is fatal, producing sudden anuria that rapidly terminates in uremic death.

Adult HUS is a disorder that is also characterized by cortical necrosis and vascular injury. HUS characteristically produces thrombosis of interlobular arteries, afferent arterioles and glomeruli together with necrosis and thickening of vessel walls ("fibrinoid necrosis") and a microangiopathic hemolytic anemia. As in DIC, the intravascular coagulation in HUS is initiated by such problems as placental hemorrhage or retained placental fragments. Like diffuse cortical necrosis, postpartum HUS has a grave prognosis, although recovery may occur in mild cases.

Eclampsia (more fully discussed in Chapter 11, Question 11) is a pregnancy-related syndrome of hypertension, proteinuria, edema, and DIC. The underlying cause is decreased uteroplacental perfusion, stimulating a number of pathophysiologic responses in the ischemic placenta. Ultimately, both arterial vasoconstriction with systemic hypertension and DIC are produced. In the kidneys, diffuse fibrin deposition in glomeruli and fibrin thrombi in capillaries typically are seen. When severe, a pattern of diffuse cortical necrosis may be produced.

A less dire but more common obstetric problem is urinary tract obstruction, a consequence of the extrinsic compression of the ureters by the enlarging uterus in normal pregnancy. Hydronephrosis, the term used to describe dilation of the renal pelvis and calyces resulting from urinary outflow obstruction, may occur but remain clinically silent. With bilateral partial obstruction, some patients with hydronephrosis may manifest symptoms of tubulointerstitial disease.

Nephrocalcinosis refers to the renal complications of hypercalcemia, namely, deposition of calcium in the kidney and the formation of calcium stones. With an extensive degree of calcinosis, chronic tubulointerstitial disease and renal insufficiency may result. The underlying causes of nephrocalcinosis include all disorders characterized by the production of hypercalcemia, such as multiple myeloma, hyperparathroidism, vitamin D intoxication, metastatic bone disease, and excess calcium intake (milk-alkali syndrome). Calcinosis is unrelated to pregnancy or delivery. *(pp. 623–624; 975; 980–982; 1081)*

**20. (B)** Hematuria is an important but nonspecific indicator of renal disease. It occurs in a larger number of disorders of either the kidney or lower urinary tract, including glomerulonephritis, nephrolithiasis, and tumors (benign or malignant), to name only a few. Although red blood cells in the urine may originate from anywhere in the urinary tract, red blood cell casts formed in the renal tubules are indicative of intrarenal disease and are useful in the differential diagnosis of hematuria. In glomerulonephritis, for example, the urine would characteristically contain red cell casts, but in nephrolithiasis casts would be lacking. Painless hematuria is a common presentation for tumors in the kidney (e.g., renal cell carcinoma) or bladder (e.g., papilloma or transitional cell carcinoma). Although some forms of cystitis typically produce mucosal hemorrhage as their major manifestation (e.g., hemorrhagic cystitis related to radiation or chemotherapy, especially with cyclophosphamide), the cystitis produced by malakoplakia is not hemorrhagic in type. Malakoplakia is a peculiar type of reaction to bacterial infection characterized by macrophage infiltrates that produce soft, raised mucosal plaques but not hemorrhage. The macrophages are filled with bacterial debris, making their cytoplasm granular and periodic acid–Schiff positive. They also contain basophilic mineralized inclusions known as Michaelis-Gutmann bodies. The reaction is thought to be related to defective macrophage phagocytic or degradative processes. Although malakoplakia occurs most commonly in the bladder, it also may affect the kidney, epididymis, or prostate (or, rarely, the colon, lungs, or bone). *(pp. 945; 985; 987; 995–997; 1002)*

**21. (D)** The fungating bladder tumor pictured in Figure 10–2 is a transitional cell carcinoma (TCC) of the bladder, by far the most common type of bladder neoplasm. Nearly all (95%) bladder tumors are epithelial in origin (i.e., carcinomas). TCC constitutes about 90% of bladder carcinomas, and squamous cell carcinoma accounts for about 5%. TCC of the bladder has been shown to be related to a number of environmental carcinogenic agents. It has been established clearly that azo dyes contain a number of chemical compounds (arylamines) that dramatically increase the incidence of TCC in exposed individuals. Azo dyes are used in textile, plastics, rubber, printing, and cable industries. Tobacco smoking also has been identified as a risk factor for bladder cancer, the incidence of bladder tumors being three to seven times greater in smokers than in nonsmokers. It has been estimated that 50 to 80% of all bladder cancers in men can be attributed to cigarette smoking. *Schistosoma haematobium* infection long has been known to increase the risk of bladder cancer. The majority (about 70%) of schistosoma-induced cancers are squamous cell carcinomas, but the rest of these tumors are TCCs. An unfortunate iatrogenic cause of TCC is heavy long-term exposure to cyclophosphamide. This immunosuppressive and cancer chemotherapeutic agent not only causes hemorrhagic cystitis (see Question 20) but increases the risk of bladder cancer about ten-fold after 12 years of exposure.

Von Hippel-Lindau disease is associated with a dramatically increased risk of developing renal cell carcinoma, often bilaterally. However, it is not associated with an increased risk of bladder cancer. *(pp. 283–284; 986–987; 1001)*

**22. (True); 23. (True); 24. (True); 25. (False); 26. (False)**

**(22, 23, 24)** Acute tubular necrosis (ATN) is a syndrome of isolated renal tubular damage (destruction of tubular epithelial cells) producing acute renal failure (acute cessation of renal function with urine output falling to <400 mL within 24 hours). ATN may occur as a result of either an ischemic or a toxic insult because tubular epithelium is both particularly sensitive to anoxia and particularly vulnerable to toxins. ATN is of great importance not only because it is the most common cause of acute renal failure, but also because it is usually completely reversible with the therapeutic intervention. Ischemic ATN occurs most commonly after an episode of shock (peripheral circulatory collapse) secondary to sepsis, acute pancreatitis, large cutaneous burns, or massive crush injuries. Nephrotoxic ATN is caused by a wide variety of agents, including heavy metals, organic solvents, antibiotics, anesthetics, chemotherapeutic agents, radiographic contrast media, insecticides, and herbicides. Histologically, toxic ATN can be differentiated from ischemic ATN by its pattern of injury, which characteristically targets the proximal tubules and generally spares the distal tubular segments of the nephron. Ischemic ATN, in contrast, is characterized by focal tubular necrosis at multiple points along the entire nephron. However, because shock and ischemia frequently complicate toxic ATN, the pattern of injury may be mixed.

**(25)** Although ATN usually produces acute renal failure with oliguria (or rarely anuria), up to 50% of patients with ATN actually have an increased urine output. Nonoliguric ATN is particularly common in nephrotoxic ATN and generally tends to have a milder clinical course.

**(26)** Recovery from ATN involves regeneration of the epithelium of the injured tubules. Because tubular cells have the capacity to divide and no stromal destruction takes place in ATN, full restoration of normal structure is possible. With tubular regeneration, normal renal function usually is restored. Of course, the underlying cause of the ATN must be reversed, and the patient must be supported with careful fluid and electrolyte management and dialysis during the oliguric phase of the injury. *(pp. 964–966)*

**27. (A); 28. (C); 29. (B); 30. (D); 31. (A); 32. (A); 33. (C)**

Rapidly progressive glomerulonephritis (RPGN) is a syndrome of glomerular damage characterized clinically by hematuria with a rapid and progressive decline in renal function and pathologically by a unique feature known as "crescents" (marked accumulation of cells in Bowman's space). RPGN can be thought of as a galloping form of acute glomerulonephritis, producing a severe nephritic syndrome (hematuria with red cell casts, azotemia, oliguria, and hypertension) that rapidly progresses to renal failure. The nephrotic syndrome is characterized clinically by massive proteinuria, hypoalbuminemia, edema, and hyperlipidemia, but, in contrast to RPGN, both the glomerular pathology and the clinical course are variable.

**(27)** Glomerular disease occurring in association with infection by nephritogenic strains of streptococcal is immunologically mediated. It typically takes the form of a nephritic syndrome (also known as syndrome of acute nephritis) rather than the nephrotic syndrome (massive proteinuria). In a small proportion of patients with poststreptococcal glomerulonephritis, however, rapid renal failure develops, and the classic clinical and pathologic features of RPGN are seen.

**(28 and 33)** Immunoglobulin A (IgA) nephropathy and systemic lupus erythematosus (SLE) (also Henoch-Schönlein purpura) are examples of diseases that may produce either a nephritic or a nephrotic syndrome. Either may cause RPGN, although SLE is more likely to do so than IgA nephropathy. IgA nephropathy (Berger's disease) is a very common form of glomerulonephritis that is characterized by prominent IgA deposits in the glomerular mesangium. It is a frequent cause of recurrent gross or microscopic hematuria but occasionally may produce either the nephrotic syndrome or RPGN. SLE is even more variable than IgA nephropathy in its renal manifestations, which range from normal renal function with minimal proteinuria and hematuria to an overt nephrotic syndrome or RPGN with corresponding differences in the associated histologic lesions.

**(29)** Penicillamine is one of several drugs, including gold (used for the treatment of arthritis) and "street heroin," that are known to cause glomerular damage and a nephrotic syndrome. **(30)** Synthetic penicillin (e.g., methicillin) is one of a long list of drugs that are associated with tubular damage or interstitial inflammation or both. It may cause either nephrotoxic acute tubular necrosis (see Questions 22 through 26) or acute drug-induced tubulointerstitial nephritis, but it is not associated with glomerular disease.

**(31 and 32)** Both Wegener's granulomatosis, a syndrome of necrotizing vasculitis, and Goodpasture's syndrome, a disease produced by autoantibodies directed against basement membranes, typically involve both the lung and kidney as their primary targets of injury. They are both well-known causes of crescentic glomerulonephritis (RPGN), and can be differentiated only on the basis of their immunofluorescent and electron microscopic characteristics. The anti–basement membrane autoantibodies of Goodpasture's syndrome produce a diagnostic pattern of linear immunofluorescence and uniform glomerular basement membrane thickening not seen in Wegener's granulomatosis. *(pp. 945–949; 956–957; 965; 972–973)*

**34. (B); 35. (C); 36. (B); 37. (D); 38. (B)**

**(34, 36, 37, and 38)** Diseases that produce cystic changes in the kidneys vary widely in their etiologies and clinical consequences. Adult polycystic kidney disease (APKD) is a relatively common autosomal dominant disorder (the gene is located on chromosome 16 in 90% of cases) in which cysts arise from any portion of the nephron. APKD accounts for 10% of patients with chronic renal failure requiring dialysis or renal transplantation. In contrast to childhood polycystic disease and medullary sponge kidney, in which cysts develop only from collecting tubules, APKD produces proximal and distal tubular cysts in addition to cysts of collecting tubule origin. The cysts initially involve only portions of the nephrons, so that renal function usually is maintained and affected individuals remain entirely asymptomatic until the fourth or fifth decade of life, when renal insufficiency commences. Patients with APKD also tend to have other congenital anomalies, the most significant of which is intracranial berry aneurysm, present in 10 to 30% of patients. As many as 10% of those with APKD succumb to the rupture of a berry aneurysm. Most patients die of renal failure or hypertension related to their chronic renal disease, however.

**(35)** In contrast to the adult and childhood polycystic diseases, which produce profound abnormalities in renal function and ultimately lead to renal failure, medullary sponge kidney rarely causes any abnormality in renal function. It usually is discovered incidentally on radiologic studies or when complications such as infection or stone formation develop. *(pp. 935–937)*

**39. (A); 40. (B); 41. (A); 42. (C); 43. (E); 44. (C); 45. (D); 46. (B); 47. (A); 48. (B); 49. (C); 50. (A)**

**(39, 41, 47, and 50)** Most forms of primary glomerular disease produce the nephrotic syndrome. They are differentiated on the basis of their clinical manifestations and morphologic patterns of injury. Lipoid nephrosis (minimal change disease, or MCD) is the most common cause of the nephrotic syndrome in children. Clinically, it may be associated with prophylactic immunizations or respiratory infections, suggesting an immunologic basis for the disease. However, affected glomeruli do not contain immunoglobulins or complement and appear normal by light microscopy. The only morphologic lesion in MCD is the fusion of glomerular epithelial cell foot processes, a nonspecific change also present in other proteinuric disorders. In contrast to the other forms of idiopathic glomerular diseases, which frequently go on to chronic glomerulonephritis and renal failure, MCD usually responds rapidly to therapy and has an excellent long-term prognosis.

**(40, 46, and 48)** Membranous glomerulonephritis (MGN) is the most common cause (40% of cases) of the nephrotic syndrome in adults. It is associated with certain malignant epithelial tumors (particularly lung cancer, colon cancer, and melanoma), autoimmune disorders (thyroiditis, systemic lupus erythematosus), inorganic salts (gold, mercury), drugs (penicillamine, captopril), infections (hepatitis B, schistosomiasis, malaria), and diabetes. The disease is mediated by the localization of antigen-antibody complexes in the glomerulus. Circulating immune complexes are found in 15 to 25% of cases, but *in situ* formation of antigen-antibody complexes (circulating antibodies combine with antigens entrapped in the glomerular basement membrane) is believed to occur in the remainder of cases. Immune complexes are seen as subepithelial dense deposits on electron microscopy and constitute the most characteristic ultrastructural feature of MGN.

**(42, 44, and 49)** Membranoproliferative glomerulonephritis (MPGN) accounts for about 10% of cases of idiopathic nephrotic syndrome in children and about 7% of cases in adults. It is characterized morphologically by basement membrane "splitting," the result of protrusion of mesangial cell processes into the basement membrane of the capillary loops (mesangial interposition). In two thirds of cases, subendothelial electron-dense deposits are seen by electron microscopy (type I MPGN). A second variant of MPGN is characterized by the deposition of electron-dense material in the lamina densa of the glomerular basement membrane (type II MPGN, or dense-deposit disease). Most patients with type II MPGN have abnormalities that suggest primary activation of the alternate complement pathway. In contrast to type I MPGN, neither C1q nor C4 is present in the glomeruli in type II MPGN.

**(45)** Immunoglobulin A (IgA) nephropathy, or Berger's disease, is a common cause of hematuria and mild proteinuria, but it also may produce either the nephrotic syndrome or RPGN (see Question 28). It is characterized by the presence of prominent IgA deposits in the mesangial regions of affected glomeruli.

**(43)** Although some patients with IgA nephropathy may present with RPGN with crescents, none of these forms of glomerulonephritis typically produces crescentic RPGN. *(pp. 948–957)*

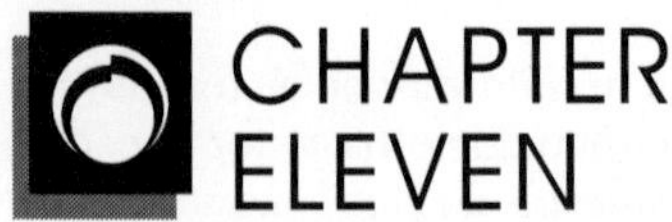

CHAPTER ELEVEN

# The Reproductive System

**DIRECTIONS:** For Questions 1 through 13, choose the ONE BEST answer to each question.

**1.** All of the following problems occur as complications of pelvic inflammatory disease EXCEPT:

A. Infertility
B. Bowel obstruction
C. Appendicitis
D. Peritonitis
E. Endocarditis

**2.** Which of the following lesions of the female genital tract is considered precancerous?

A. Cystic atrophy of the endometrium
B. Endocervical polyps
C. Condyloma acuminatum of the vulva
D. Endometrial polyps
E. Atypical hyperplasia of the endometrium

**3.** Uterine leiomyomas:

A. Are the most common gynecologic tumor
B. Never metastasize
C. Require progesterone for growth
D. Usually regress during pregnancy
E. Are the precursor lesions of most uterine leiomyosarcomas

**4.** Endometrial carcinoma is NOT associated with:

A. Diabetes mellitus
B. Infertility
C. Oral contraceptive steroid use
D. Hypertension
E. Obesity

**5.** Factors that predispose to the development of ectopic pregnancy include all of the following EXCEPT:

A. Previous appendicitis
B. Endometriosis
C. Previous pelvic surgery
D. Gonorrheal salpingitis
E. Fetal chromosomal abnormalities

**6.** The tumor pictured in Figure 11–1 is characterized by all of the following features EXCEPT:

A. Origin from primordial germ cells
B. Poor prognosis
C. Lack of endocrine function
D. Lymphocytic infiltration of the tumor stroma
E. High degree of radiosensitivity

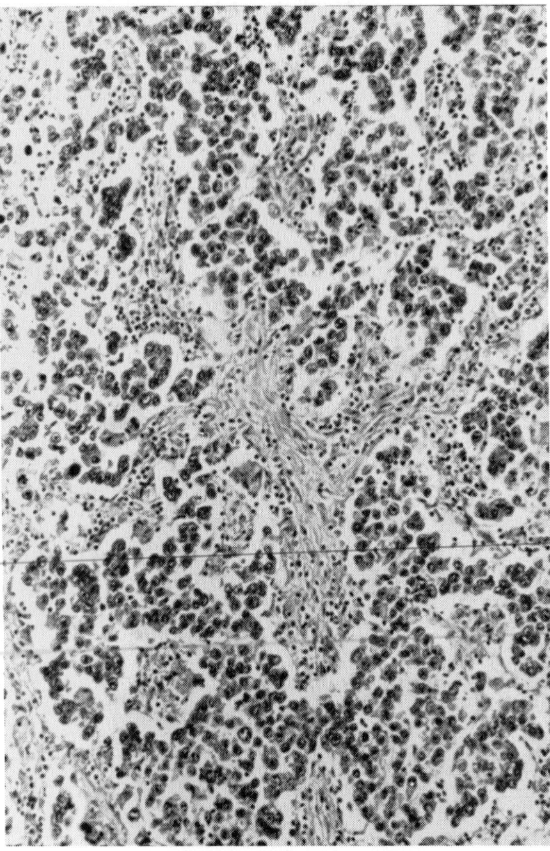

Figure 11–1

**7.** Which of the following statements about nodular hyperplasia of the prostate (benign prostatic hypertrophy) is INCORRECT?

A. It is related to dihydrotestosterone stimulation.
B. It occurs in about 90% of males over 70 years of age.
C. It typically involves the periurethral region of the prostate.
D. Hyperplasia of both glands and stroma is seen histologically.
E. It is a risk factor for prostatic adenocarcinoma.

**8.** Factors associated with high risk for cervical carcinoma include all of the following EXCEPT:

A. Early age at first intercourse
B. Multiple sexual partners
C. High-dose estrogen therapy
D. Male partner with multiple previous sexual partners
E. Human papillomavirus type 16

**9.** All of the following statements about invasive cervical carcinoma are true EXCEPT:

A. It is occurring at an increasingly younger age.
B. It is on the decline as a cause of cancer death.
C. It originates from cervical intraepithelial neoplasia (CIN) in most cases.
D. It is the end result of most CIN.
E. Its stage at discovery largely determines the prognosis.

**10.** Causes of abnormal uterine bleeding include all of the following EXCEPT:

A. Endometrial infection
B. Endometrial hyperplasia
C. Endometrial atrophy
D. Anovulatory cycle
E. Adenomyosis·

**11.** Factors that contribute to the development of toxemia of pregnancy (eclampsia) include all of the following EXCEPT:

A. Increased placental thromboxane production
B. Decreased placental prostaglandin production
C. Increased placental renin production
D. Increased placental angiotensin production
E. Increased maternal catecholamine production

**12.** All of the following diseases of the male genitalia are associated with human papillomavirus EXCEPT:

A. Bowenoid papulosis
B. Condyloma acuminatum
C. Penile squamous cell carcinoma
D. Balanoposthitis
E. Giant condyloma (Buschké-Lowenstein tumor)

**13.** All of the following factors are associated with an increased risk of testicular carcinoma EXCEPT:

A. Testicular irradiation
B. Klinefelter syndrome
C. Complete androgen insensitivity syndrome (testicular feminization)
D. Cryptorchidism
E. A sibling with testicular carcinoma

**DIRECTIONS:** For Questions 14 through 34, you are to decide whether EACH choice is TRUE or FALSE.

For each of the following statements about the normal menstrual cycle, choose whether it is TRUE or FALSE.

**14.** The basal third of the endometrium does not shed during menstruation.
**15.** Following ovulation, endometrial glands undergo marked proliferation.
**16.** Following ovulation, subnuclear vacuolization of endometrial glandular epithelium is seen.
**17.** Following ovulation, estrogen levels rise to their highest peak.
**18.** The length of the postovulatory phase of the menstrual cycle is the same in all women.

For each of the following statements about acute prostatitis, choose whether it is TRUE or FALSE.

**19.** It is the most common pathologic process of the prostate.
**20.** It most commonly is caused by bacterial infection.
**21.** The most commonly associated infectious agents are gram-negative bacilli.
**22.** Diagnosis depends on prostatic biopsy.
**23.** Progression to chronic disease predisposes to prostatic carcinoma.

For each of the following statements about the lesion pictured in Figure 11–2, choose whether it is TRUE or FALSE.

**24.** It is a rare complication of gestation.
**25.** It is usually accompanied by a developing fetus.
**26.** It typically has a normal female karyotype.
**27.** Its entire chromosome complement comes from the sperm.
**28.** It is the most common precursor of choriocarcinoma.
**29.** It produces higher serum levels of human chorionic gonadotropin than does choriocarcinoma.

For each of the following statements about prostate cancer, choose whether it is TRUE or FALSE.

**30.** It is the most common cancer in males.
**31.** Most tumors originate from the periurethral region of the gland.
**32.** Prognosis correlates well with the histologic grade of the tumor.
**33.** Tumor mass correlates with serum concentrations of prostate-specific antigen.
**34.** Osteoblastic bone lesions are virtually diagnostic of metastatic disease.

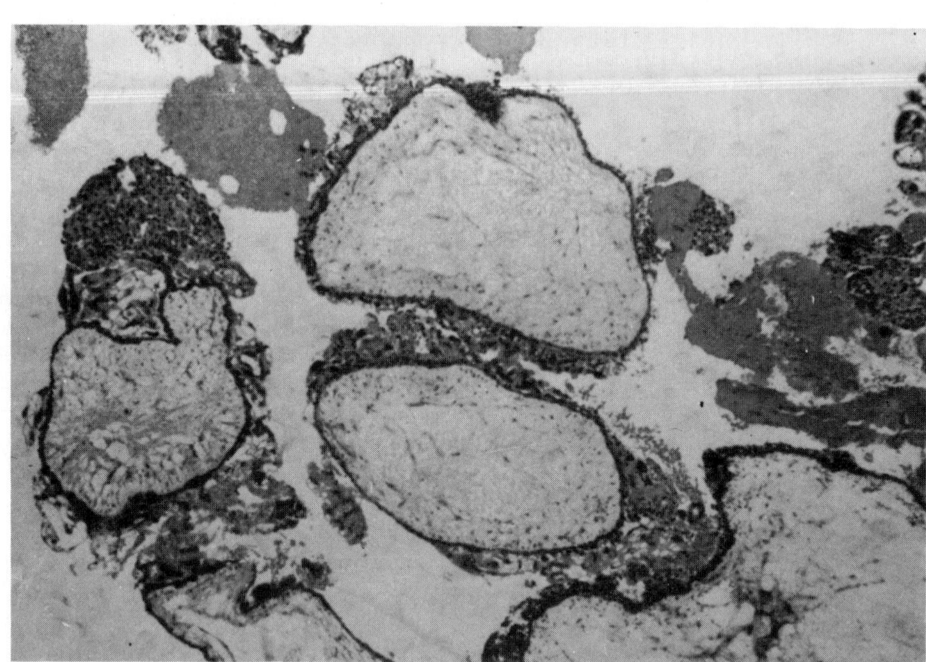

**Figure 11–2**

**DIRECTIONS:** For questions 35 through 53, the set of lettered headings is followed by a list of numbered words or phrases. For each numbered word or phrase choose:

A—if the item is associated with (A) only
B—if the item is associated with (B) only
C—if the item is associated with *both* (A) and (B)
D—if the item is associated with *neither* (A) nor (B)

For each of the features listed below, choose whether it describes adenomyosis, endometriosis, both, or neither.

A. Adenomyosis
B. Endometriosis
C. Both
D. Neither

**35.** Characterized by endometrial tissue in an abnormal location
**36.** Almost never occurs in women over age 50
**37.** Often produces dysmenorrhea
**38.** Sometimes results in infertility
**39.** Caused by increased estrogen exposure

For each of the characteristics listed below, choose whether it describes serious ovarian tumors, mucinous ovarian tumors, both, or neither.

A. Serous tumors of the ovary
B. Mucinous tumors of the ovary
C. Both
D. Neither

**40.** Oral contraceptive steroid use is a predisposing factor.
**41.** The majority of tumors exhibit cystic growth.
**42.** The majority of tumors are malignant.
**43.** Malignant tumors are more often bilateral than benign tumors.
**44.** "Borderline" variants of low malignant potential are recognized.
**45.** Simultaneous endometrial carcinoma is an associated complication.
**46.** Malignant variants tend to spread by direct seeding throughout the peritoneal cavity.
**47.** Pseudomyxoma peritonii is an associated complication.
**48.** The expression of high levels of HER-2/*neu* oncogene correlates with poor prognosis in malignant tumors.

For each of the characteristics of ovarian stromal tumors listed below, choose whether it describes granulosa-theca cell tumors, Sertoli-Leydig cell tumors, both, or neither.

A. Granulosa-theca cell tumors
B. Sertoli-Leydig cell tumors
C. Both
D. Neither

**49.** Usually cause virilization
**50.** Greatly predispose to endometrial carcinoma
**51.** Typically exhibit cystic growth
**52.** Seldom exhibit malignant biologic behavior
**53.** Are often associated with ascites

**DIRECTIONS:** Questions 54 through 63 are matching questions. For each numbered item, choose the most likely associated lettered item from those provided. Each numbered item has ONLY ONE answer. Within each group, each lettered item may be the answer to one, more than one, or none of the numbered items.

For each of the descriptions below, decide whether it refers to a Gartner's duct cyst, a Nabothian cyst, a Bartholin's cyst, a hydatid cyst of Morgagni, or none of these.

A. Gartner's duct cyst
B. Nabothian cyst
C. Bartholin's cyst
D. Hydatid cyst of Morgagni
E. None of these

**54.** Inflamed vulvovaginal gland with blocked duct
**55.** Mesonephric duct remnant of the vagina
**56.** Inflamed endocervical gland with a blocked duct
**57.** Endometriosis of the ovary
**58.** Wolffian duct remnant of the fallopian tube

For each of the characteristics of germ cell tumors listed below, choose whether it describes teratoma, choriocarcinoma, embryonal carcinoma, yolk sac tumor, or none of these.

A. Teratoma
B. Choriocarcinoma
C. Embryonal carcinoma
D. Yolk sac tumor
E. None of these

**59.** Is the most common malignant germ cell tumor in men
**60.** Is the most common benign germ cell tumor in women
**61.** Has as a specialized variant known as struma ovarii
**62.** Elaborates only α-fetoprotein
**63.** Elaborates only human chorionic gonadotropin

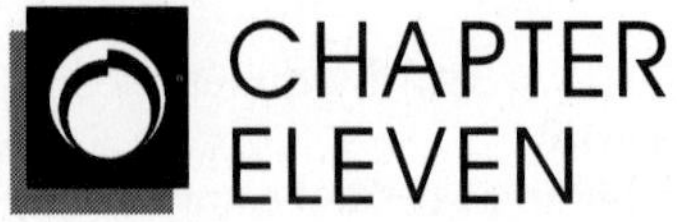

CHAPTER ELEVEN

# The Reproductive System

## ANSWERS

**1. (C)** Pelvic inflammatory disease (PID) is a common disorder caused by ascending infection of the female genital tract that may be transmitted sexually or occur as a septic complication of abortion or delivery. The severity of the disease depends somewhat on the causal organism and the route of infection. Postabortion and postpartum infections are typically the most difficult to control and ultimately may necessitate surgical removal of the involved organs. The consequences of uncontrolled PID, especially that caused by destructive pyogenic organisms, can be severe. Local complications include peritonitis, bowel obstruction (caused by adhesions between the inflamed pelvic organs and the adjacent intestinal loops), and infertility (caused by adhesions and scarring of the genital organs). With septicemia, systemic complications such as infective endocarditis, meningitis, or suppurative arthritis may ensue.

The pelvic pain caused by PID sometimes may be severe enough to present as an acute abdomen mimicking acute appendicitis. However, PID is not a cause of acute appendicitis. *(pp. 1038–1039)*

**2. (E)** Endometrial hyperplasia refers to a spectrum of excessive proliferative changes in the endometrial glands and stroma. It is caused by prolonged estrogenic stimulation, with diminished or absent progesterone production. It often occurs around the time of menopause or in association with persistent anovulation in younger women and produces abnormal uterine bleeding. It also may occur as a result of an underlying disease, such as an adrenal or ovarian disorder (see Question 50), in which excess estrogen is produced or as a consequence of iatrogenic administration of estrogenic substances.

Beyond its production of abnormal uterine bleeding, endometrial hyperplasia is especially important because of the association of the more complex and atypical forms with endometrial carcinoma. In general, the greater the degree of atypia, the greater the risk of malignancy. Lower grade hyperplasias uncommonly progress to adenocarcinoma. These include both simple (also known as "cystic") hyperplasia, the mildest form, and complex hyperplasia (also known as adenomatous hyperplasia without atypia). In simple hyperplasia, the proliferated glands are architecturally abnormal but lack cytologic atypia. This form of hyperplasia rarely progresses to endometrial carcinoma. In complex hyperplasia, the proliferated glands are more crowded and tortuous and may exhibit "budding" into the surrounding stroma. Conspicuous cytologic atypia is absent, but some stratification of the glandular epithelium may be seen. Less than 5% of these lesions progress to malignancy. Higher grade hyperplasias are known either as atypical hyperplasias or adenomatous hyperplasias with atypia. In these lesions, both architectural and cytologic atypicality are present and severe cases may resemble frank carcinoma. Such lesions are considered precancerous because about 25% of these lesions evolve into malignancy.

Cystic atrophy of the endometrium is a change in the endometrial glands that occurs with anovulatory cycles and, thus, is most common after menopause. It can be confused with simple endometrial hyperplasia because the glands are cystically dilated in both conditions. However, in contrast to simple hyperplasia, the endometrial glandular epithelium is flattened (versus tall in hyperplasia) and the stroma is atrophic. Most importantly, cystic atrophy is not believed to have malignant potential.

Endocervical polyps are completely benign inflammatory lesions consisting of hypertrophied endocervical glands in inflamed fibromyomatous stroma. They may cause irregular vaginal bleeding but are cured by simple curettage.

Condylomata acuminata of the vulva are sexually transmitted, benign warty lesions caused by human papillomavirus. These lesions often regress spontaneously and, except in immunosuppressed individuals, are not considered to be precancerous.

Endometrial polyps are sessile masses of either functional endometrium or hyperplastic endometrium, usually of the simple type. Although malignant change in an initially benign endometrial polyp may occur, it is extremely rare. Thus, endometrial polyps generally are not considered precancerous lesions. *(pp. 1041; 1047; 1057–1059)*

**3. (A)** Uterine leiomyomas ("fibroids") are the most common gynecologic tumors, occurring in at least 25% of premenopausal women. These benign smooth muscle tumors are well-circumscribed masses that usually arise within the myometrium of the uterine corpus and are often multiple. Leiomyomas are known to be hormone-dependent tumors that require estrogen for growth and regress following menopause or castration. Conversely, they tend to increase rapidly in size during pregnancy and may cause spontaneous abortion or other gestational or puerperal problems. Malignant transformation of leiomyomas is extremely rare. This class of tumors is also noteworthy because it sometimes breaks one of the cardinal rules of pathology: "benign tumors never metastasize." A rare variant of uterine leiomyoma known as "benign metastasizing leiomyoma" is a tumor of benign histology that grows into vessels, breaks off and metastasizes to other sites, most commonly the lung. However, uterine leiomyomas rarely, if ever, undergo transformation to a truly malignant tumor. Leiomyosarcomas of the uterus almost always arise directly from the myometrium and not from malignant transformation of a pre-existing benign leiomyoma. *(pp. 1059–1060)*

**4. (C)** Endometrial carcinoma is the most common invasive malignancy of the female genital tract and now accounts for about 7% of all invasive cancer in women. A number of important risk factors for this disease have been defined: diabetes mellitus, infertility, hypertension, obesity, estrogen-secreting tumors, and (an iatrogenic cause) estrogen replacement therapy. Overt diabetes mellitus is present in about 10% of patients with endometrial carcinoma and abnormal glucose tolerance in over 60%. Infertility and a clinical history of functional menstrual irregularities consistent with anovulatory cycles tend to be common among those who develop this disease. Fifty per cent of patients with endometrial carcinoma have hypertension, and 50% weigh more than 180 pounds.

There is substantial evidence that endometrial carcinoma is related to prolonged estrogen stimulation in many patients. In the past, an increased risk of endometrial carcinoma was reported with sequential contraceptive regimens that included estrogens in high dose, but these compounds are no longer in use. Present formulations of oral contraceptive steroids to not increase the risk for development of endometrial carcinoma. *(pp. 1060–1062)*

**5. (E)** Ectopic pregnancy refers to implantation of the fetus in any site other than the normal uterine location. It occurs most commonly in the fallopian tubes, usually the consequence of an acquired postinflammatory tubal abnormality. The most important predisposing condition is pelvic inflammatory disease (PID) (see Question 1) of any etiology (e.g., gonorrheal). Up to 50% of patients have PID-related chronic salpingitis. Less commonly, previous appendicitis, surgery, or endometriosis produce peritubal fibrous adhesions that interfere with tubal function. Intrauterine contraceptive devices also may increase the risk of ectopic pregnancy.

In contrast to these maternal abnormalities, fetal abnormalities do not contribute appreciably to the development of ectopic pregnancy. However, they are responsible for the majority of spontaneous abortions. *(p. 1078–1079)*

**6. (B)** The tumor pictured in Figure 11–1 could be either a seminoma or a dysgerminoma because these two tumors are morphologically indistinguishable. Seminoma and dysgerminoma are the most common types of malignant germinal tumors occurring in men and women, respectively. Despite their different names, they are identical in biologic type and are believed to arise from primordial germ cells. They are composed of sheets of uniform, undifferentiated cells that are divided into poorly demarcated lobules by lymphocyte-laden, fibrous tissue septa. The tumor cells themselves lack endocrine function. Occasionally, however, syncytiotrophoblastic cells, which produce human chorionic gonadotropin, may occur within the tumor.

In addition to their histologic similarities, seminomas and dysgerminomas share biologic traits. They have an excellent prognosis when excised while still localized within the gonad. Furthermore, because they are both highly radiosensitive, neoplasms that extend beyond the gonad can be well controlled or even eradicated by radiation therapy in most cases. *(pp. 1016–1017; 1073–1074)*

**7. (E)** Nodular hyperplasia of the prostate or benign prostatic hypertrophy (BPH) refers to a process of stromal and glandular hyperplasia that originates from and is most severe within the periurethral portion of the prostate. It is an extremely common disorder in men over the age of 50 and increases in frequency with increasing age. Thus, about 90% of men over age 70 have BPH. Because of its strategic location, it often produces symptoms related to urination (e.g., pain, overflow dribbling, difficulties stopping and starting the stream of urine) or urinary tract obstruction (e.g., bladder distention, urinary tract infection). Although it once was thought that BPH predisposed to prostatic carcinoma, most recent studies refute this. Thus, BPH has been exonerated and is no longer considered to be a risk factor for prostate cancer. *(pp. 1118–1121)*

**8. (C)** The risk of developing cervical carcinoma is strongly related to sexual history. Early age at first intercourse, multiple sexual partners, and male partner(s) with multiple previous sexual partners are the most potent of all risk factors for cervical carcinoma. These associations strongly implicate sexually transmitted agents in the etiology of cervical cancer. There is now strong evidence that one such agent is human papillomavirus (HPV). In particular, certain strains of this virus are associated with high risk for cervical cancer: types 16, 18, 31, and 33. A low risk is associated with types 6, 11, 42, and 44. In 85% of cervical cancers, HPV DNA can be found integrated into the host genomic DNA. Nevertheless, 15% of cervical cancers do not appear to be related to HPV infection, suggesting that HPV may not be the only important factor in this disease.

In contrast to endometrial carcinoma (and breast cancer), estrogen exposure is not related to the pathogenesis of cervical carcinoma. Thus, use of high-dose estrogenic supplements during or after menopause is not associated with increased risk of cervical carcinoma. *(pp. 340; 1048)*

**9. (D)** The realization that epithelial malignancies could arise from precursor lesions of increasingly disordered epithelial growth and differentiation (dysplasia) came from studies of cervical carcinoma. It is clear that invasive squamous cell carcinoma is the end stage of a continuum of progressive cervical intraepithelial neoplasia (CIN) in the vast majority of cases. The progression to invasive malignancy is usually a slow process, allowing for regular medical surveillance with early diagnosis and ablative treatment of the precursor lesions before invasive disease has a chance to develop. This approach has improved the cure rate for cervical cancer greatly and resulted in a dramatic decline in the death rate from invasive cervical carcinoma despite the increasing frequency of CIN. The peak incidence of both CIN III and invasive cervical carcinoma is occurring at an increasingly younger age, making it important to begin Papanicolau smear ("Pap test") screening at earlier ages in sexually active women.

Although most CIN progresses to higher stage lesions with time, the rates of progession are highly variable. Furthermore, progression is not inevitable; some lesions may even regress. About one third and two thirds of CIN I and CIN II, respectively, persist or progress to CIN III. However, the likelihood of developing invasive carcinoma once the lesion has progressed to CIN III (the highest grade; denotes carcinoma *in situ*) is increased. Even so, with current screening and treatment methods, only about 1 in 500 patients with treated CIN III ever develops invasive cancer. The prognosis and survival for invasive cancer, once established, is largely determined by the stage of disease at the time of discovery. *(pp. 1047–1053)*

**10. (A)** Abnormal uterine bleeding may be caused by a large number of disorders that can be categorized generally as either organic lesions, ovulatory dysfunction, endocrine dysfunction, or complications of pregnancy. Among pre- and perimenopausal woman, ovulatory abnormalities include anovulatory cycles and inadequate progesterone production by the corpus luteum (inadequate luteal phase). Adenomyosis, a disorder characterized by deep extension of normal endometrium into the myometrium, is an example of an organic lesion occurring in the reproductive age group. Endometrial atrophy is an example of an organic lesion occurring in the postmenopausal age group. Endometrial hyperplasia is an example of an organic lesion occurring in either age group.

Infections of the endometrium are usually related to ascending spread of organisms from the lower genital tract in pelvic inflammatory disease. The presentation of infection is not one of abnormal uterine bleeding but of pain, fever, and discharge. *(pp. 1038; 1055–1056)*

**11. (E)** Toxemia of pregnancy refers to a syndrome of hypertension, proteinuria, and edema (pre-eclampsia) that occurs in about 6% of pregnant women. A subset of these patients become seriously ill, developing coma or convulsions, a situation known as eclampsia. Patients with eclampsia develop disseminated intravascular coagulation.

The pathogenesis of toxemic hypertension appears to be related largely to decreased placental perfusion, the underlying reasons for which may be varied and are not well defined. Hypoperfusion leads to a number of abnormal physiologic responses by the placental tissues, including decreased prostaglandin E production and increased placental renin and angiotensin production. The result is a loss of the normal physiologic adaptations of the renin-angiotensin system that usually occur during pregnancy and protect against hypertension. The normal pregnant woman is resistant to the vasoconstrictive and hypertensive effects of angiotensin because of the protective effect of prostaglandins of the E series, which are produced in the uteroplacental vascular bed. With the loss of this protection and the added effect of increased renin and angiotensin, hypertension results. Placental ischemia also leads to the output of other vasoconstrictor substances besides angiotensin that contribute to the generation of systemic hypertension in toxemia. These include thromboxane (a product of arachidonic acid metabolism that is a potent platelet aggregating agent and vasoconstrictor) and endothelin.

Catecholamines, with their strong vasoconstrictor effects, are well known to increase blood pressure, but cathecholamines of either maternal or fetal-placental origin are not known to contribute to the pathogenesis of toxemia. *(pp. 68; 1079–1081)*

**12. (D)** A spectrum of diseases of the penis, from inflammatory to precancerous to malignant, are believed to be causally related to human papillomavirus (HPV) infection. Among them are condyloma acuminatum, giant condyloma (Buské-Lowenstein tumor), bowenoid papulosis, and squamous cell carcinoma of the penis.

Bowenoid papulosis is a penile lesion that appears clinically as multiple pigmented papules and histologically as a squamous cell carcinoma *in situ*. It is a premalignant lesion associated with HPV type 16 infection. DNA sequences of HPV type 16 can be detected in virtually all lesions with polymerase chain reaction amplification.

Like condylomata acuminata (benign venereal warts), giant condylomas (Buské-Lowenstein tumors) are believed to be causally related to HPV types 6 and 11. In contrast to condylomata acuminata, however, giant condylomas are locally invasive tumors that tend to recur but do not metastasize. Thus, the biologic behavior of Buské-Lowenstein tumors is midway between warts and squamous cell carcinoma.

Squamous cell carcinomas of the penis, like those of the female cervix, have been linked with HPV type 16 and, to a lesser degree, type 18. It has been hypothesized that the protective effect of circumcision in preventing penile carcinoma may be related to improved penile hygiene and reduced likelihood of infection by HPV.

Balanoposthitis is a bacterial infection of the glans penis and/or prepuce. It is not related to HPV. *(pp. 1008–1011)*

**13. (A)** Testicular germ cell tumors occur with greatly increased frequency in pathologic conditions associated with gonadal maldevelopment, among which testicular dysgenesis and cryptorchidism are the two most important. Testicular dysgenesis (failure of development of the seminiferous tubules) occurs in both the Klinefelter syndrome (sex chromosomal disorder with two or more X and one or more Y chromosomes) and the complete androgen insensitivity (or "testicular feminization") syndrome. The risk is highest in testicular feminization, a disorder caused by mutations in the gene for the androgen receptor.

Cryptorchidism (undescended testis) represents failure of descent of the intra-abdominal testis into the scrotal sac. It occurs in up to 0.8% of the male population and is unilateral in most cases. Cryptorchidism increases the risk of developing testicular carcinoma about tenfold above that in normal subjects. In patients with unilateral cryptorchidism, both testes are at increased risk of developing a malignancy, although the risk is significantly higher in the undescended testis. Nevertheless, this suggests that an underlying intrinsic defect in testicular development and cellular differentiation may be present that is unrelated to anatomic position. Surgical correction of the undescended testis does not eliminate the risk of malignancy, further suggesting the presence of an underlying defect.

Another risk factor of apparent importance to testicular cancer is genetic predisposition. Even though there are no well-defined patterns of inheritance in testicular cancer, having a sibling with testicular carcinoma apparently increases an individual's risk of testicular cancer about ten-fold above that of the normal population.

Testicular irradiation, like cryptorchidism, causes testicular atrophy but, in contrast to cryptorchidism, it is not associated with an increased risk of testicular carcinoma. *(pp. 159; 162; 1011–1012; 1016)*

**14. (True); 15. (False); 16. (True); 17. (False); 18. (True)**

The cyclic rise and fall of ovarian hormones normally produces a regular sequence of histologic changes in the endometrium. **(14)** The basal third (deep aspect) of the endometrium does not respond to ovarian hormones, so it remains behind after the menstrual flow and gives rise to the regenerated surface epithelium during the next cycle. **(15)** Before ovulation takes place, the regenerating endometrial glands undergo marked proliferation. Following ovulation, proliferation ceases and the glands become secretory.

**(16)** A phenomenon that is particularly characteristic of the postovulatory endometrium is subnuclear vacuolization of the endometrial gland epithelium. It begins immediately after ovulation and peaks on the third day after ovulation. The presence of this feature confirms that ovulation has taken place. **(17)** Endometrial growth in the proliferative phase of the cycle is stimulated by the estrogen production of the enlarging ovarian follicle. Estrogen rises progressively, reaches a peak just prior to ovulation, and then falls. Following ovulation, estrogen levels again rise briefly at the end of the first postovulatory week, but the level is never as high as the preovulatory peak. In contrast, progesterone, produced by the corpus luteum, rises progressively after ovulation until just before menstruation, when it falls to basal levels.

**(18)** Although the preovulatory phase of the menstrual cycle varies in length from woman to woman or even in the same woman during different cycles, postovulatory events occur according to a fixed physiologic schedule 14 days in length. Thus, glandular secretions, stromal predecidualization, and menstruation all normally occur in a highly predictable temporal sequence following ovulation. *(pp. 1035–1037)*

**19. (False); 20. (True); 21. (True); 22. (False); 23. (False)**

**(19)** Prostatitis may be either acute (highly symptomatic) or chronic (vaguely symptomatic), bacterial or abacterial. All types taken together are still not as common a prostatic problem as nodular hyperplasia (see Question 7).

**(20 and 21)** Acute prostatitis is virtually always the result of a bacterial infection, most often caused by *Escherichia coli* or other gram-negative bacilli (fecal in origin). In contrast, bacterial infection may or may not be present in chronic prostatitis. In fact, the abacterial form of chronic prostatitis is the most common type of prostatitis encountered overall.

**(22)** Diagnosis of prostatitis and differentiation among the three types (i.e., acute bacterial, chronic bacterial, and chronic abacterial) depend largely on microscopic examination and culture of expressed prostatic secretions acquired via transrectal prostatic massage. Biopsy is not required.

**(23)** In contrast to the many other chronic inflammatory processes in the body that are well known to predispose to epithelial malignancy in the involved organ (e.g., chronic esophagitis, gastritis, or colitis), chronic prostatitis does not predispose to prostatic carcinoma. *(pp. 1023–1024)*

**24. (False); 25. (False); 26. (True); 27. (True); 28. (True); 29. (False)**

**(24)** The lesion pictured in Figure 11–2 is a complete hydatidiform mole. Moles are common complications of gestation that occur about once in every 1,000 births in the United States. They represent benign tumorous proliferations of pregnancy-associated trophoblastic tissue. Two types are recognized: complete moles and partial moles. The two forms have different karyotypes (46,XX and triploid in complete and partial moles, respectively) and are characterized by different amounts of trophoblast proliferation, villous edema, and tissue expression of human chorionic gonadotropin (hCG) (more of each in complete moles compared to partial moles). Only complete moles have distinct malignant potential (2.5% develop into choriocarcinoma). As shown in the micrograph, a complete mole is characterized by cystic swelling of all or most of the chorionic villi. This is accompanied by diffuse trophoblastic proliferation. Patients usually present in the fourth or fifth month of pregnancy with uterine bleeding and an abnormally large uterus for the gestational stage. **(25)** Complete moles almost always lack fetal tissues. **(26)** Cytogenetic studies have shown that over 90% of complete moles have a normal female karyotype and **(27)** that the entire chromosome complement comes from the sperm, a phenomenon known as androgenesis. Thus, they are believed to originate from fertilization by a single sperm of an ovum that has lost its chromosomes. Less commonly, empty egg fertilization by two sperm results in complete moles with 46,XY karyotypes.

**(28)** Although moles are benign neoplasms, they are the most common precursors of choriocarcinoma. About 1 in 40 hydatidiform moles give rise to a choriocarcinoma, whereas only about 1 in 150,000 normal pregnancies results in choriocarcinoma. **(29)** Serum levels of hCG are often helpful in distinguishing between a benign mole and a choriocarcinoma, because the latter usually produces significantly higher serum levels of this hormone. Although it is the most dreaded complication of hydatidiform mole, gestational choriocarcinoma now can be cured with chemotherapy in almost all cases. *(pp. 1081–1086)*

**30. (True); 31. (False); 32. (True); 33. (True); 34. (True)**

**(30)** Prostatic carcinoma is the most commonly occurring cancer in males. Its incidence exceeds that of lung cancer, but lung cancer causes more deaths than prostate cancer. **(31)** In contrast to nodular hyperplasia of the prostate (see Question 7), a much more common disorder and one from which prostatic carcinoma must be differentiated (indeed, the two often coexist), prostatic carcinoma most often arises in the posterior peripheral region of the gland, rather than the periurethral zone. In this location, it can be palpated on digital rectal examination, a useful direct method of detection of early cancers.

**(32)** In prostate cancer, the grade of the tumor is of particular importance in determining the prognosis, because the correlation between the degree of differentiation of the tumor and its biologic behavior is fairly good.

**(33)** Prostate-specific antigen (PSA) is the most useful biochemical marker for prostatic carcinoma. It is a serine protease of prostatic epithelial origin that normally is secreted into the semen but is present in serum only in minute amounts. In both nodular hyperplasia and prostatic carcinoma, serum PSA levels are elevated. Although the serum concentrations of PSA are typically higher in prostatitic carcinoma than in nodular hyperplasia, some overlap exists, especially in the early stages of tumor development. Serum PSA levels increase proportionately with tumor growth. Tumor mass correlates with serum concentrations of PSA, so monitoring of serum PSA levels is useful in determining responses to therapy and in detecting the presence of metastatic tumor following prostatectomy. Conversely, in patients presenting with metastatic disease, the prostatic origin of the tumor can be determined by the finding of PSA within tumor cells on immunohistochemical stains of biopsy tissue.

**(34)** Metastatic spread of prostate cancer chiefly involves bones, particularly the vertebral bodies. Metastatic lesions are characteristically osteoblastic, in contrast to most other forms of metastatic carcinoma, which are osteolytic. Therefore, osteoblastic bone lesions in men with known prostate cancer are virtually diagnostic of metastatic disease. *(pp. 1026–1031)*

**35. (C); 36. (B); 37. (C); 38. (B); 39. (D)**

**(35)** Adenomyosis refers to a pathologic process within the uterus characterized by the presence of endometrial tissue deep within the myometrial wall. Endometriosis is also characterized by the presence of endometrial tissue in an abnormal location, but it involves extrauterine sites such as the ovaries, uterine ligaments, rectovaginal septum, or pelvic peritoneum. The two processes are biologically and clinically distinct.

**(36)** Adenomyosis may occur at any stage of adult life. It can be quite common among postmenopausal women and has been reported to occur in 10 to 15% of uteri examined at autopsy. In contrast, endometriosis is primarily a disease of women in active reproductive life and rarely occurs in women over the age of 50.

**(37)** Premenopausal women with either of these processes frequently have dysmenorrhea and other functional pain. **(38)** Although both disorders may produce significant discomfort, only endometriosis is associated with serious complications. In long-standing disease with tubal and ovarian involvement, repeated bleeding of the ectopic endometrium with menstrual cycles leads to progressive scarring that may disrupt reproductive function. Infertility is the presenting complaint in 30 to 40% of women with endometriosis.

**(39)** Although the pathogenesis of both of these conditions is still somewhat controversial, neither of these processes is believed to be related to increased estrogen exposure. Although the pathogenesis of adenomyosis is unknown, it most often occurs in the presence of normal or low estrogen levels. Theories about the pathogenesis of endometriosis include: (1) regurgitation of endometrial tissue through the fallopian tubes, (2) metaplasia of celomic epithelium, and (3) lymphatic or vascular dissemination. *(pp. 1054–1055)*

**40. (D); 41. (C); 42. (D); 43. (C); 44. (C); 45. (D); 46 (C); 47. (C); 48. (C)**

Tumors of the surface epithelium of the ovary are the most common types of ovarian neoplasms, and among these, serous and mucinous tumors are the two most common variants. **(40)** Although the risk factors for ovarian carcinoma are much less clear than for other genital malignancies, it is at least apparent that the use of oral contraceptive steroids decreases rather than increases the risk of developing this malignancy. Nulliparity and family history are the two most important risk factors presently recognized.

**(41)** Both mucinous and serous carcinomas are cystic tumors in the majority of cases and cannot be differentiated definitively from one another by gross examination. **(42)** Both are more likely to be benign than malignant. Eighty per cent of mucinous tumors and 75% of serous tumors are either benign or of borderline malignant potential. **(43)** Malignant tumors of either type are more likely to be bilateral than their benign counterparts. Overall, the incidence of bilaterality in both benign and malignant forms is greater with serous tumors than with mucinous tumors. **(44)** "Borderline" tumors are lesions that by histopathologic criteria show greater cytologic complexity and atypia than benign tumors but lack the destructive infiltrative growth patterns of clearly malignant tumors. They represent a group of slow-growing tumors having a protracted course. Borderline tumors comprise about 15% of serous neoplasms and 10% of mucinous tumors.

**(45)** Simultaneous occurrence of an endometrial carcinoma in a significant number of cases is a property associated with endometrioid carcinomas of the ovary, another type of ovarian surface epithelial tumor. Neither serous nor mucinous tumors have this association.

**(46)** Malignant variants of both serous and mucinous tumors have many similarities in their biologic behavior, the strongest being their tendency to spread by direct seeding throughout the peritoneal cavity. For both tumors, metastasis by lymphatic or hematogenous routes is much less common.

**(47)** A unique feature of mucinous tumors is the production of a situation known as pseudomyxoma peritonii ("jelly belly"), in which the peritoneal cavity becomes filled with the mucinous secretions of tumor cells that have seeded the peritoneal wall. Pseudomyxoma peritonii is primarily a complication of borderline or malignant neoplasms.

**(48)** Although histopathologic classification is the most important determinant of prognosis in ovarian adenocarcinomas, molecular tumor markers may provide useful information. Approximately 30% of ovarian adenocarcinomas, including both serous and mucinous types, express high levels of HER-2/*neu* oncogene, which correlates with poor prognosis. *(pp. 1065–1070)*

**49. (B); 50. (A); 51. (D); 52. (C); 53. (D)**

Ovarian stromal tumors are of particular interest because of their ability to elaborate hormones. **(49)** Sertoli-Leydig cell tumors predominantly synthesize androgens, so they usually cause masculinization with hirsutism, voice changes, and clitoral enlargement. **(50)** Granulosa-theca cell tumors, in contrast, are predominantly estrogen-producing and greatly predispose to endometrial carcinoma (see Question 4) as well as breast cancer. About 10 to 15% of patients with estrogen-producing granulosa cell tumors eventually develop endometrial carcinoma.

**(51)** Typically, both of these tumor types are composed of solid masses of neoplastic cells, although granulosa-theca cell tumors may show focal microscopic cystification. Their characteristically solid growth makes them easily distinguishable from the far more common cystic epithelial neoplasms of the ovary (i.e., serous and mucinous tumors; see Questions 40 through 48).

**(52)** Although occasionally troublesome or even dangerous (see Question 50) because of their hormone-producing capacity, both of these tumor types tend to be benign in their biologic behavior. Granulosa-theca cell tumors exhibit malignant behavior in 5 to 25% of cases, and less than 5% of Sertoli-Leydig cell tumors are malignant.

**(53)** The occurrence of ascites is a curious associated finding in theca-fibromas of the ovary, not granulosa-theca cell or Sertoli-Leydig cell tumors. Theca-fibromas are another type of sex-cord stroma tumor of the ovary, but these usually are composed predominantly of fibroblasts and are hormonally inactive. However, large (>6 cm in diameter) theca-fibromas produce ascites in 40% of cases for unknown reasons. The ascites also may be accompanied by hydrothorax (usually right sided), and the triad of ascites, hydrothorax, and ovarian tumor is known as Meigs' syndrome. *(pp. 1074–1077)*

**54. (C); 55. (A); 56. (B); 57. (E); 58. (D)**

Benign cystic lesions are extremely common in the female genital tract. They are commonly the result of cystic dilation of either an inflamed normal gland or a remnant of an embryologic structure. **(54)** Bartholin's cysts arise from inflamed vulvovaginal glands and usually are associated with infection. They are unilocular and may be large (3 to 5 cm in diameter). They typically cause pain and local discomfort. They require surgical excision or marsupialization, by which they are opened permanently.

**(56)** Similarly, Nabothian cysts originate from chronically inflamed endocervical glands and are usually small and multiple. They are a typical feature of chronic cervicitis, a common inflammatory process related to bacterial colonization or infection of cervical mucosa.

**(55)** Among the developmental structures that may persist as remnants and undergo cystic change are the Gartner's duct cysts of the vagina, which represent mesonephric ductal structures, and **(58)** hydatid cysts of Morgagni of the fallopian tube, which arise from wolffian duct remnants.

**(57)** Endometriosis of the ovary (see Question 38) may, with repeated bleeding, undergo cystic change. These cysts have a distinctive gross appearance characterized by a brown, hemosiderin-laden wall and turbid hemorrhagic cyst fluid. On the basis of this appearance, they have become known as "chocolate cysts." *(pp. 1039; 1046; 1055; 1064)*

**59. (E); 60. (A); 61. (A); 62. (D); 63. (B)**

Whereas germ cell tumors represent only 15 to 20% of all ovarian cancers, they comprise the vast majority (about 95%) of testicular malignancies. **(59)** Among the malignant germ cell tumors in both sexes, the most biologically primitive (the dysgerminoma in the female and the seminoma in the male) are the most common (see Question 6). **(60)** Overall, testicular germ cell tumors are almost always malignant, and ovarian germ cell tumors are almost always benign. Benign cystic teratomas or "dermoid cysts" constitute about 95% of ovarian germ cell tumors. These teratomas are very well differentiated. Although they contain primarily ectodermal structures, mesodermal and endodermal elements also are encountered and are also well differentiated. **(61)** Occasionally, a single histologic element of an ovarian teratoma will comprise the entire tumor, a phenomenon known as monodermal or specialized teratoma. One of the most interesting of these is a tumor composed entirely of mature thyroid tissue known as struma ovarii. These tumors may hyperfunction, so they may be a rare cause of hyperthyroidism.

**(62)** Like fetal tissues arising from germ cells, germ cell tumors synthesize embryonic and trophoblastic polypeptides, which serve as useful tumor markers. α-Fetoprotein (AFP), the major serum protein of the early fetus, is synthesized by the yolk sac as well as the fetal intestine and liver. Analogously, yolk sac tumors synthesize AFP almost exclusively. Embryonal carcinoma and teratomas may both synthesize AFP, but these tumors usually produce both AFP and human chorionic gonadotropin (hCG) simultaneously. **(63)** At the other end of the spectrum, choriocarcinoma usually produces only hCG, like its normal counterpart, the trophoblast. Frequently, especially in testicular neoplasms, mixtures of these "pure" patterns of tumor differentiation will occur simultaneously and, in turn, cause mixed patterns of oncofetal antigen and hormone elaboration. *(pp. 1015–1021; 1071–1074)*

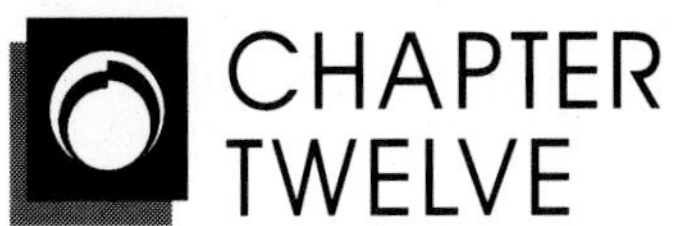

# CHAPTER TWELVE

# The Breast

**DIRECTIONS:** For Questions 1 through 19, choose the ONE BEST answer to each question.

**1.** The most important prognostic feature in invasive breast cancer is:

A. The histologic type of the tumor
B. The grade of the tumor
C. The size (diameter) of the tumor
D. The status of the draining lymph nodes
E. The presence or absence of estrogen receptors on tumor cells

**2.** Terminal duct lobular units increase in size during all of the following events EXCEPT:

A. Menstruation
B. Lactation
C. Proliferative phase of the menstrual cycle
D. Secretory phase of the menstrual cycle
E. Menarche

**3.** Poor prognosis in breast cancer is associated with:

A. Overexpression of the *erb*B2/*neu* oncogene
B. Absence of estrogen receptors
C. Presence of aneuploidy
D. Extensive angiogenesis
E. All of the above

**4.** All of the following statements about intraductal carcinoma of the breast are true EXCEPT:

A. It is usually undetectable on palpation.
B. It is usually detectable by mammography.
C. It is metastatic in a small percentage of cases.
D. It is a precursor of invasive carcinoma.
E. It often can be cured by surgical excision (lumpectomy).

**5.** Gynecomastia is associated with all of the following conditions EXCEPT:

A. Alcoholic cirrhosis
B. Prostatic carcinoma
C. Cimetidine ingestion
D. Leydig cell tumor
E. Klinefelter's syndrome

**6.** All of the following statements about sclerosing adenosis are true EXCEPT:

A. It is a variant of fibrocystic disease.
B. It typically lacks cysts.
C. Florid cases resemble carcinoma clinically.
D. Florid cases resemble carcinoma histologically.
E. It is not associated with increased risk of cancer.

**7.** All of the following are risk factors for breast cancer EXCEPT:

A. Close relatives with breast cancer
B. Early menarche
C. Early menopause
D. Endometrial carcinoma
E. Obesity

**8.** All of the following statements about phyllodes tumors are true EXCEPT:

A. They are named for their lobulated growth pattern.
B. They are tumors of myoepithelial cells.
C. They occur only in the breast.
D. Metastases are typically hematogenous rather than lymphatic.
E. Overall, they have a worse prognosis than ductal carcinoma.

**9.** Microscopic features of gynecomastia include all of the following EXCEPT:

A. Ductal hyperplasia
B. Stromal hyalinization
C. Stromal hyperplasia
D. Lobular hyperplasia
E. Nuclear monomorphism

**10.** Types of breast cancer associated with a much better overall prognosis (twofold greater survival rate or more), compared to infiltrating ductal carcinoma (the most common type), include all of the following EXCEPT:

A. Tubular carcinoma
B. Paget's disease
C. Colloid (mucinous) carcinoma
D. Medullary carcinoma
E. Infiltrating lobular carcinoma

**11.** All of the following statements about carcinoma of the male breast are true EXCEPT:

A. It is about 100 times less common than female breast cancer.
B. It has a worse overall prognosis than female breast cancer.
C. It metastasizes in the same pattern as female breast cancer.
D. It usually is preceded by gynecomastia.
E. It occurs at an older age relative to female breast cancer.

**12.** Paget's disease of the breast:

A. Is caused by dermal lymphatic invasion from an underlying ductal carcinoma
B. Seldom is associated with a palpable breast mass
C. Usually requires mammogram for detection
D. Typically is accompanied by an osteolytic-osteoblastic process in bone
E. Has the same prognosis as infiltrating ductal carcinoma of comparable stage

**13.** Benign histologic lesions that are associated with an increased risk of breast carcinoma include all of the following EXCEPT:

A. Atypical ductal hyperplasia
B. Multiple intraductal papillomas
C. Atypical lobular hyperplasia
D. Apocrine metaplasia
E. Sclerosing adenosis

**14.** A high level of estrogen receptors in a breast cancer is likely to be associated with:

A. A low degree of tumor cell differentiation
B. Previous exposure to estrogenic drugs
C. Therapeutic response of the tumor to tamoxifen
D. Therapeutic response of the tumor to Adriamycin (doxorubicin)
E. A poorer prognosis overall compared to estrogen receptor–negative tumors

**15.** Lesions of the breast that are characteristically tender or painful include all of the following EXCEPT:

A. Acute mastitis
B. Infiltrating ductal carcinoma
C. Mammary duct ectasia
D. Fibrocystic disease
E. Paget's disease

**16.** The breast lesion pictured in Figure 12–1:

A. Is a sharply circumscribed lesion on palpation
B. Represents a clonal proliferation of both stromal and glandular cells
C. Is rare before age 30
D. Often harbors an occult carcinoma
E. Does not change in size with menses

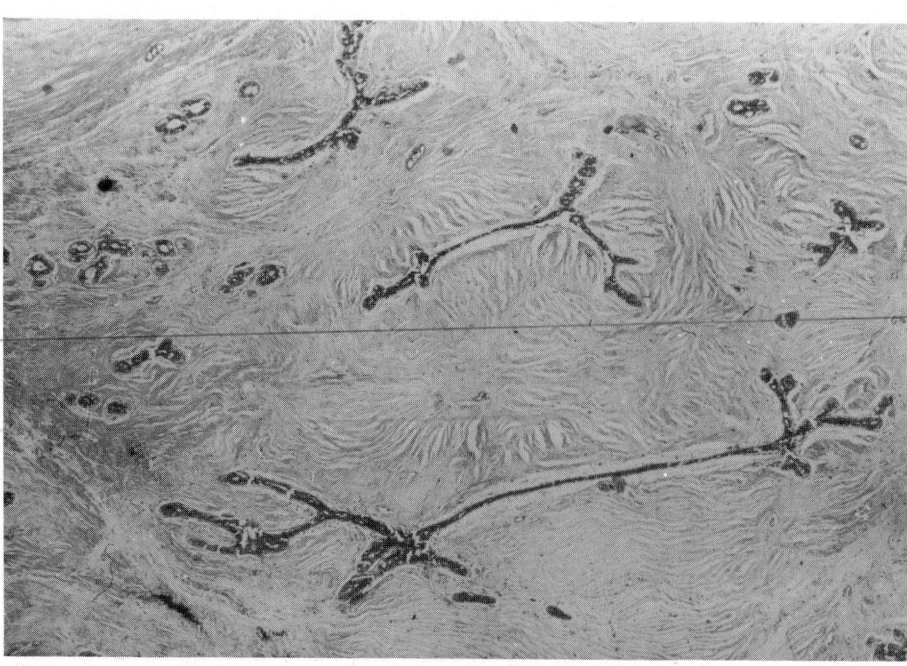

**Figure 12–1**

**17.** Histologic changes occurring in fibrocystic disease include all of the following EXCEPT:

A. Stromal proliferation
B. Proliferation of small ductules
C. Acute inflammation
D. Proliferation of ductal epithelium
E. Ductal dilation

**18.** A 40-year-old woman notices a lump in the upper outer quadrant of the left breast that does not fluctuate in size with her menstrual cycle. This clinical behavior is compatible with all of the following EXCEPT:

A. Fibroadenoma
B. Fat necrosis
C. Multiple intraductal papillomas
D. Infiltrating ductal carcinoma
E. Infiltrating lobular carcinoma

**19.** A 50-year-old woman has a brownish discharge from the nipple but has no palpable mass in the breast. This clinical situation describes all of the following EXCEPT:

A. Intraductal papilloma
B. Mammary duct ectasia
C. Paget's disease
D. Nipple adenoma
E. Galactorrhea

**DIRECTIONS:** For Questions 20 through 37, the set of lettered headings is followed by a list of numbered words or phrases. For each numbered word or phrase choose:
A—if the item is associated with (A) only
B—if the item is associated with (B) only
C—if the item is associated with *both* (A) and (B)
D—if the item is associated with *neither* (A) nor (B)

For each of the characteristics listed below, choose whether it describes ductal carcinoma, lobular carcinoma, both, or neither.

A. Ductal carcinoma
B. Lobular carcinoma
C. Both
D. Neither

**20.** Occurs most frequently in the upper outer quadrant of the breast
**21.** Is commonly palpable in the *in situ* state
**22.** Commonly produces scirrhous tumors
**23.** Produces Paget's disease in the nipple
**24.** Tends to arise multicentrically in the same breast
**25.** Occurs bilaterally in approximately 20% of cases
**26.** Commonly is associated with calcifications on mammography

For each of the characteristics listed below, choose whether it describes medullary carcinoma, colloid (mucinous) carcinoma, both, or neither.

A. Medullary carcinoma
B. Colloid (mucinous) carcinoma
C. Both
D. Neither

**27.** Represents a variant of lobular carcinoma
**28.** Occurs bilaterally twice as frequently as usual ductal carcinoma
**29.** Typically feels soft on palpation
**30.** Is composed of anaplastic tumor cells with a high mitotic rate
**31.** Is characterized histologically by a lymphocytic infiltrate
**32.** Commonly contains numerous large foci of necrosis and hemorrhage

For each of the characteristics listed below, choose whether it describes inflammatory carcinoma of the breast, acute mastitis, both, or neither.

A. Inflammatory carcinoma of breast
B. Acute mastitis
C. Both
D. Neither

**33.** The involved breast is usually red and hot.
**34.** The process is usually unilateral.
**35.** Skin retraction is a common clinical finding.
**36.** The process is more common in women over age 50.
**37.** Neutrophils are found in affected ducts.

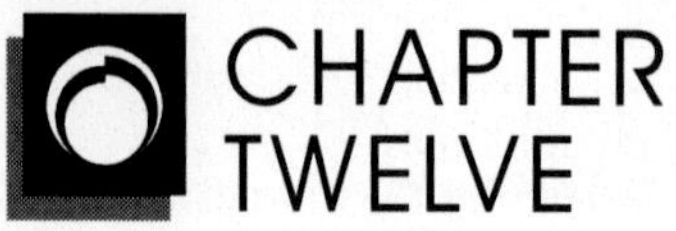

CHAPTER TWELVE

# The Breast

## *ANSWERS*

**1. (D)** Overall, the status of the draining lymph nodes of the breast containing malignancy is the most important prognostic factor in breast cancer once the tumor has become invasive ("infiltrating" rather than *in situ* carcinoma) and largely determines the survival rate. The size (transverse diameter) of the tumor and the fixation of nodes or the tumor to the skin or deeper structures are all factors considered in the assessment of stage. Although the histologic type of the tumor and its grade are significant prognostic factors, neither as accurately reflects the clinical course and survival rates of breast cancer patients as the degree of nodal involvement. *(p. 1108)*

**2. (A)** Under the influence of estrogen and progesterone, the terminal ducts and ductules (terminal duct lobular units) of the normal breast undergo proliferation. Conversely, when these hormones are withdrawn, involution or atrophy occurs. Thus, the increasing estrogen secretion occurring during the proliferative phase of the menstrual cycle (referring to proliferation of the endometrium) and the increasing progesterone occurring during the secretory phase both induce ductal proliferation in the breast. It is only with the fall in estrogen and progesterone levels during the menstrual phase of the cycle that ductal involution occurs. Both menarche and lactation, with their strong increases in hormonal output, are associated with dramatic increases in ductal proliferation in the normal breast. *(pp. 1036; 1089)*

**3. (E)** On the whole, invasive breast cancers with high levels of estrogen and/or progesterone receptors have a better prognosis than those with low levels or no receptors. The presence of these receptors correlates with both a high degree of tumor differentiation and a high tumor response rate to therapeutic hormonal manipulation. Oncogenes such as *erb*B2, *int*-2, c-*ras*, and c-*myc* and suppressor genes such as *p53* and *Rb* have been found to be activated or overexpressed in some, but not all, breast cancers. At present, the usefulness of most of these genes as prognostic markers in breast cancer has not yet been defined fully. However, it is now known that the *erb*B2/*neu* oncogene is associated with poor prognosis in patients with lymph node–positive metastatic disease. Aneuploidy (randomly increased DNA content) and high proliferative rate in breast cancers also have been correlated with poor prognosis in some studies. More recently, high degrees of intra- and peritumoral angiogenesis have been shown to correlate strongly with poor prognosis in breast cancer. Nevertheless, none of these features as a single finding presently is thought to be as strongly predictive of outcome (survival) in patients with breast cancer as lymph node status (See Question 1). *(pp. 275; 1107–1108)*

**4. (C)** Intraductal carcinoma of the breast is, by definition, an *in situ* malignancy of ductal epithelium. At this stage, the malignant ductal cells have grown vertically into the duct lumen and/or horizontally along the length of the duct, but they have not yet penetrated the ductal basement membrane. They have not gained access to the lymphatics or blood vessels of the periductal stroma and cannot metastasize. Thus, draining lymph nodes are always free of tumor. Unfortunately, however, intraductal tumors are difficult, if not impossible, to feel on palpation, and special screening techniques such as mammography are required to detect them. Intraductal carcinoma is believed to be the precursor of invasive breast cancer and, as such, increases the risk of invasive tumor in the involved breast (recurrence or invasion in the same region as the original tumor). However, at this early stage of progression, the tumor can be cured in most cases by excisional biopsy (lumpectomy) alone. *(pp. 1102; 1107)*

**5. (B)** Elevated serum levels of either estrogen or prolactin in the male may cause gynecomastia (see Question 9). Conditions that cause hyperestrogenism in males are diverse. Cirrhosis causes hepatic parenchymal destruction that leads to decreased catabolism of estrogenic compounds. A small percentage of patients treated with cimetidine for peptic ulcer disease develop gynecomastia as a consequence of elevated serum levels of prolactin caused by the drug. Leydig (interstitial) cell tumors of the testis are often hormonally active and may secrete a large variety of steroid hormones, including estrogens. Patients with Klinefelter's syndrome have atrophic testes and primary hypogonadism. The levels of circulating androgens in these patients are drastically reduced, and relative hyperestrogenism with gynecomastia results. Gynecomastia may occur in puberty or in the very aged as a result of changes in the ratios of circulating androgens and estrogens. It also may occur with chronic marijuana or heroin use or may occur without apparent cause.

Carcinoma of the prostate does not itself cause gynecomastia. However, therapies for this disease that involve hormonal manipulations, such as estrogen administration or castration, may lead to the subsequent development of gynecomastia. *(pp. 1109–1110)*

**6. (E)** Sclerosing adenosis is a benign condition characterized by proliferation of both intralobular connective tissue and small ductules or acini. Although sclerosing adenosis is considered a variant of fibrocystic disease, it typically lacks cysts. Rather, the lumens of the glandular elements are either small or lacking altogether. Sclerosing adenosis is also distinctive because it often resembles carcinoma both clinically and histologically. Like carcinoma, it often presents as a mass that is hard and poorly localized on palpation. Histologically, the proliferation of small glandular structures and nests or cords of cells within a densely fibrous stroma closely resembles infiltrating carcinoma. Although long believed to be a completely innocuous lesion, recent studies have demonstrated a slightly increased risk of subsequent breast cancer in women with sclerosing adenosis. *(p. 1095)*

**7. (C)** Although the etiology of human breast cancer is still unknown, epidemiologic studies have shown that certain clinical factors are associated with development of the disease and are now considered significant risk factors. Major categories of risk factors include: (1) genetic background (race and family history); (2) endogenous hormonal factors related to reproductive history; and (3) premalignant pathologic lesions in the breast tissue, specifically epithelial hyperplasia. Women with a strong family history of breast cancer (carcinoma developing in first-degree female relatives) are at exceptionally high risk. The greater the number of first-degree relatives with breast cancer, the younger the relatives at the time of developing cancer, and the higher the frequency of bilateral cancers, the greater the risk. With regard to the influence of hormonal environment on breast cancer development, endogenous estrogen excess (hormonal imbalance) plays a significant role. In general, the longer the uninterrupted exposure to endogenous estrogens, the greater the risk of developing breast carcinoma. Therefore, nulliparity, first parity after age 30, early menarche, and late menopause are all risk factors. In contrast, early menopause, by ending the estrogen peaks of the menstrual cycle, decreases the risk of breast cancer. Endometrial carcinoma is another malignancy associated with uninterrupted estrogen stimulation (of endometrial glands). Because breast cancer and endometrial carcinoma share this common risk factor, the development of endometrial carcinoma often is accompanied by the development of a breast malignancy in the same patient, and a history of endometrial carcinoma represents a risk factor for breast cancer. Less well understood is the relationship of obesity to increased risk of breast cancer. Estrogen metabolism is altered in obese women (the synthesis of estrone is increased). In postmenopausal women especially, the relatively increased synthesis of estrogens from adrenal and ovarian androgen precursors with age and obesity is believed to contribute to increased risk of estrogen-related tumors such as breast cancer and endometrial cancer. *(pp. 1100–1101; 1060)*

**8. (B)** Like fibroadenomas, which they may resemble histologically, phyllodes tumors arise from the interlobular stroma of the breast, not ductal myoepithelial cells. In contrast to fibroadenomas, however, phyllodes tumors are not always benign. They may recur after excision (low- or high-grade lesions) or even metastasize (high-grade lesions). Histologically, high-grade lesions typically appear more frankly sarcomatous, with high mitotic rates, dense cellularity, and cytologic pleomorphism, and sometimes are called cystosarcoma phyllodes (even though they are not always cystic). *Phyllodes* is a Greek term that refers to the "leaf-like" or lobulated gross configuration of these locally expansile tumors. Although they may grow to enormous size, occasionally filling the entire breast with pressure necrosis of the overlying skin, phyllodes tumors are usually biologically indolent. Even malignant phyllodes tumors may remain localized for long periods of time before metastasizing. When metastatic spread does occur, however, it is typically via hematogenous rather than lymphatic routes. Simple mastectomy is usually the treatment of choice. *(p. 1098–1099)*

**9. (D)** Gynecomastia refers to enlargement of the male breast in response to hyperestrogenism or increased prolactin. The major histologic component of the normal male breast is fibrostromal tissue. The glandular component consists exclusively of major mammary ducts and secondary branches, but lobular elements are not present at all. As in the female, breast elements in the male are responsive to hormonal stimulation and will undergo hyperplasia when exposed to excessive estrogens. Microscopically, gynecomastia is characterized by proliferation of ductal epithelium (epithelial hyperplasia), stromal hyperplasia, and stromal hyalinization. The proliferating epithelial cells are typically quite uniform, with a cuboidal or columnar shape and small, regular nuclei. They lack the cytologic pleomorphism of carcinoma. Since lobules are not a component of the male breast, lobular hyperplasia is not a feature of gynecomastia. *(p. 1109)*

**10. (E)** Tubular carcinoma of the breast is a form of ductal carcinoma displaying a high degree of differentiation. It behaves less aggressively than infiltrating ductal carcinoma and has a low incidence of axillary lymph node metastasis. Paget's disease is infiltration of nipple skin by underlying ductal carcinoma, usually arising from the main excretory duct. The prognosis of this lesion is directly related to the stage of the underlying carcinoma, but, because it is found most often in association with an *in situ* cancer, its overall prognosis is relatively good. Papillary carcinoma, colloid (mucinous) carcinoma, and medullary carcinoma are variants of ductal carcinoma that also have a relatively good prognosis because they tend to metastasize to axillary lymph nodes less frequently than the usual infiltrating ductal carcinoma. The long-term survival rates for papillary, medullary, and colloid carcinomas are about 65%, 58%, and 58%, respectively—about twice the survival rate for infiltrating ductal carcinoma (29%). The reason for this difference in behavior is unknown, however. Infiltrating lobular carcinoma, like infiltrating ductal carcinoma, is considered to be a moderately to highly metastasizing tumor type, with survival rate largely dependent on tumor stage at discovery. The long-term survival rate for infiltrating lobular carcinoma is about 34%, only slightly better than that for infiltrating ductal carcinoma. *(pp. 1102–1107)*

**11. (D)** Carcinoma of the male breast is a very rare entity and, compared with carcinoma of the female breast, has an incidence ratio of 1:100. Unlike female breast cancer, it occurs almost exclusively in individuals of advanced age. Furthermore, carcinoma of the male breast has a worse prognosis than carcinoma of the female breast. Because males have only a small amount of breast tissue, tumors can infiltrate the underlying chest wall or the overlying skin rapidly. Thus, skin involvement by fixation, ulceration, and microscopic Paget's disease is relatively much more common in males than in females. Overall, however, dissemination of male breast cancer follows the same pattern as in the female, and axillary lymph node metastases are present at the time of discovery in about 50% of cases. Although the predisposing factors for carcinoma in the male breast remain obscure, there is no evidence that gynecomastia is related to the development of carcinoma. Carcinoma does not develop with increased frequency in patients with gynecomastia. Conversely, patients with carcinoma rarely have a history of preceding or coexisting gynecomastia. *(p. 1202)*

**12. (E)** Paget's disease of the breast is a form of ductal carcinoma arising in the major excretory ducts beneath the nipple and extending outward along the duct toward the skin surface, directly invading the nipple epidermis (not dermal lymphatics, as in inflammatory breast cancer). The primary tumor is usually noninvasive (intraductal), with invasive ductal carcinoma occurring less commonly. Although Paget's disease may appear in the absence of a palpable breast mass, an underlying lump (possible contributions to which include distended excretory duct, periductal tumor infiltration, and/or inflammation resulting from disrupted nipple skin) is detectable in 50 to 60% of cases. Even in the absence of a palpable mass, however, Paget's disease is readily recognizable on physical examination by the striking gross findings of nipple fissuring, ulceration, and/or oozing characteristic of this lesion. Consequently, it may constitute the only form of *in situ* breast cancer that can be detected on patient self-exam. Overall, however, the prognosis for Paget's disease is determined by the extent of the underlying tumor, and patients with Paget's disease have the same prognosis as those with usual infiltrating ductal carcinoma of comparable stage.

Although the eczematous appearance of the skin in Paget's disease may resemble inflammatory carcinoma of the breast clinically, the two lesions can be differentiated from one another by their histologic appearance. Inflammatory carcinoma of the breast corresponds to dermal lymphatic invasion from an underlying breast carcinoma (see Question 33), whereas Paget's disease refers exclusively to epidermal involvement.

Paget's disease of the breast is not to be confused with Paget's disease of bone (osteitis deformans), a totally unrelated disorder. Paget's disease of bone is a benign disorder of unknown etiology that is characterized by an osteolytic-osteoblastic process in the bones of affected individuals. *(pp. 1105; 1106; 1223–1225)*

**13. (D)** Epithelial hyperplasias of either ductal or lobular origin are the two forms of benign breast disease that are associated with a significantly increased (five-fold) risk of development of carcinoma. The more severe and atypical the hyperplasia, the greater the risk of carcinoma. Although intraductal papillomas are benign growths within lactiferous ducts that are usually solitary and do not give rise to papillary carcinoma, multiple intraductal papillomas (florid papillomatosis) behave more like epithelial hyperplasias and are associated with a slightly increased (1.5 to 2 times) risk of carcinoma. Likewise, sclerosing adenosis recently has been shown to be associated with a slightly increased (1.5 to 2 times) risk of breast cancer. In contrast, apocrine metaplasia is a very common, completely innocuous feature of fibrocystic disease of the breast and is not associated with increased cancer risk. *(p. 1096)*

**14. (C)** The therapeutic response of a breast cancer to hormonal manipulation (hormone ablation by oophorectomy and adrenalectomy or competitive inhibition by synthetic, hormonally inactive hormone analogues) is proportional to the quantity of estrogen and progesterone receptors expressed by the tumor cells. Thus, quantitative analysis of estrogen and progesterone receptor protein often is performed on fresh tissue from a surgically excised tumor to determine whether recurrent or concurrent disease would be responsive to this form of adjuvant therapy. In general, the greater the differentiation of the tumor, the greater the number of estrogen receptors. Although estrogen is known to act as a promoter in breast carcinogenesis, previous exposure to exogenous estrogen is not known to influence the estrogen receptor positivity of the breast tumors developing under this influence. Despite the tight correlation between estrogen receptor positivity of a tumor and its response to antiestrogenic drugs such as tamoxifen (a synthetic estrogen analogue), estrogen receptor positivity has no predictive value in the response of the tumor to nonhormonal chemotherapeutic agents such as Adriamycin (doxorubicin). Nevertheless, the high degree of differentiation and therapeutic response to hormonal manipulation give breast cancers with high levels of estrogen receptors a better overall prognosis compared to malignancies with intermediate levels or no estrogen receptors. *(p. 1107)*

**15. (B)** Pain (or tenderness to palpation) is a symptom more often associated with benign rather than malignant diseases of the breast and is characteristic of such lesions as acute mastitis, galactocele, mammary duct ectasia, and fibrocystic disease. Although infiltrating ductal carcinoma rarely may present as a painful lesion, the tumor most often comes to the patient's or physician's attention as a firm but painless mass in the breast. Paget's disease may constitute a notable exception to the typical painlessness of malignancy, because the disruption (fissuring, ulceration) of the nipple epidermis caused by the infiltrating cancer cells often is associated with a painful, secondary inflammatory response. *(pp. 1092–1094; 1105)*

**16. (A)** Figure 12–1 is a micrograph of a fibroadenoma of the breast. Fibroadenoma is the most common benign tumor of the female breast and is found most frequently in women under the age of 30. It contains both stromal and glandular elements, but cytogenetic studies have shown that only the stromal component is clonal. The lesion is typically hormonally responsive, increasing in size during the late phase of the menstrual cycle and during pregnancy. Although it may be confused clinically with a cyst, a fibroadenoma is usually easy to differentiate clinically from carcinoma because of its sharply circumscribed borders and rubbery consistency. The overwhelming majority of fibroadenomas are completely benign. Although, in principle, the epithelial component of a fibroadenoma should be as likely as ductal cells elsewhere in the breast to give rise to a carcinoma, the occurrence of malignancy within a fibroadenoma is an extremely rare event. *(pp. 1097–1098)*

**17. (C)** Fibrocystic disease of the breast is a very common condition caused by an exaggerated response of stromal and glandular breast elements to hormonal imbalances such as relative estrogen excess or progesterone deficiency during the menstrual cycle. Both stromal and epithelial elements may undergo proliferative changes, although the proportionate changes vary from case to case. Stromal hyperplasia with increased collagen production (stromal sclerosis or fibrosis) may be the predominant feature, and it may be accompanied by various degrees of epithelial hyperplasia. Ductal dilation with cyst formation is common. The types of hyperplastic epithelial responses that may occur in fibrocystic disease include proliferation of small ductules or acinar structures (adenosis) or proliferation of ductal lining cells (intraductal hyperplasia). Fibrocystic disease is not an inflammatory condition and is not characteristically associated with the presence of acute inflammation on histologic examination, unless infection has been superimposed on the process. However, nonspecific chronic inflammation, in the form of stromal lymphocytic infiltrates, is a common finding in fibrocystic disease. *(pp. 1093–1094)*

**18. (A)** In the fluctuating hormonal environment produced by the normal menstrual cycle, cyclical variation in the size of hormonally responsive benign proliferative lesions of the breast such as fibroadenomas and fibrocystic disease is common and helps to differentiate these lesions from malignancies. Not all benign lesions have this property, however. For example, multiple intraductal papillomas (neoplastic papillary growths that are associated with increased risk of carcinoma) usually form poorly delineated masses in peripheral regions of the breast that are not known to fluctuate noticeably with hormonal cycles. Carcinomas of either the infiltrating ductal or infiltrating lobular type occur most commonly in the upper outer quadrant of the breast and tend to increase relentlessly in size without fluctuation in response to hormonal cycles. Fat necrosis, a consequence of breast trauma, may occur anywhere in the breast but is not responsive to hormones. *(pp. 1092; 1097–1098; 1099–1106)*

**19. (E)** Nipple discharge in a middle-aged woman may result from either a benign or malignant neoplastic process involving the major excretory ducts of the breast. Intraductal papilloma of the nipple is a benign epithelial proliferative lesion that usually affects the major lactiferous ducts in the subareolar region and often causes bloody nipple discharge. It is not a cancer precursor. Its more ominous look-alike, known as nipple adenoma or florid papillomatosis of the nipple, is also a neoplastic growth of the lactiferous duct epithelium intermixed with fibrosis and also causes bloody nipple discharge. However, this lesion is not innocuous because it is associated with concomitant or subsequent carcinoma in 16% of cases. Mammary duct ectasia, an inflammatory disorder principally involving the major excretory ducts, tends to occur in the fifth or sixth decade of life. It often causes discharge from the nipple as well as pain and induration. Paget's disease of the breast is the principal malignant process causing nipple discharge that must be differentiated from benign conditions producing this symptom. Paget's disease represents a form of ductal carcinoma involving the major excretory ducts and the skin of the overlying nipple. In addition to an oozy, bloody discharge, the nipple often shows eczematous changes and fissuring or ulceration with surrounding inflammatory hyperemia and edema. Galactorrhea or nonpuerperal lactation usually is caused by inappropriate prolactin secretion (e.g., hormone-secreting tumor or ingestion of drugs that decrease the inhibitory dopaminergic control of hypothalamic secretion). Although the amount of milk produced varies, the secretions in this condition are not qualitatively abnormal (not bloody). *(pp. 1092; 1099; 1105; 1117)*

**20. (C); 21. (D); 22. (A); 23. (A); 24. (B); 25. (B); 26. (C)**

**(20)** Both ductal and lobular carcinomas of the breast occur with greatest frequency in the upper outer quadrant, which is the region of greatest concentration of glandular tissue in the breast. **(21)** In general, neither ductal carcinoma *in situ* nor lobular carcinoma *in situ* is palpable. Rather, it is the infiltrating tumor with its sclerotic stromal response that presents clinically as a firm lump. **(22)** Infiltrating tumors of ductal origin classically induce marked stromal sclerosis. Such tumors have a hard, cartilaginous consistency on palpation and are known as "scirrhous" carcinomas. Although the great majority of scirrhous tumors are infiltrating ductal carcinomas, any given scirrhous malignancy may be of either ductal or lobular origin. Most invasive lobular carcinomas, however, are rubbery and typically are not scirrhous. **(23)** Paget's disease of the breast is produced only by ductal carcinoma that arises in a major excretory duct and extends to involve the skin of the nipple (see Question 12).

Lobular carcinoma is associated with two clinically important features: **(24)** a tendency to be multicentric within the same breast and **(25)** a high incidence of bilaterality. Bilaterality and multicentricity are not unique to lobular carcinoma but occur about twice as frequently with lobular carcinomas (about 20% of cases) as with ductal carcinoma (about 10% of cases). **(26)** Because early breast cancers are often nonpalpable, special techniques such as radiologic imaging (e.g., mammography) are needed for breast cancer screening. Mammography can detect the microcalcifications that are associated with invasive (and sometimes *in situ*) breast cancer of either ductal or lobular origin. Although calcifications are found in more than half of cancers by this technique, the finding is not diagnostic of malignancy. Many benign lesions contain calcifications as well. Thus, biopsy or cytologic studies usually are needed for definitive diagnosis. *(pp. 1102–1107)*

**27. (D); 28. (D); 29. (C); 30. (A); 31. (A); 32. (A)**

**(27)** Both medullary carcinoma and colloid carcinoma of the breast arise from ductal epithelial cells and represent variants of ductal carcinomas. **(28)** The incidence of bilaterality in patients with either of these tumor types is not significantly different from that in patients with usual ductal carcinoma. **(29)** Unlike usual ductal carcinomas, medullary carcinoma and colloid carcinoma induce little stromal response. Thus, they typically feel soft on palpation and may resemble each other clinically. Histologically, however, the two variants are distinctly different. Medullary carcinomas are characterized by solid, syncytium-like sheets of large pleomorphic cells, **(30)** a high mitotic rate, and **(31)** an abundant lymphocytic infiltrate between the sheets of tumor cells. **(32)** In addition, medullary carcinomas typically contain foci of hemorrhage and necrosis that are large and numerous, whereas colloid carcinomas create large, pale, gray-blue gelatinous masses that typically are not associated with hemorrhage or necrosis. *(pp. 1103–1105)*

**33. (C); 34. (C); 35. (C); 36. (A); 37. (B)**

**(33)** Although inflammatory carcinoma of the breast shares some clinical features with acute mastitis, it is not truly an inflammatory process. Inflammatory carcinoma is actually an infiltrating ductal carcinoma of the breast with a characteristic tendency to extensively invade the lymphatics of the breast and overlying skin. Acute mastitis is a true inflammatory process caused by bacteria (usually *Staphylococcus aureus*), which gain access to the breast substance through cracks in the nipple skin created during nursing. The involved breast in both inflammatory carcinoma and acute mastitis is usually reddened, swollen, and warm to touch. **(34)** In both processes, the involvement is typically unilateral and **(35)** produces skin retraction or nipple retraction as a result of the accompanying marked edema. **(36)** Inflammatory carcinoma is more common in women over 50 (because infiltrating ductal carcinoma itself is more common in this age group), whereas acute mastitis is a disease of young lactating women. **(37)** Histologically, the presence of numerous neutrophils within affected ducts is characteristic only of acute mastitis. *(pp. 1092; 1106)*

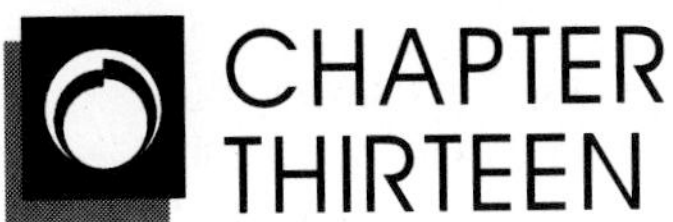

CHAPTER THIRTEEN

# The Skin

**DIRECTIONS:** For Questions 1 through 25, choose the ONE BEST answer to each question.

**1.** Typical characteristics of basal cell carcinoma include:

A. Rapid growth
B. Early metastasis
C. Occurrence in deeply pigmented individuals
D. Association with papillomavirus infection
E. Occurrence in basal cell nevus syndrome

**2.** A healthy 20-year-old woman develops hives when she eats nuts. All of the following statements about this situation are true EXCEPT:

A. The development of the skin lesions is mediated by immunoglobulin E.
B. Mast cell degranulation occurs within the lesions.
C. Complement activation occurs during formation of the lesions.
D. The lesions typically regress within 24 hours.
E. Aspirin administration is contraindicated.

**3.** All of the following statements about the excised lesion shown in Figure 13–1 are true EXCEPT:

A. It is a very common lesion.
B. The cell of origin is a melanocyte.
C. The dermal infiltration indicates aggressive biologic behavior.
D. Mitoses rarely are found in these lesions.
E. Malignant transformation is exceedingly rare.

**4.** A patient notices a deeply pigmented, raised nodule with indefinite borders on the upper extremity. Although a nodular melanoma is suspected, none of the following lesions can be ruled out on clinical inspection EXCEPT:

A. Basal cell carcinoma
B. Seborrheic keratosis
C. Blue nevus
D. Dermatofibroma
E. Lentigo simplex

**5.** All of the following statements about malignant melanoma are true EXCEPT:

A. It is etiologically related to sun exposure.
B. It is typically uniformly pigmented.
C. It does not metastasize during its horizontal growth phase.
D. Risk of metastasis increases with depth of dermal infiltration.
E. Increased early diagnosis has improved survival rates.

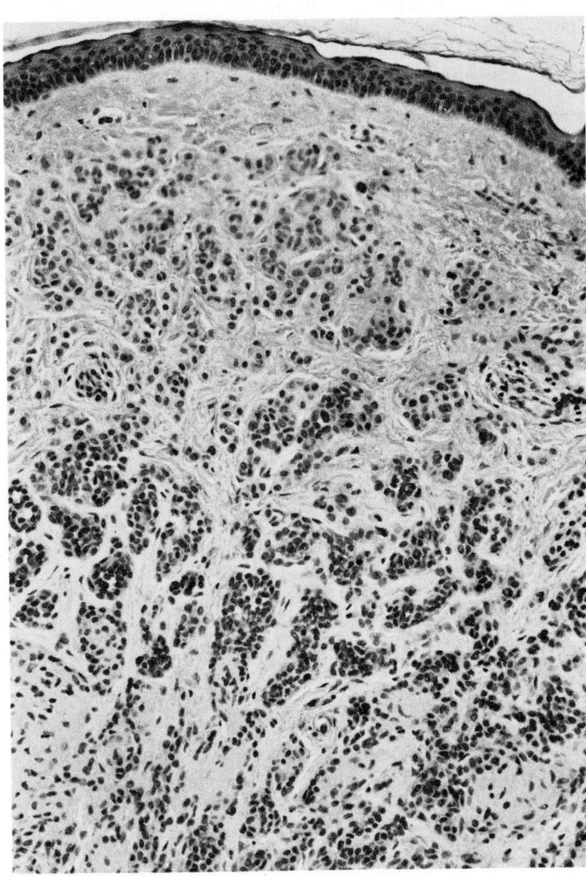

Figure 13–1

**6.** Which of the following statements about mycosis fungoides is TRUE?

A. Lesions resemble superficial fungal infection.
B. The causative agent is an atypical mycobacterium.
C. Lesions contain suppressor T cells with convoluted nuclei.
D. Hematogenous involvement is known as Sézary's syndrome.
E. Munro's microabscesses are diagnostic.

**7.** All of the following statements about dysplastic nevi are true EXCEPT:

A. They typically originate from nondysplastic precursor lesions.
B. They occur almost exclusively on sun-exposed body surfaces.
C. They predispose to intralesional melanoma formation.
D. They predispose to melanoma formation in unaffected skin.
E. They occur in individuals with the heritable melanoma syndrome.

**8.** Which of the following would be the LEAST likely cause of thrombocytopenia-induced purpuric lesions developing in a patient with promyelocytic leukemia?

A. Hypersplenism
B. Bone marrow replacement by tumor
C. Intercurrent infection
D. Disseminated intravascular coagulation
E. Administration of drugs

**9.** Langerhans' cells are:

A. Giant cells in tubercular granulomas
B. Pancreatic islet cells
C. Melanocyte precursors
D. Antigen-presenting dendritic cells
E. Transformed lymphocytes

**10.** All of the following statements regarding actinic keratosis are true EXCEPT:

A. It is a premalignant skin condition
B. It is caused by sun exposure
C. Cytologic atypia of basal cells is characteristic
D. Proliferating basal cells typically disrupt the basement membrane
E. Elastosis of the subjacent dermis is characteristic

**11.** Which of the following skin disorders is LEAST likely to occur in an individual with a diffuse B-cell lymphoma?

A. Xanthoma
B. Acanthosis nigricans
C. Squamous cell carcinoma
D. Cutaneous vasculitis
E. Mycosis fungoides

**12.** All of the following statements are true of psoriasis EXCEPT:

A. The epidermal mitotic rate is increased.
B. Other organ systems often are involved.
C. Lesions often are precipitated by trauma.
D. Epidermal microabscesses are seen histologically.
E. The disorder is usually self-limited.

**13.** Dysplastic nevi differ from common acquired nevi in all of the following ways EXCEPT:

A. They are generally larger.
B. They are generally more unevenly pigmented.
C. They are more likely to occur on sun-protected body sites.
D. They are more likely to occur as solitary lesions.
E. They are more likely to undergo malignant transformation.

**14.** All of the following statements about benign fibrous histiocytomas are true EXCEPT:

A. They represent fibroblastic proliferations.
B. They sometimes are termed sclerosing hemangiomas.
C. They cause hyperpigmentation of the overlying epidermis.
D. They are slow-growing, indolent lesions.
E. They are caused by viral infection.

**15.** Malignancy-associated skin disorders include all of the following EXCEPT:

A. Erythema induratum
B. Acanthosis nigricans
C. Erythema multiforme
D. Erythema nodosum
E. Seborrheic keratosis

**16.** A patient being treated for acute myelogenous leukemia develops palpable purpura. Likely causes include:

A. Malignancy-associated vasculitis
B. Drug sensitivity
C. Leukemia infiltration of the skin
D. All of the above
E. None of the above

**17.** Factors strongly implicated in the genesis of acne vulgaris include all of the following EXCEPT:

A. Androgenic hormones
B. Bacteria
C. Sebum output
D. Heredity
E. Diet

**18.** All of the following statements about dermatitis herpetiformis are true EXCEPT:

A. Lesions are very pruritic.
B. Subepidermal blisters are produced.
C. Lesions are bilaterally symmetrical in distribution.
D. It is caused by herpesvirus infection.
E. It is associated with celiac disease.

**19.** Cutaneous horns are produced with all of the following skin disorders EXCEPT:

A. Actinic keratosis
B. Verruca vulgaris
C. Seborrheic keratosis
D. Squamous cell carcinoma
E. Malignant melanoma

**20.** A patient taking sulfonamides has an increased probability of developing all of the following cutaneous lesions EXCEPT:

A. Melasma
B. Erythema multiforme
C. Erythema nodosum
D. Urticaria
E. Eczematous dermatitis

**21.** All of the following statements about glomus cells are true EXCEPT:

A. They are smooth muscle cells.
B. They regulate arterial blood flow in the skin.
C. They are found most commonly in facial skin.
D. They are responsive to temperature changes.
E. They give rise to extremely painful tumors.

**22.** Xeroderma pigmentosum is associated with an increased incidence of which of the following neoplasms?

A. Malignant melanoma
B. Lung cancer
C. Colon cancer
D. All of the above
E. None of the above

**23.** Characteristics of keratoacanthoma include all of the following EXCEPT:

A. Viral inclusions in nuclei
B. Histologic resemblance to squamous cell carcinoma
C. Rapid growth
D. Extension of the lesion into the dermis
E. Spontaneous regression

**24.** Characteristics typical of lichen planus include all of the following EXCEPT:

A. Pruritic lesions
B. Purple lesions
C. Association with underlying malignancy
D. Self-limited (spontaneously regressing) lesions
E. Band-like lymphoid infiltrates in the upper dermis

**25.** All of the following statements about mastocytosis are true EXCEPT:

A. It is characterized by increased numbers of mast cells in the skin.
B. It is the cause of urticaria pigmentosa.
C. It is associated with dermatographism.
D. It represents metastatic spread from a bone marrow malignancy.
E. Darier's sign is a finding on physical examination.

**DIRECTIONS:** For Questions 26 through 47, the set of lettered headings is followed by a list of numbered words or phrases. For each numbered word or phrase choose:

A—if the item is associated with (A) only
B—if the item is associated with (B) only
C—if the item is associated with *both* (A) and (B)
D—if the item is associated with *neither* (A) nor (B)

For each of the characteristics listed below, choose whether it describes Spitz nevus, nodular malignant melanoma, both, or neither.

A. Spitz nevus
B. Nodular malignant melanoma
C. Both
D. Neither

**26.** Lesions consist of pleomorphic proliferations of melanocytes with a high mitotic rate.
**27.** Deep infiltration of the underlying dermis by the tumor cells is a prominent feature.
**28.** Infiltration of the overlying epidermis by the tumor cells is a common feature.
**29.** Lesions occur only in adults.
**30.** Lesions typically show variegated pigmentation.

For each of the following statements, choose whether it describes molluscum contagiosum, verruca vulgaris, both, or neither.

A. Molluscum contagiosum
B. Verruca vulgaris
C. Both
D. Neither

**31.** The lesion is caused by a virus.
**32.** Children and young adults are affected most commonly.
**33.** The process spares mucous membranes.
**34.** Cytoplasmic vacuolization (koilocytosis) is a characteristic feature.
**35.** Lesions are self-limited (regress spontaneously).

For each of the following characteristics, choose whether it describes pemphigus vulgaris, bullous pemphigoid, both, or neither.

A. Pemphigus vulgaris
B. Bullous pemphigoid
C. Both
D. Neither

**36.** Subepidermal blisters are characteristic.
**37.** Acantholysis in the blistered epidermis is typical.
**38.** Injury is mediated by autoantibodies.
**39.** Oral involvement is common.
**40.** Scalp and face lesions are common.

For each of the following characteristics, choose whether it describes squamous cell carcinoma, basal cell carcinoma, both, or neither.

A. Squamous cell carcinoma
B. Basal cell carcinoma
C. Both
D. Neither

**41.** It is more common than malignant melanoma.
**42.** It is etiologically related to sun exposure.
**43.** It has significant metastatic potential.
**44.** Its incidence increases with immunosuppression.
**45.** Its incidence is high in xeroderma pigmentosum.
**46.** It appears as leukoplakia on mucosal surfaces.
**47.** *In situ* lesions are red and scaly.

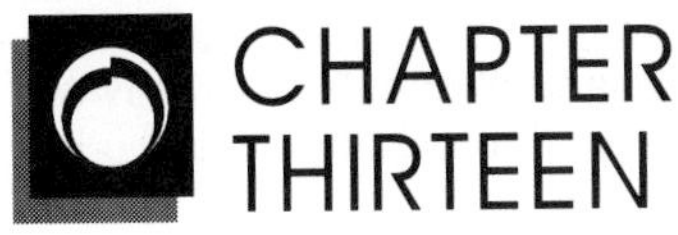

# CHAPTER THIRTEEN

# The Skin

## ANSWERS

**1. (E)** Basal cell carcinomas are common, slow-growing malignant epidermal tumors that rarely metastasize. They tend to occur in lightly pigmented individuals, although the tumors themselves may be deeply pigmented and may be difficult to differentiate clinically from a nevocellular nevus or melanoma. Histologically, the tumors are composed of small, dark "basaloid" cells with scant cytoplasm usually growing in nests with peripheral palisading (radial orientation of nuclei), an appearance easily distinguished from their clinical look-alikes. The early development of numerous basal cell carcinomas is characteristic of a rare, dominantly inherited disorder known as the basal cell nevus syndrome, a disorder also associated with skeletal, neural, and reproductive abnormalities.

As with squamous cell carcinomas, basal cell carcinomas are linked etiologically to sun exposure. In contrast to squamous cell carcinomas, however, no etiologic link with human papillomavirus infection has been established. *(p. 1187)*

**2. (C)** Urticaria, otherwise known as "hives," is a very common skin disorder characterized by focal swelling and itching (pruritic wheals). It is caused by localized mast cell degranulation and resultant dermal microvascular hyperpermeability. The pathogenesis of urticaria includes both immunologic and nonimmunologic mechanisms. In immunoglobulin E (IgE)–mediated immunologic urticaria (allergic type), specific antigen sensitivity to foods, pollens, or drugs produces a type I hypersensitivity immune response, with mast cell degranulation and a histamine-induced increase in venular permeability. In IgE-independent urticaria, direct stimulation of mast cell degranulation can be produced in sensitive individuals by drugs such as opiates, curare, radiographic contrast agents, or certain antibiotics. In either case, resolution of the lesions typically occurs within hours.

Complement activation is not involved in the pathogenesis of either IgE-dependent or IgE-independent allergic urticaria, and vasculitis is not produced. This contrasts with immunologic urticaria resulting from type III hypersensitivity responses, which are mediated by immune complexes. Acute necrotizing vasculitis is produced as a result of immune complex deposits and complement activation in the walls of small vessels. The associated urticaria is understandably much more persistent than that produced by type I reactions, and underlying vasculitis should be suspected in individuals in whom urticarial reactions do not resolve within 24 hours.

Prostaglandins retard IgE-dependent release of mast cell granules. Agents that act as arachidonic acid metabolism inhibitors, such as aspirin, tend to potentiate or may even cause IgE-mediated urticaria by impairing prostaglandin synthesis. Therefore, aspirin would be contraindicated in the clinical situation described here. *(pp. 178–182; 184–187; 1192–1193)*

**3. (C)** The lesion pictured in Figure 13–1 is an acquired intradermal nevocellular nevus. Nevocellular nevi are extremely common benign tumors of melanocytes that may be either congenital or acquired. Typically, neval cells are round to oval in shape and contain uniform nuclei. They grow in nests, which may be present at the dermal-epidermal junction (junctional nevus), only within the dermis (intradermal nevus), or in both places simultaneously (compound nevus). They arise at the dermal-epidermal junction and typically migrate downward with time. Infiltration of the deep dermis, therefore, does not indicate aggressive biologic behavior. On the contrary, neval cells tend to become more cytologically and histochemically "mature" with downward progression into the dermis. They cluster, become spindle shaped, and lose their tyrosinase activity, coming more to resemble neural tissue than melanocytes. The process of "neuralization" can be diagnostically helpful in distinguishing some forms of nevi from malignant melanoma. Typical intradermal nevi rarely show mitoses on histologic examination and have little malignant potential. They usually are distinguished readily from dysplastic nevi, lesions with distinct malignant potential. Dysplastic nevi are compound (rather than intradermal) nevi with both cytologic and architectural atypia and are known to be precursors of malignant melanoma. Characteristically, however, the progression to malignancy in dysplastic nevi virtually always begins with the junctional component. Thus, mature intradermal nevi lacking a junctional component typically are considered innocuous. *(pp. 1176–1179)*

**4. (E)** Basal cell carcinomas, seborrheic keratoses, nevocellular nevi, or dermatofibromas all can appear as nodular hyperpigmented lesions. When deeply pigmented, any of these lesions, including the darkly pigmented blue nevus (a histologic variant of a nevocellular nevus), may be confused clinically with malignant melanoma. In contrast, lentigo simplex is never nodular and is usually relatively lightly pigmented. Lentigenes are benign hyperplasias of melanocytes. They are macular lesions that are usually tan-brown and, unlike freckles, do not darken with exposure to sunlight. *(pp. 1176–1177; 1181; 1187; 1188)*

**5. (B)** Malignant melanoma is a relatively common, highly aggressive neoplasm. Like most cutaneous malignancies, it is related etiologically to sun exposure. Hereditary factors and the development of precursor lesions (dysplastic nevi; see Questions 7 and 13) are also important in its pathogenesis. Melanomas are typically asymptomatic, but the lesions can be recognized on clinical inspection by their typically variegated pigmentation (a mixture of shades of brown, black, blue, red, gray, or even white) and irregular "notched" borders. Increased recognition of these features has resulted in earlier diagnosis and excision. Thus, despite the increasing incidence of melanoma, the overall survival rate for this disease has improved greatly. The prognosis in individual cases correlates closely with the tumor stage at excision. Melanomas tend to grow horizontally within the epidermis and superficial dermis for prolonged periods of time before infiltrating vertically. During the horizontal growth phase, melanomas do not have the capacity to metastasize and can be cured with surgical resection. When the tumor develops vertical growth, it becomes nodular in appearance and acquires metastatic potential. The deeper the invasion, the greater the probability of metastasis. In fact, the probability of metastasis can be predicted by measuring (using an ocular micrometer) the depth of invasion of the malignancy in the resection specimen. *(pp. 1179–1181)*

**6. (D)** Mycosis fungoides is a T-cell lymphoma that arises primarily in the skin but may evolve into generalized systemic disease with involvement of lymph nodes and viscera. The development of a leukemia-like picture with seeding of the blood by malignant T cells accompanied by diffuse erythroderma and cutaneous scaling is known as Sézary's syndrome.

Although the name is suggestive of fungal infection, mycosis fungoides neither clinically resembles nor has any association with mycotic infection of the skin. The etiology of mycosis fungoides is the subject of vigorous investigation, and there is increasing evidence that at least some cases may be related to retroviral infection. (There is certainly no association with atypical mycobacterial infection, however.)

The early lesions of mycosis fungoides resemble eczema both clinically and histologically, but even at this stage, karyotypic abnormalities of lymphocytes in the blood and lymph nodes can be observed. Plaque-like lesions develop as the disease progresses and are characterized by an intensification of the features of the eczematous phase with the addition of Pautrier's microabscesses (collections of Sézary-Lutzner cells) in the epidermis. These are not to be confused with the Munro's microabscesses of psoriasis, which are collections of neutrophils in the stratum corneum. The diagnosis of mycosis fungoides depends on the identification of tumor cells (Sézary-Lutzner cells) within the characteristic superficial dermal band–like inflammatory infiltrates and Pautrier's abscesses of the skin lesions. Sézary-Lutzner cells are CD4+ helper T cells with hyperchromatic, highly convoluted "cerebriform" nuclei. *(pp. 1190–1192)*

**7. (B)** Dysplastic nevi (also known as "BK moles") constitute a distinct subset of nevocellular nevi that evolve into lesions with a high degree of cytologic atypicality and undergo transformation to malignant melanoma with significant frequency. They are considered true precursors of malignant melanoma. Unlike ordinary acquired nevocellular nevi, dysplastic nevi tend to be variably pigmented (variegated), have irregular borders, and occur on non–sun-exposed as well as sun-exposed skin sites (see Question 13). They are associated with an increased risk of melanoma in the clinically unaffected as well as the lesional skin. The occurrence of dysplastic nevi in the heritable melanoma syndrome (dysplastic nevus syndrome), in which the trait is autosomal dominant and associated with a susceptibility gene located on the short arm of chromosome 1, suggests that genetic factors may play a strong role in the development of these lesions. For persons with the dysplastic nevus syndrome, the actuarial probability of developing melanoma is 56% at age 59. Thus, the importance of identification and prophylactic surveillance of such individuals is obvious. *(pp. 1177–1179)*

**8. (A)** A reduction in the platelet count is the most common cause of generalized bleeding and is manifested most commonly by petechial skin lesions. Thrombocytopenia will result from any condition causing either decreased platelet production, increased platelet destruction, sequestration of platelets, or dilution of platelets (massive transfusions). The risk of developing thrombocytopenia through one or more of these mechanisms is increased in patients with acute leukemia. Leukemic infiltration of the bone marrow replaces normal hematopoietic elements and causes decreased production of platelets. Administration of drugs, particularly chemotherapeutic agents, will reduce normal hematopoiesis even further. Immunopathologic mechanisms associated with drugs or intercurrent infection also may cause increased platelet destruction. Patients with promyelogenous leukemia are especially prone to increased platelet destruction from disseminated intravascular coagulation, because the cytoplasmic granules that characterize the neoplastic promyelocytes are rich in a thromboplastin-like substance capable of activating the coagulation cascade. Although patients with *chronic* myelogenous leukemia may develop massive splenomegaly leading to platelet sequestration (hypersplenism), splenomegaly usually is not a feature of the acute forms of leukemia. *(pp. 616–618; 649–654)*

**9. (D)** Langerhans' cells are bone marrow–derived, antigen-presenting cells of the epidermis. They are dendritic in shape and have clear cytoplasm. Langerhans' cells can be identified unequivocally in the electron microscope by their pathognomonic pentilaminar cytoplasmic granules (Birbeck granules), some of which have dilated tips and resemble tiny matchsticks or tennis rackets. Langerhans' cells contain hydrolytic enzymes and exhibit cell surface markers (such as class II human lymphocyte antigens) characteristic of monocytes and macrophages, so it is likely that they are descendants of this cell line. They interact with cutaneous T cells in the presentation of antigens, but Langerhans' cells themselves are not lymphocytes. Although the terminology is sometimes confusing, Langerhans' cells have nothing to do with the pancreatic islets of Langerhans or with the Langhans' giant cells of tubercular granulomata. *(pp. 81; 173; 907; 1173)*

**10. (D)** Actinic (solar) keratosis is a premalignant condition caused by chronic exposure to sunlight in which progressively dysplastic epidermal changes precede the development of squamous cell carcinoma. Although the lesions are often hyperplastic and hyperkeratotic, epidermal atrophy also may be seen. Deposition of abnormal, thickened, blue-gray elastic fibers in the subjacent dermis (elastosis) is also characteristic. However, the essential microscopic feature of actinic keratosis is cytologic atypia of the epidermis, characteristically seen first and most prominently in the lowermost layers. The atypia may progress to involve the full thickness of the epidermis, becoming squamous cell carcinoma *in situ*. With penetration of the underlying basement membrane by the proliferating cells, the process evolves to invasive squamous cell carcinoma (and is no longer classified as a mere actinic keratosis). *(pp. 1185–1187)*

**11. (E)** Xanthomas, lesions composed of lipid-laden foamy histiocytes, may occur in normal individuals or in association with hyperlipidemic disorders (either acquired or familial), but also are known to develop in association with malignancies (especially lympho- or myeloproliferative neoplasms). Likewise, acanthosis nigricans, a lesion characterized by epidermal thickening and hyperpigmentation, has both a benign and a malignancy-associated form. It usually occurs either as a heritable trait or in association with obesity or endocrinopathies, but it also can be associated with an underlying tumor. Patients with lymphoma, perhaps as a result of endogenous or chemotherapeutic immunosuppression, are prone to develop second malignancies, especially cutaneous squamous cell carcinomas.

Numerous conditions are associated with cutaneous vasculitis: lymphomas, leukemias, carcinomas, infections, drug sensitivities, C2 deficiency, and collagen vascular diseases.

Mycosis fungoides is itself a T-cell lymphoma originating in the skin and is not a paraphenomenon of a lymphoproliferative disorder. *(pp. 295; 1284; 1288; 1291; 1293)*

**12. (E)** Psoriasis is a common chronic inflammatory dermatosis that persists for years (i.e., it is not self-limited). It is characterized by scaling lesions that occur primarily on elbows, knees, scalp, and lumbosacral regions and appear as salmon-colored plaques covered by silver-white scale. The disease may involve other organs besides the skin, such as the musculoskeletal system (e.g., psoriatic arthritis and myopathy). Psoriatic skin lesions are characterized by increased epidermal cell turnover (mitotic rate) with epidermal thickening, elongation of rete ridges, and numerous mitotic figures seen microscopically. The stratum granulosum is typically thinned or absent, the overlying stratum corneum is parakeratotic, and small neutrophilic abscesses are present in the superficial epidermis (spongiform pustules) and stratum corneum (Munro's microabscesses). The etiology of the disease is still unknown, but its association with certain HLA types suggests a genetic predisposition. The genesis of the lesions is thought to be linked to aberrant inflammatory and/or immune reactions to epidermal antigens, perhaps involving abnormal cytokine-mediated cellular responses. Epidermal injury appears to set these responses in motion, because lesions may be precipitated in susceptible individuals by trauma (the "Koebner phenomenon"). *(pp. 1197–1198)*

**13. (D)** In contrast to common acquired nevocellular nevi, which rarely (if ever) undergo malignant transformation, the less common but much more ominous dysplastic nevi have a marked propensity to undergo malignant transformation and are recognized as true precursors of malignant melanomas. Thus, it is of the utmost importance to be able to recognize these lesions both clinically and histologically and to differentiate them from innocuous nevocellular lesions. Compared to acquired nevocellular nevi, dysplastic nevi are, as the name implies, more cytologically pleomorphic and hyperchromatic (dysplastic). They tend to be larger (greater than 5 mm in diameter) than acquired nevi (usually less than 6 mm in diameter) and more unevenly pigmented (variegated). In contrast to acquired nevi, they tend to occur on sun-protected body sites as well as sun-exposed sites. However, like acquired nevi, they tend to be multiple. Thus, the discovery of a single dysplastic nevus should prompt a careful search for additional concomitant lesions and careful lifelong follow-up of the patient for subsequent development of new lesions. *(pp. 1176–1179)*

**14. (E)** Benign fibrous histiocytomas are intradermal tumors of fibroblasts and histiocytes, the most common form of which is called a dermatofibroma. The histologic variant that contains numerous blood vessels and hemosiderin deposits is known as a sclerosing hemangioma. These lesions are completely benign in their biologic behavior. They are neither locally aggressive nor rapidly growing. The dermal lesions have poorly demarcated borders and are accompanied by hyperplasia and hyperpigmentation of the overlying epidermis, which can cause confusion with melanoma clinically. The etiology of these lesions is unknown, but no evidence for viral infection exists. Many cases are associated with previous local trauma, and it has been hypothesized that the lesions may represent an abnormal repair (scarring) response. *(p. 1188)*

**15. (A)** Acanthosis nigricans, erythema multiforme, erythema nodosum, and xanthomas are all benign cutaneous lesions that may be associated with underlying malignancy. Acanthosis nigricans is a hyperplastic, hyperpigmented epidermal lesion (a sort of epidermal overgrowth) that commonly affects flexural areas (skin folds). It may be seen in benign conditions such as puberty (arguably a benign condition), diabetes, or obesity, but it also occurs in association with malignancy, usually adenocarcinoma. It may, in fact, precede the recognition of an underlying tumor and serve as a sentinel sign of malignant disease. Erythema multiforme is a self-limited immune-mediated cytotoxic disorder associated with infection, certain drugs, collagen-vascular diseases, and malignancies (carcinomas and lymphomas). Erythema nodosum is a common form of panniculitis that is most often idiopathic in origin but may be associated with certain infections, drugs, or malignancies. Seborrheic keratoses are common benign lesions, usually unassociated with underlying disease. However, the sudden appearance of large numbers of seborrheic keratoses may occur as a paraneoplastic syndrome known as the sign of Leser-Trélat.

Erythema induratum, in contrast to erythema nodosum, is an uncommon form of panniculitis seen mostly in adolescents and postmenopausal females that has no association with malignancy. *(pp. 1181–1182; 1195–1196)*

**16. (D)** Purpura represents hemorrhage into the skin and, when caused by inflammatory damage to vessel walls, will produce palpable induration. An important cause of palpable purpura is cutaneous necrotizing vasculitis. This disorder produces fibrinoid necrosis of venular walls with extravasation of red blood cells and serum. Neutrophils and cellular debris are present in and around the walls of the damaged vessels. The lesions are believed to be produced by an immune complex–mediated mechanism (type III hypersensitivity) in which complement is activated. Numerous diverse conditions are associated with this type of vasculitis. In many cases, the source of the inciting antigen is well defined; drugs, foreign proteins (serum sickness), viruses, and bacteria (intercurrent infections) are common examples. In other disorders, although the known association with vasculitis may be well established, the precise antigen is unknown, or multiple diverse antigens may be involved. Examples of such situations include vasculitis associated with malignancy (leukemias, lymphomas, and carcinomas), collagen vascular disease, Henoch-Schönlein purpura, and C2 deficiency. Although it is not mediated by immunologic mechanisms, leukemic infiltration of the skin can be purpuric in nature and always must be included in the differential diagnosis of palpable purpura in this setting. The histopathology of these lesions is not that of a necrotizing vasculitis, however, but that of a dense dermal infiltrate of myeloid cells, including numerous immature forms. *(pp. 184–187)*

**17. (E)** Acne vulgaris is a common chronic inflammatory dermatosis involving the pilosebaceous unit. Its tendency towards familial occurrence has suggested a hereditary factor contributing to the risk of development of the disorder, but developmental influences also are known to contribute. Principal among them are hormonal factors, especially androgens (e.g., castrated individuals do not develop acne; the hormonal fluctuations of puberty are linked to onset of acne). Essential to the production of the follicular lesions is the output of sebum, which is, in turn, degraded by bacterial lipases to inflammation-inducing free fatty acids. Thus, antibacterial treatment, either topical or systemic, is used to target the *Proprionibacterium acnes* and/or other bacteria that may contribute to this process. In contrast to common beliefs about chocolate and French fries, diet is not thought to play any significant role in the pathogenesis of acne vulgaris. *(pp. 1201–1202)*

**18. (D)** Dermatitis herpetiformis (DH) is a rare but very distinctive blistering disease having a strong association with celiac disease (gluten enteropathy or sprue). Although not all patients with celiac disease have DH, it appears that nearly all patients with DH have celiac disease (often clinically latent). It is believed that the immunologic response to gluten in these individuals constitutes the underlying pathogenesis of both diseases. The lesions of DH consist of urticarial plaques and vesicles that are characteristically extremely pruritic (itchy). They typically are distributed over extensor surfaces in a bilaterally symmetrical fashion. The vesicles of DH frequently are grouped like those seen in herpesvirus infection (hence the name of the disease), but the etiology of DH is not at all related to viral infection. The blisters of DH are subepidermal, caused by a separation of the dermo-epidermal junction beginning at the tips of the dermal papillae (between rete ridges). By immunofluorescence, granular deposits of immunoglobulin A are localized in the tips of the involved papillae. *(pp. 1203–1204)*

**19. (E)** Exuberant conical excrescences of keratin known as cutaneous horns may be the predominant clinical feature of several diverse epidermal lesions. Warts (human papillomavirus lesions), actinic keratoses, seborrheic keratoses, and squamous cell carcinomas all may appear clinically as cutaneous horns and require biopsy for definitive diagnosis. Seborrheic keratosis is a common benign tumor of basaloid keratinocytes growing in cords and sheets and superficially forming horned cysts. It is usually exophytic, but occasionally grows inward, extending into the dermis ("inverted seborrheic keratosis"). Occasionally, seborrheic keratoses may be difficult to distinguish clinically from malignant melanoma because of their pigmented appearance. However, because melanomas do not form horn cysts, this feature will readily differentiate the two lesions on gross inspection with a hand lens. *(pp. 1181–1182; 1185–1187; 1205–1206)*

**20. (A)** Erythema multiforme is an uncommon, self-limited dermatosis that causes a cytotoxic pattern of injury in the epidermis. In many cases it is believed to represent a hypersensitivity response to certain infections or drugs. Its association with specific drugs is well established, and sulfonamides, penicillin, barbiturates, salicylates, hydantoins, and antimalarial drugs are among the primary offenders. Erythema nodosum is a type of panniculitis (i.e., inflammation of the subcutaneous fat). Like erythema multiforme, it also is associated commonly with infections or the administration of certain drugs, especially sulfonamides. Urticaria (hives) may develop in an individual taking antibiotics such as sulfonamides, either as a result of an immunologically mediated hypersensitivity response to the drug or as a direct action of the drug on mast cells, causing their degranulation. Drug-related eczematous dermatitis is a hypersensitivity-mediated spongiotic dermatitis caused by systemic administration of a drug such as an antibiotic, which acts as an antigen or hapten. Typically, eruption occurs with administration of the drug and resolves with drug withdrawal.

Melasma is a mask-like zone of facial hyperpigmentation commonly occurring during pregnancy. It is thought to result from enhanced transfer of pigment from melanocytes to keratinocytes in response to hormonal changes. It also may occur with the administration of some drugs such as oral contraceptives or hydantoins, but is not associated with antibiotic use. *(pp. 1192–1194; 1195; 1196)*

**21. (C)** Glomus bodies are specialized smooth muscle cells that regulate arterial blood flow through arteriovenous shunts in the skin in response to temperature changes. Tumors of these cells commonly occur on the distal portions of the fingers and toes, where glomus bodies are most numerous. Tumors of glomus cells are characteristically exquisitely painful and bothersome but have virtually no malignant potential. *(pp. 507–508)*

**22. (A)** Xeroderma pigmentosum is an autosomal recessive disorder characterized by predisposition to chromosomal breakage secondary to defective excision repair of DNA. Several distinct subsets of this disease have been defined, each with a specific enzymatic defect. The major subset lacks dimeric endonucleases. Because of their inability to repair acquired cellular mutations induced in the skin by ultraviolet irradiation, affected individuals have a markedly increased predisposition to skin cancers. All sunlight-induced epidermal malignancies (basal cell carcinomas, squamous cell carcinomas, and melanomas) occur with greatly increased frequency in individuals with xeroderma pigmentosum. However, there is no increased predisposition to major visceral malignancies such as cancers of the lung, colon, or breast. This suggests that the mutagenic effects of sunlight on the skin far exceed the effects of all other environmental mutagens on the body. *(pp. 285; 1186–1187)*

**23. (A)** Keratoacanthomas are rapidly growing but benign tumors of keratinocytes. These lesions may resemble squamous cell carcinomas closely both clinically and histologically. They may deeply penetrate the underlying dermis but never extend beyond the depth of adjacent hair follicles. Differentiation from squamous cell carcinoma depends on the overall symmetrical, smooth contour of the lesion and the mature, homogenous "glassy" appearance of its component squamous cells. Although alarming in appearance, keratoacanthomas regress spontaneously and heal without treatment. The etiology of keratoacanthomas is unknown. Their cells do not contain viral inclusions, nor are these lesions known to be related to viral infection in any way. *(p. 1183)*

**24. (C)** Lichen planus is a chronic inflammatory dermatosis that is characterized by "pruritic, purple, polygonal papules." Histologically, the lesions typically show degeneration and necrosis of the basal keratinocytes and a bandlike ("lichenoid") infiltrate of lymphocytes along the dermoepidermal junction. Although the etiology of lichen planus is unknown, an immune response is suggested by the cellular responses in the disorder (T cell predominance of the lymphoid infiltrate and Langerhans' cell hyperplasia in the epidermis). The lesions occur on both the skin and the mucous membranes. Although oral lesions may persist for years, lichen planus is a self-limited disorder, resolving spontaneously within 12 to 24 months. There is no association of the lesion with underlying malignancy. *(pp. 1198–1199)*

**25. (D)** Mastocytosis represents a spectrum of disease in which increased numbers of mast cells occur in the skin and sometimes in other organs as well. The most common subset of mastocytosis is known as urticaria pigmentosa, a localized cutaneous form of the disease that predominantly affects children. However, mastocytosis may be systemic in distribution, with mast cell infiltration of many organs (e.g., bone marrow, liver, spleen, lymph nodes) in addition to skin involvement. Systemic mastocytosis may have a poor prognosis because of the physiologic effects of mast cell degranulation. In all forms of the disease, the clinical signs of mastocytosis are related to the effects of mast cell products such as histamine and heparin. Two common signs related to skin involvement are dermatographism (dermal edema resembling a hive resulting from localized stroking of uninvolved skin) and Darier's sign (dermal edema resulting from stroking of lesional skin). It is unclear whether mastocytosis is a true neoplasm or whether the defect results from altered mast cell maturation or proliferation in response to abnormalities of the local microenvironment. However, it does not represent metastatic disease from an underlying malignancy in the bone marrow. *(p. 1192)*

**26. (C); 27. (C); 28. (B); 29. (D); 30. (B)**

**(26 through 30)** The Spitz nevus, once termed "juvenile melanoma," is an uncommon nevocellular nevus that occurs predominantly in childhood but also can arise adults. Spitz nevi are benign in their biologic behavior but are characterized by histologic features usually associated with malignancy. The neval cells typically show striking nuclear irregularities, and mitoses may be numerous, causing confusion with malignant melanoma. In addition, the lesions are often highly infiltrative and extend deep into the dermis. In contrast to most malignant melanomas, however, their pigmentation is usually sparse, and the nevi appear clinically as pink-tan papules or nodules.

In nodular malignant melanoma dermal infiltration is not an innocuous feature. In fact, its extent is the most important factor in determining prognosis in this disease. Malignant melanoma can occur in any age group, although it is most common between the ages of 40 and 60. In contrast to Spitz nevi, malignant melanomas are most often heavily but variably pigmented with shades of black, brown, blue, red, or other hues. Histologically, melanomas are composed of markedly atypical neoplastic melanocytes that show frequent mitoses. Helpful features in the diagnosis of malignant melanoma include the involvement of the overlying epidermis and the presence of atypical mitoses; these features are typically lacking in Spitz nevi. *(pp. 1178–1181)*

**31. (C); 32. (C); 33. (D); 34. (B); 35. (C)**

**(31 and 32)** Molluscum contagiosum and verruca vulgaris are the two most common viral lesions of skin. Molluscum contagiosum is caused by a pox virus, whereas verruca vulgaris is caused by papillomaviruses of the papovavirus group. Both occur most frequently in children and young adults and are characterized by epidermal hyperplasia. **(33)** Both may occur on mucous membranes. **(34)** Virally infected keratinocytes in both conditions exhibit characteristic histologic changes. Verrucal keratinocytes typically show marked cytoplasmic vacuolization known as "koilocytosis" and zones of pallor surrounding infected nuclei. Virally infected keratinocytes in molluscum contagiosum are uniquely characterized by large, homogenous eosinophilic cytoplasmic inclusions (molluscum bodies) containing replicating virions that compress the nucleus to one side of the cell. **(35)** Both molluscum contagiosum and verruca vulgaris are contagious diseases, caused by direct contact, and both are self-limited, regressing spontaneously within 6 months to 2 years. *(pp. 1205–1206)*

**36. (B); 37. (A); 38. (C); 39. (C); 40. (A)**

**(36 through 38)** Pemphigus vulgaris and bullous pemphigoid are both uncommon autoimmune blistering (bullous) diseases. Pemphigus vulgaris is characterized by antibody-mediated damage to intercellular cement substances in the epidermis causing dissolution or lysis of the epithelium (acantholysis). Bullous pemphigoid, in contrast, is characterized by subepidermal blisters mediated by autoantibodies to basal lamina and hemidesmosomal antigens. **(39 and 40)** Both diseases may involve mucosal as well as cutaneous surfaces, but the characteristic distribution of lesions differs in the two diseases. Pemphigus vulgaris typically involves the scalp and face as well as the axilla, groin, trunk, and points of pressure. Bullous pemphigoid lesions occur predominantly on the inner aspects of the thighs, flexor surfaces of the forearms, groin, axilla, and lower abdomen but spare the face and scalp. *(pp. 1201–1203)*

**41. (C); 42. (C); 43. (A); 44. (C); 45. (C); 46. (A); 47. (A)**

**(41)** Both squamous cell carcinoma (SCC) and basal cell carcinoma (BCC) are more common than the considerably more aggressive malignant melanoma. **(43)** Of the two epithelial neoplasms, only SCC has significant metastatic potential (BCC rarely, if ever, metastasizes). **(42)** Both are related to sun exposure which, for both, is the single most common etiologic agent with which they are associated. **(44)** For both, tumorogenesis is favored by immunologic suppression as a result of chemotherapy or organ transplantation. Sunlight itself has depressive effects on epidermal Langerhans' cells and may contribute to immunosuppressive permissive conditions for SCC and BCC development in otherwise normal, immunocompetent individuals. **(45)** In xeroderma pigmentosum, a disease characterized by defective DNA repair, the incidence of both SCC and BCC (as well as malignant melanoma) is high.

**(46)** Curiously, BCC occurs exclusively in epidermis and never involves squamous mucosal surfaces. In contrast, SCC arises in squamous mucosal epithelium fairly commonly. Mucosal SCC usually has the appearance of white patches called leukoplakia, an appearance that also may be produced by benign conditions. Thus, biopsy may be needed to differentiate benign from malignant leukoplakia.

**(47)** Although the concept is somewhat illogical and perhaps results only from arbitrary definition, BCC is not recognized as having an *in situ* stage. Even exuberant basal cell hyperplasia like that occurring in actinic lesions is not given the label of "BCC *in situ*." Thus, BCC is diagnosed only after penetrating the epidermal basement membrane and penetrating the underlying dermis. Then, it most commonly appears as pearly papules. *In situ* lesions of SCC, in contrast, are well recognized entities that typically appear as red scaly plaques on the skin or as leukoplakia on mucosal surfaces. *(pp. 1185–1187)*

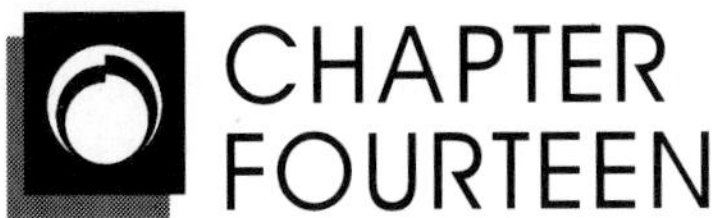

CHAPTER FOURTEEN

# The Endocrine System

**DIRECTIONS:** For Questions 1 through 17, choose the ONE BEST answer to each question.

**1.** A woman fails to lactate or menstruate after giving birth. Which of the following is the most likely cause?

A. Sheehan's syndrome
B. Nonsecretory pituitary adenoma
C. Empty sella syndrome
D. Hypothalamic glioma
E. Prolactinoma

**2.** Simple goiter is associated with all of the following conditions EXCEPT:

A. Fluorides in the water supply
B. Puberty
C. Androgenic steroid therapy
D. Dietary iodine deficiency
E. Pregnancy

**3.** The most common cause of the "syndrome of inappropriate antidiuretic hormone" secretion is:

A. Subdural hematoma
B. Radiation injury to the hypothalamus
C. Meningitis
D. Oat cell carcinoma of the lung
E. Pituitary adenoma

**4.** A goitrogen is a substance that:

A. Mimics the action of tri-iodothyronine ($T_3$)
B. Mimics the action of thyroxine ($T_4$)
C. Suppresses $T_3$ and $T_4$ synthesis
D. Mimics the action of thyroid-stimulating hormone
E. Depletes the body of iodine

**5.** A 30-year-old female recovering from a bout of influenza suddenly develops a painful, enlarged thyroid. The most likely diagnosis is:

A. Subacute lymphocytic thyroiditis
B. Reidel's thyroiditis
C. Thyroid abscess
D. Subacute granulomatous thyroiditis
E. Hashimoto's thyroiditis

**6.** Thyroid enlargement is greatest in:

A. Grave's disease
B. Simple goiter
C. Hashimoto's thyroiditis
D. Multinodular goiter
E. de Quervain's thyroiditis

**7.** A lobe of thyroid removed from a male with thyrotoxicosis contained the 2.0-cm nodule pictured in Figure 14–1. It is most likely:

A. A medullary carcinoma
B. A papillary carcinoma
C. A multinodular goiter
D. A follicular carcinoma
E. A follicular adenoma

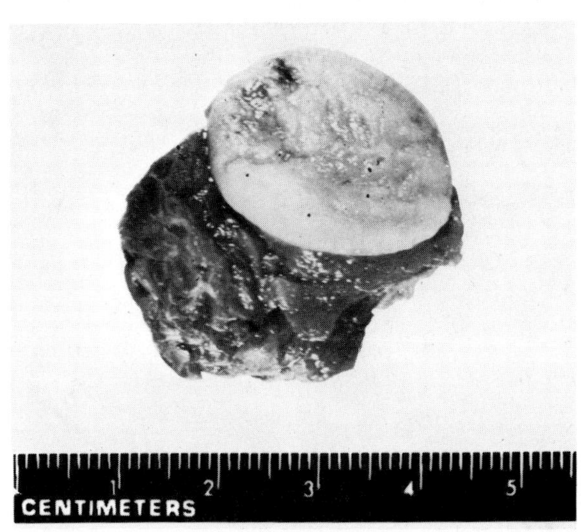


Figure 14–1

**8.** All of the following characteristics are associated with the thyroid lesion pictured in Figure 14–2 EXCEPT:

A. Aggressive biologic behavior and poor prognosis
B. Multifocality within the thyroid gland
C. Preference for lymphatic rather than hematogenous spread
D. Strong association with external irradiation
E. Appearance as a "cold" nodule on thyroid scan

**9.** Parathyroid hormone increases serum calcium by all of the following mechanisms EXCEPT:

A. Reducing renal calcium excretion
B. Increasing intestinal absorption of calcium
C. Blocking calcitonin secretion from the thyroid
D. Lowering serum phosphate levels
E. Mobilizing calcium from bone

**10.** On a check-up visit to his physician, a 50-year-old man who has noticed some muscular weaknesses and fatigability is found to have hypercalcemia by routine laboratory tests. Statistically, it is most likely that this man has:

A. Primary parathyroid hyperplasia
B. Secondary parathyroid hyperplasia
C. A parathyroid adenoma
D. A parathyroid carcinoma
E. A nonparathyroid carcinoma

**11.** Hyperaldosteronism associated with an adrenal adenoma is known as:

A. Bartter's syndrome
B. Nelson's syndrome
C. Conn's syndrome
D. Cushing's syndrome
E. None of these

**12.** Somatostatin exerts inhibitory control over all of the following EXCEPT:

A. Insulin
B. Thyrotropin
C. Prolactin
D. Glucagon
E. Growth hormone

**13.** All of the following statements correctly describe the disease of the thyroid pictured in Figure 14–3 EXCEPT:

A. It is the most common cause of hyperthyroidism.
B. It is a major cause of nonendemic goiter in children.
C. It is associated with suppressor T-cell deficiency.
D. It is associated with thyroid-stimulating hormone receptor antibodies.
E. It is associated with antibodies to thyroid peroxidases.

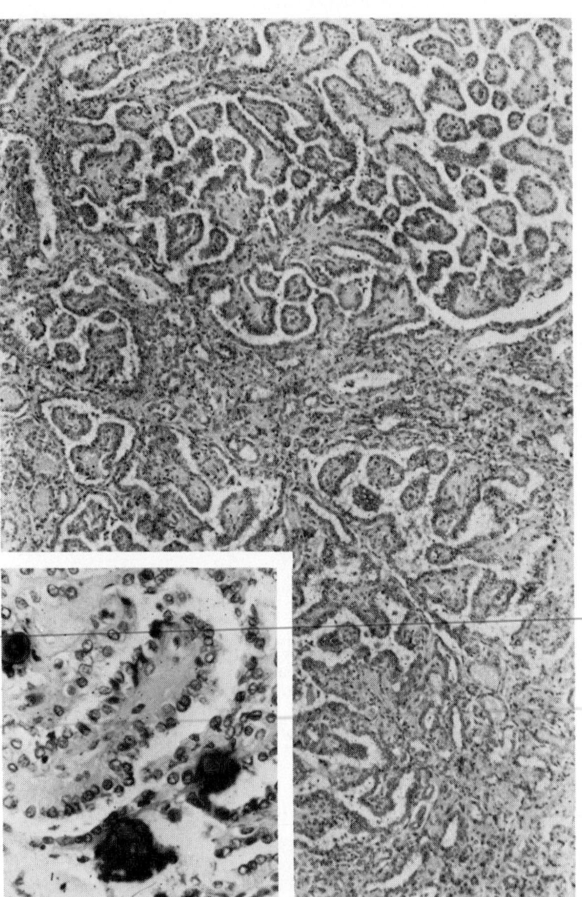

**Figure 14–2**

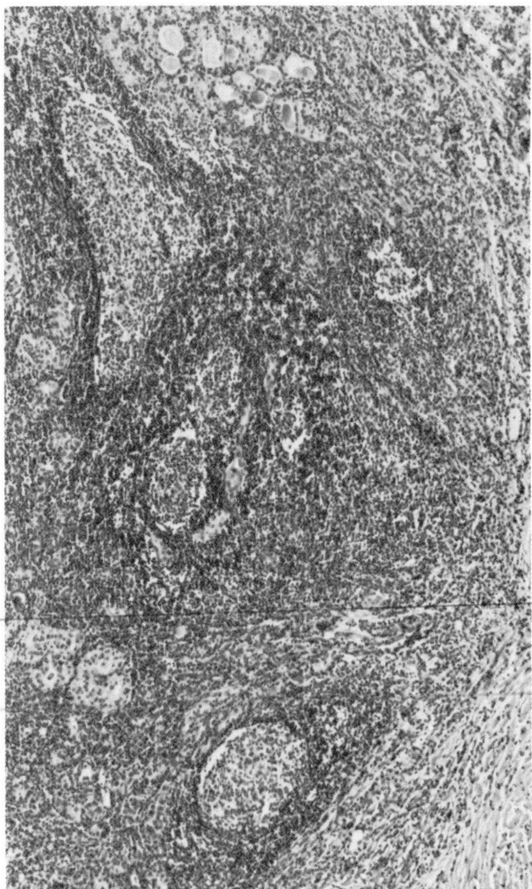

**Figure 14–3**

**14.** All of the following statements about medullary carcinoma of the thyroid (MCT) are true EXCEPT:

A. Neurosecretory granules are found within the tumor cells.
B. Amyloid is deposited within the tumor.
C. Thyroglobulin is the major tumor cell product.
D. Tumors occurring in the familial MCT syndrome are biologically indolent.
E. Sporadically occurring tumors are biologically aggressive.

**15.** Most females born with 21-hydroxylase deficiency would be expected to have all of the following EXCEPT:

A. Clitoral hypertrophy
B. Reduced levels of aldosterone
C. Elevated adrenocorticotrophic hormone levels
D. Gene mutation within the human lymphocyte antigen complex
E. Hypernatremia

**16.** The possible occurrence of pheochromocytoma should be expected in patients with:

A. Medullary carcinoma of the thyroid
B. Pituitary adenoma
C. Pancreatic islet cell adenoma
D. All of the above
E. None of the above

**17.** Which of the following statements about thymomas is correct?

A. They are composed of neoplastic T-cells (thymocytes).
B. They often are associated with myasthenia gravis.
C. They are most often aggressive tumors with a poor prognosis.
D. They often occur in children.
E. They often result in immunodeficiency syndromes.

**DIRECTIONS:** For Questions 18 through 22, you are to decide whether EACH choice is TRUE or FALSE.

For each of the following statements about Graves' disease, choose whether it is TRUE or FALSE.

**18.** It can be distinguished from all other forms of thyrotoxicosis by the presence of proptosis.
**19.** Nodular enlargement of the thyroid is characteristic.
**20.** Virtually all patients have antibodies to thyroid-stimulating hormone receptors.
**21.** It shares a human lymphocyte antigen genotype association with Hashimoto's thyroiditis.
**22.** Localized myxedema is an associated clinical feature.

**DIRECTIONS:** For Questions 23 through 51, the set of lettered headings is followed by a list of numbered words or phrases. For each numbered word or phrase choose:

A—if the item is associated with (A) only
B—if the item is associated with (B) only
C—if the item is associated with *both* (A) and (B)
D—if the item is associated with *neither* (A) nor (B)

For each of the following characteristics, choose whether it describes Cushing's syndrome, acromegaly, both, or neither.

A. Cushing's syndrome
B. Acromegaly
C. Both
D. Neither

**23.** Is caused most commonly by a pituitary adenoma
**24.** Is caused by lung cancer
**25.** Produces truncal obesity
**26.** Produces hyperglycemia
**27.** Produces hypertension
**28.** Produces osteoporosis
**29.** Produces changes in the facial appearance

For each of the characteristics listed below, choose whether it describes myxedema (hypothyroidism), Addison's disease (hypoadrenalism), both, or neither.

A. Myxedema (hypothyroidism)
B. Addison's disease (hypoadrenalism)
C. Both
D. Neither

**30.** Most commonly is caused by an autoimmune process
**31.** Commonly causes fatigability and constipation
**32.** Commonly is associated with hypertension
**33.** Characteristically produces cardiomyopathy
**34.** Characteristically produces hyperpigmentation
**35.** Commonly is associated with mental dysfunction
**36.** Sometimes is associated with mucocutaneous candidiasis and hypoparathyroidism

For each of the characteristics listed below, choose whether it describes pheochromocytoma, neuroblastoma, both, or neither.

A. Pheochromocytoma
B. Neuroblastoma
C. Both
D. Neither

**37.** Tumors characteristically elaborate catecholamines.
**38.** Young adults are affected most commonly.
**39.** Tumors are virtually always malignant.
**40.** Extra-adrenal tumors carry a better prognosis.
**41.** Deletion of part of chromosome 1 is a characteristic karyotypic abnormality.

For each of the statements below, choose whether it describes insulin-dependent diabetes mellitus, non–insulin-dependent diabetes mellitus, both, or neither:

A. Insulin-dependent diabetes mellitus
B. Non–insulin-dependent diabetes mellitus
C. Both
D. Neither

**42.** Underutilization of glucose is characteristic.
**43.** Cellular insulin resistance is a major pathogenetic factor.
**44.** Obesity is a commonly associated feature.
**45.** Autoantibodies against pancreatic islet cells are characteristic.
**46.** Insulitis is a characteristic histopathologic feature.
**47.** Strong associations with specific human lymphocyte antigens types exist.
**48.** Viral infection of the islet cells is causally related in some cases.
**49.** Most affected individuals develop retinopathy.
**50.** Most treated individuals now enjoy a normal life expectancy.
**51.** Ketoacidosis is the most common cause of death.

**DIRECTIONS:** Questions 52 through 69 are matching questions. For each numbered item, choose the most likely associated lettered item from those provided. Each numbered item has ONLY ONE answer. Within each group, each lettered item may be the answer to one, more than one, or none of the numbered items.

For each of the endocrine organs listed below, choose whether its embryologic origin is from Rathke's pouch, the foramen cecum, pharyngeal pouches, or none of these.

A. Rathke's pouch
B. Foramen cecum
C. Pharyngeal pouches
D. None of these

**52.** Thyroid gland
**53.** Parathyroid glands
**54.** Thymus gland
**55.** Anterior pituitary gland
**56.** Posterior pituitary gland
**57.** Pineal gland

For each of the characteristics listed below, choose whether it describes prolactin, growth hormone, corticotropin, thyrotropin, or none of these.

A. Prolactin
B. Growth hormone
C. Corticotropin
D. Thyrotropin
E. None of these

**58.** Is produced in the hypothalamus
**59.** Is derived from the same precursor as melanocyte-stimulating hormone
**60.** Causes the most common pituitary endocrinopathy
**61.** Is rarely elaborated by pituitary tumor adenomas
**62.** Is frequently secreted by pituitary carcinomas
**63.** Causes the most common pituitary hormone deficiency syndrome
**64.** Causes hypogonadism (in both sexes) with overproduction

For each of the characteristics listed below, choose whether it describes pituitary dwarfism, cretinism, achondroplastic dwarfism, or none of these.

A. Pituitary dwarfism
B. Cretinism
C. Achondroplastic dwarfism
D. None of these

**65.** Has an inherited mode of transmission
**66.** Produces mental retardation
**67.** Produces a disproportionately large head and body
**68.** Is associated with a broad, flat nose and large tongue
**69.** Cannot currently be prevented with treatment

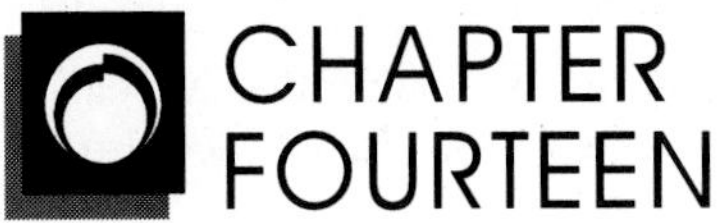

# The Endocrine System

## ANSWERS

**1. (A)** Postpartum pituitary necrosis, also known as Sheehan's syndrome, is one of the three most common causes of pituitary hypofunction. During pregnancy, the pituitary enlarges to almost twice its normal size, compressing its own venous vasculature and causing relative ischemia. Sudden systemic hypotension, such as that which may occur from blood loss during delivery, precipitates ischemic necrosis of much or all of the anterior lobe. The posterior pituitary, which is less vulnerable to anoxia, is spared. Other causes of pituitary hypofunction include nonsecretory (chromophobe) pituitary adenomas and the empty sella syndrome, most often caused by herniation of the arachnoid through a defect in the diaphragma sellae. In both of these situations, hypofunction is caused by pressure atrophy of the surrounding normal pituitary by the space-occupying lesion. Hypothalamic suprasellar tumors such as gliomas can cause anterior pituitary hypofunction but do so far less commonly than the disorders mentioned above. Other than the fact that Sheehan's syndrome with total pituitary necrosis ultimately may produce an empty sella syndrome, there is no direct relationship of any of the other causes of hypopituitarism (besides Sheehan's syndrome) with pregnancy.

In contrast to all of these disorders, prolactinomas would be associated with a syndrome of hyper- rather than hypofunction of the pituitary. Although prolactinomas are associated with amenorrhea (one of this patient's problems), they most often induce lactation with no relationship to childbirth (i.e., inappropriate lactation termed galactorrhea). *(pp. 1118–1120)*

**2. (C)** Diffuse nontoxic (simple) goiter is thyroid enlargement caused by compensatory hypertrophy and hyperplasia. It diffusely involves the entire gland without producing nodularity and does not usually produce thyroid function abnormalities (i.e., affected individuals are typically euthyroid). It is very common throughout the world and traditionally has been the most common thyroid abnormality in the United States. The disorder either arises sporadically in association with altered physiologic (e.g., hormonal) factors, occurs as an hereditary defect in iodine metabolism or hormone transport, or, far more commonly, occurs as an endemic disorder related either to deficient iodine intake or to ingested goitrogens (i.e., dietary substances that promotes goiter formation). Fluorides and calcium in the water supply are known to promote goiter formation, as do many vegetables in the Brassica and Crucifera families (e.g., brussels sprouts, cabbage, cauliflower).

In the sporadic variety of simple goiter, a minimal iodine deficiency may be present that leads to disease only in the presence of increased physiologic demands on thyroid function (e.g., with puberty, pregnancy, or stress). Contributory physiologic mechanisms may be multiple in these circumstances. For example, estrogen-induced increases in serum levels of thyroid-binding globulin (TBG) during pregnancy or oral contraceptive steroid use decreases the amount of unbound (active) tri-iodothyronine and thyroxine. Decreased serum concentrations of free hormones, in turn, reduce feedback inhibition of the anterior pituitary, resulting in thyroid-stimulating hormone release and thyroid stimulation. Androgenic steroids produce the opposite effect of estrogens on thyroid activity by lowering serum levels of TBG, and, therefore, are antigoiterogenic. *(pp. 1131–1132)*

**3. (D)** The syndrome of inappropriate antidiuretic hormone (SIADH) secretion is a condition characterized by antidiuretic hormone (ADH) secretion that is unrelated to plasma osmolarity. Under normal conditions, the posterior lobe of the pituitary is the source of ADH, but in SIADH secretion, the source of the ADH is usually a tumor. Approximately 80% of all cases are caused by bronchogenic carcinoma, especially oat cell carcinoma. Other neoplasms associated with SIADH secretion include thymoma, pancreatic carcinoma, and lymphoma. Although intracranial hemorrhage (e.g., subdural hematoma) or infection of the central nervous system (e.g., meningitis) occasionally may cause SIADH secretion, this is relatively uncommon.

In contrast to conditions causing an overproduction of ADH, inflammatory injury or neoplastic involvement of the hypothalamic-hypophyseal axis (e.g., by radiation or a pituitary adenoma) usually leads to ADH deficiency and diabetes insipidus. Although an uncommon cause of increased ADH secretion, (as mentioned above), meningitis is also known to result in decreased ADH secretion and produce diabetes insipidus occasionally. *(p. 1121)*

**4. (C)** A goitrogen is any chemical agent that suppresses or otherwise reduces the synthesis of tri-iodothyronine and thyroxine. With the reduction in thyroid hormone, feedback inhibition to the hypothalamus (producer of thyrotropin-releasing hormone) and pituitary (producer of thyroid-stimulating hormone, or TSH) is reduced. As a result, increased amounts of TSH are released, causing hypertrophic and hyperplastic enlargement of the thyroid gland, a condition known as goiter. *(pp. 1123; 1131)*

**5. (D)** The sudden development of an enlarged painful thyroid in association with some form of viral infection (e.g., influenza, measles, mumps, adenovirus, or echovirus) is characteristic of a self-limited inflammation of the thyroid gland known as subacute granulomatous thyroiditis or de Quervain's thyroiditis. This entity is three times more common in females than in males, and its peak incidence is in the second to fifth decades of life.

In contrast to de Quervain's thyroiditis, subacute lymphocytic thyroiditis (a self-limited idiopathic lymphocytic infiltration of the thyroid) and Reidel's thyroiditis (an idiopathic fibrosing reaction) are painless processes and have no association with prior viral infections. Hashimoto's thyroiditis, an autoimmune thyroiditis that occasionally may be painful and usually occurs in females, has no known association with viral illness. Whereas thyroid abscesses may occur from direct extension of a local infectious process or even by metastatic spread of infection, this is extremely uncommon and would not be expected in the setting of a viral illness such as influenza. *(pp. 1125–1128)*

**6. (D)** Multinodular goiter, the consequence of longstanding simple goiter (see Question 2), is associated with the most extreme enlargement of the thyroid gland and may increase thyroid weight to 2000 gm or more (normal thyroid weight is about 25 gm). Although Graves' disease, simple goiter, Hashimoto's thyroiditis, and de Quervain's thyroiditis all produce thyroid enlargement, it is usually modest in comparison, in the range of two- to threefold greater than normal. *(pp. 1126–1132)*

**7. (E)** A discrete, encapsulated single nodule is apparent in the otherwise normal thyroid lobe pictured in Figure 14–1. The patient has thyrotoxicosis, so it is most likely that this nodule represents a functioning thyroid adenoma. Most adenomas do not function and appear as "cold" nodules on thyroid scan, but some adenomas actively produce hormone. These functioning or hyperfunctioning adenomas accumulate radioiodine and appear as "warm" or "hot" nodules, respectively, on scintiscans. Along with Graves' disease and toxic multionodular goiter, toxic adenomas are one of the three most common causes of thyrotoxicosis. Only rarely do well-differentiated (papillary or follicular) thyroid carcinomas secrete sufficient thyroid hormone to cause clinical hyperthyroidism. Moreover, in such instances, the tumor is usually widely metastatic. Medullary carcinomas originate from the neurosecretory calcitonin-producing C cells (not from follicular cells) of the thyroid and do not secrete thyroid hormones. Multinodular goiter (toxic type), although a major cause of thyrotoxicosis, is characterized by multiple thyroid nodules with enlargement of the entire gland and would not correspond to a single nodule within a normal thyroid as pictured. *(pp. 1124; 1132–1136)*

**8. (A)** A papillary carcinoma of the thyroid with characteristic psammoma bodies is shown in the photomicrograph in Figure 14–2. Papillary adenocarcinoma is the most common form of thyroid cancer, but, fortunately, the great majority of these are biologically indolent and have an excellent prognosis. Among the salient features of this tumor are its tendency to be multifocal within the thyroid gland as a result of intraglandular spread and its preference for local lymphatic rather than hematogenous metastasis. Many cases of papillary thyroid carcinoma are associated with prior exposure to ionizing radiation, which is now known to cause thyroid carcinoma in 4 to 9% of exposed individuals. Although papillary tumors are not the only radiation-associated thyroid cancers, they are the most common. Papillary carcinomas are usually nonfunctioning and, therefore, appear as cold nodules on thyroid scintiscans. *(pp. 1136–1140)*

**9. (C)** Parathyroid hormone, the most important physiologic regulator of serum calcium levels, has several modes of action. It acts to raise serum calcium by reducing renal excretion and increasing intestinal absorption of calcium. It also mobilizes calcium from the bone through stimulation of osteoclast activity. In addition, PTH lowers levels of serum phosphate (to which calcium might bind) by enhancing renal phosphate excretion. However, PTH has no known direct effect on the secretion of calcitonin, the calcium-lowering hormone produced by the C cells of the thyroid. *(p. 1243)*

**10. (E)** Overtly symptomatic hypercalcemia much more often results from paraneoplastic syndromes related to nonparathyroid malignancies than from hyperparathyroidism. Hypercalcemia is the most common paraneoplastic syndrome associated with nonendocrine malignancies. Two mechanisms may be involved: (1) local osteolysis caused by the paracrine effects of cytokines secreted by tumor cells that are in contact with bone (bony metastases) and (2) skeletal osteolysis caused by a parathyroid hormone–like hormone(s) that the tumor releases into the systemic circulation.

Primary hyperparathyroidism is caused by parathyroid adenomas and primary parathyroid hyperplasia in 95% of cases. Secondary hyperparathyroidism is most commonly the result of renal insufficiency and, in contrast to the primary form, is characterized by hypocalcemia. Parathyroid carcinoma, although a cause of primary parathyroid hyperfunction, is quite rare. *(pp. 295; 1144–1147)*

**11. (C)** Conn's syndrome is caused by an adrenal adenoma producing large amounts of aldosterone. This syndrome is characterized by sodium retention and potassium wasting, which in turn cause hypertension and neuromuscular abnormalities.

Bartter's syndrome is a form of secondary hyperaldosteronism caused by overproduction of renin by the kidneys. In contrast to other forms of secondary hyperaldosteronism, which typically increase blood pressure, the blood pressure in Bartter's syndrome is usually low.

Nelson's syndrome has little to do with the adrenals. It is caused by hypersecretion of adrenocorticotrophic hormone (ACTH) from a pituitary tumor that cannot be eradicated and, therefore, necessitates removal of the end organs. Following bilateral adrenalectomy, the feedback inhibition of cortisol on the pituitary adenoma is removed, and intense hyperpigmentation related to excess production of ACTH and melanotropin ensues.

Cushing's syndrome is caused by overproduction of glucocorticoids. It may be caused by a hyperfunctioning adrenal adenoma, but it would be the result of a cortisol-producing rather than aldosterone-producing tumor. *(pp. 1150–1153)*

**12. (C)** Somatostatin is an intriguing inhibitory hormone that is produced in the hypothalamus as well as in many other tissues throughout the body. It exerts inhibitory control over (inhibits secretion of) a number of other hormones, including insulin, glucagon, gastrin, thyrotropin (thyroid-stimulating hormone, or TSH) and growth hormone (GH). Thus, it plays a number of physiologic roles in addition to its well-known function as a factor that inhibits the release of GH and TSH from the anterior pituitary. Prolactin secretion is under hypothalamic dopaminergic inhibitory control. Somatostatin does not affect prolactin secretion. *(pp. 909; 1117)*

**13. (A)** Figure 14–3 is a histologic section from the thyroid of a patient with Hashimoto's thyroiditis, the most common cause of goitrous hypothyroidism (not hyperthyroidism) in regions that have sufficient iodine supplies. The characteristic follicular atrophy (small clusters of persistent thyroid follicles are present at the top center of photograph) and extensive infiltration by lymphoid cells (focally forming germinal centers) are seen in the micrograph. Hashimoto's thyroiditis is an organ-specific autoimmune disorder thought to be caused by a deficiency in thyroid antigen–specific suppressor T cells. This suppressor cell deficit permits the emergence of antithyroid, CD4+ helper T cells, which promote the generation of thyroid-specific autoantibodies. It is believed that cell-mediated cytotoxic responses also are involved in the autoimmune follicular injury that is the hallmark of this disease. The autoantibodies most commonly isolated from patients with Hashimoto's thyroiditis are those directed against thyroid-stimulating hormone (TSH) receptors and thyroid peroxidases (formerly known as antimicrosomal antibodies). Some of the anti–TSH receptor autoantibodies appear to mimic the stimulatory action of TSH (some patients may be hyperthyroid initially until gland destruction supervenes), whereas others simply block the hormone receptor site. *(pp. 1126–1127)*

**14. (C)** Medullary carcinomas of the thyroid (MCT) are neuroendocrine tumors derived from the C cells of the thyroid, which are the only cells in the thyroid derived from the neural crest. As in other neuroendocrine neoplasms, neurosecretory dense core granules can be identified in the cytoplasm of medullary carcinoma cells when examined by electron microscopy. Histologically, one of the most distinctive features of MCT is amyloid deposition in the stroma. The presence of amyloid is unique among thyroid malignancies and is virtually pathognomonic of MCT. The amyloid is believed to be derived from the polypeptide hormonal products of the tumor cells. Most MCTs elaborate the major hormonal product of their cell of origin (i.e., the calcium-lowering hormone calcitonin). Less frequently, MCTs elaborate other products, such as somatostatin, prostaglandins, adrenocorticotrophic hormone, vasoactive intestinal polypeptide, neuron-specific enolase, histaminase, carcinoembryonic antigen, or serotinin. Sporadically occurring MCTs, as well as those associated with the multiple endocrine neoplasia syndrome IIb (see Question 16) are biologically aggressive (having a 10-year survival rate of 30 to 50%) and have a much less favorable prognosis than MCT occurring in the familial medullary carcinoma syndrome. In this syndrome, tumors tend to be indolent and the 10-year survival rate approaches 90%. *(pp. 234; 1140–1142)*

**15. (E)** The most common cause of congenital adrenal virilism (one of a group of distinctive clinical syndromes known collectively as "congenital adrenal hyperplasia" or "adrenogenital syndrome") is 21-hydroxylase deficiency. This defect impairs the synthesis of both cortisol and aldosterone and shunts the precursors of these hormones into the alternate pathway of androgen production. Because of the block in cortisol synthesis, feedback inhibition to the pituitary is reduced, and adrenocorticotrophic hormone secretion consequently is increased. As a result of increased androgens, females with this syndrome show signs of virilization, such as clitoral hypertrophy, that can be recognized easily at birth. Because of the block in aldosterone synthesis, a salt-wasting syndrome with hyponatremia and hyperkalemia develops. This is usually the basis of recognition of 21-hydroxylase deficiency in infant males. *(p. 1155–1157)*

**16. (A)** Pheochromocytoma is a neoplasm of the adrenal medulla that usually occurs sporadically but is also known to occur in several different familial syndromes. The tumor has at least four hereditary patterns, two of which are part of a multiple endocrine neoplasia syndrome. In multiple endocrine neoplasia syndrome, type IIa (MEN IIa or Sipple's syndrome), pheochromocytoma is associated with medullary carcinoma of the thyroid and with parathyroid adenomas or hyperplasia. In this syndrome, which is transmitted by autosomal dominant inheritance (germ line mutation of the *RET* proto-oncogene on chromosome 10), the pheochromocytomas are bilateral in about 70% of cases. Other hereditary patterns of pheochromocytoma include: (1) multiple endocrine neoplasia syndrome, type IIb (MEN IIb), in which the pheochromocytoma is associated with mucosal neuromas and a marfanoid habitus; (2) Sturge-Weber syndrome with associated cavernous hemangiomas in the fifth cranial nerve distribution; (3) von Recklinghausen's neurofibromatosis with associated neural and neural sheath tumors; and (4) von Hippel-Lindau disease with associated renal, hepatic, and pancreatic cysts, angiomatosis, cerebellar hemangioblastomas and renal cell carcinoma.

Pituitary adenomas and pancreatic islet cell adenomas are part of the spectrum of MEN syndrome, type I (Wermer's syndrome), in which they occur in association with parathyroid and adrenocortical adenomas. Neither of these lesions is part of the constellation of endocrine abnormalities associated with pheochromocytoma. *(pp. 148–149; 1162–1165; 1168–1170)*

**17. (B)** Thymomas, although rare, are the most common neoplasm of the thymus gland and one of the most common anterior mediastinal tumors. The neoplastic element of a thymoma is not the thymic lymphocyte but rather the thymic epithelial cell. In the normal gland, this cell is the source of a humoral factor known as thymosin that influences the differentiation of thymocytes (T cells). Patients with thymomas have a striking predisposition to the development of myasthenia gravis, an autoimmune disorder characterized by autoantibodies to acetylcholine receptors in skeletal muscle motor end plates (see Chapter 15, Question 3). Approximately 50% of patients with symptomatic thymoma come to clinical attention because of the associated myasthenia gravis, and, conversely, thymic abnormalities are present in the majority of patients with myasthenia gravis. Thymomas occur in about 15% of patients with myasthenia gravis, and thymic hyperplasia is present in most of the remaining patients. The relationship between these two disease processes is still unclear.

The great majority of thymomas occur in adults, usually older than 40 years. Thymomas rarely occur in children. The great majority (about 75%) of thymomas are benign and can be cured by surgical excision. Malignant thymomas are less common and have a poor prognosis. Although thymomas occasionally may be associated with autoimmune-type paraneoplastic syndromes (other than or in addition to myasthenia gravis), such as Grave's disease, Cushing's syndrome, pernicious anemia, or dermatomyositis-polymyositis, they are not associated with decreased immune responses (immunodeficiency syndromes). *(pp. 1167–1168; 1291)*

**18. (True); 19. (False); 20. (True); 21. (True); 22. (True)**

Graves' disease is a syndrome of thyrotoxicosis caused by a hyperfunctioning, diffusely hyperplastic thyroid accompanied by infiltrative ophthalmopathy and sometimes infiltrative dermopathy. It is unique among the goiters. Like simple goiter, Graves' disease is diffuse rather than nodular, but simple goiter does not cause hyperfunction. Multinodular goiter may be hyperfunctioning but, as the name indicates, the thyroid enlargement is nodular rather than diffuse. In contrast to both simple and nodular goiter, Graves' disease is not caused by goitrogens or inborn errors of metabolism (see Question 6). Like Hashimoto's thyroiditis, Graves' disease is an autoimmune form of goiter. However, Hashimoto's thyroiditis typically causes hypo- rather than hyperfunction.

**(18)** Other forms of thyrotoxicosis may have eye changes, such as retraction of the upper eyelid and lid lag, but only Graves' disease causes protrusion of the globe (proptosis) caused by autoimmune and inflammatory processes.

**(19)** In addition to Graves' disease and functioning thyroid adenomas, toxic nodular goiter is one of the three major causes of thyrotoxicosis. However, as emphasized, Graves' disease refers only to *diffuse* hyperfunctioning goiter without nodularity.

**(20)** In Graves' disease, autoantibodies to thyroid-stimulating hormone (TSH) receptors on thyroid follicular cells are produced because of a defect in organ-specific suppressor T-cell function. The major class of anti–TSH receptor antibodies found in this disease mimics the action of TSH, inducing thyroid growth and hyperfunction. These antibodies are known as thyroid-stimulating immunoglobulins (TSI). Blocking antibodies also are identified that prevent the binding of TSH to the cell and are called thyrotropin-binding inhibitor immunoglobulin. TSH autoantibodies can be identified in virtually all patients with Graves' disease.

**(21)** Graves' disease and Hashimoto's thyroiditis are both thyroid-specific autoimmune disorders. Although they are quite distinctive histopathologically, they may have overlapping clinical features and common genotype associations. Although the HLA-D8 haplotype in Graves' disease and the HLA-DR5 haplotype in Hashimoto's thyroiditis are nonoverlapping genotype associations, the HLA-DR3 haplotype is linked to both diseases. Presumably, this difference in genotypic association is related to the difference in the type of TSH receptor autoantibodies produced in each of these diseases. In Graves' disease the autoantibodies are predominantly stimulatory, whereas in Hashimoto's thyroiditis blocking antibodies are more common. Nevertheless, some patients with Hashimoto's thyroiditis present with hyperthyroidism, and TSI such as those found in Grave's disease, are identified.

**(22)** Infiltrative dermopathy taking the form of localized skin edema over the dorsa of the legs or feet is especially characteristic of Graves' disease. However, it is present in about 10 to 15% of patients. Although ironically referred to as "localized myxedema," this change has nothing to do with true myxedema (which is hypothyroidism in the older child or adult). *(pp. 1126; 1129–1130)*

**23. (B); 24. (A); 25. (A); 26. (C); 27. (C); 28. (C); 29. (C)**

**(23)** Cushing's syndrome and acromegaly are syndromes of hormonal excess caused by cortisol and growth hormone (GH), respectively. Acromegaly is virtually always related to direct elaboration of GH by an endocrine tumor, almost always a functioning pituitary adenoma. In contrast, Cushing's syndrome may be caused by either a cortisol-producing neoplasm in the adrenal cortex or by hyperstimulation of the normal adrenal by adrenocorticotrophic hormone (corticotropin; ACTH) produced by a tumor. Although pituitary adenomas are the most common source of elevated ACTH in Cushing's syndrome, ectopic production of ACTH by nonencodrine neoplasms accounts for about 15% of cases (see Question 24).

**(24)** About 70% of all cases of Cushing's syndrome are caused by pituitary adenomas secreting ACTH. A less common cause is ACTH production by nonendocrine cancers with Cushing's syndrome occurring as a paraneoplastic phenomenon. The most common ACTH-producing tumors are bronchogenic carcinomas (particularly oat cell carcinomas), which account for about 60% of cases of "ectopic Cushing's syndrome." Although ectopic hormone production is a relatively common paraneoplastic phenomenon, acromegaly is notably absent from the list of endocrinopathies caused by nonendocrine cancers. In some cases, GH may be elaborated by endocrine neoplasms such as pancreatic endocrine tumors or carcinoid tumors, but, even in these cases, acromegaly rarely, if ever, results.

**(25)** The most common clinical feature of Cushing's syndrome is "central" obesity involving the trunk and upper back. This feature in combination with the typical "moon facies" of Cushingoid patients, makes them fairly easy to recognize. Acromegaly affects only the head, hands, and feet (i.e., the acral rather than central parts of the body) and is not associated with obesity.

**(26)** Hyperglycemia and **(27)** hypertension are clinical characteristics of both Cushing's syndrome and acromegaly. In both of these conditions, glucose intolerance may be severe enough to produce overt diabetes mellitus. **(28)** Another feature common to both of these disorders is osteoporosis caused by the effects of GH and ACTH on bone metabolism.

**(29)** Both Cushing's syndrome and acromegaly cause characteristic changes in the facial appearance of affected individuals. In Cushing's syndrome, with its characteristic central obesity, rounding of the face (moon facies) and thickening of the neck occur. Acromegaly causes bone growth in the head and extremities, with striking coarsening of the facial features and enlargement of the hands and feet. *(pp. 295; 1116–1117; 1150–1151)*

**30. (C); 31. (C); 32. (D); 33. (A); 34. (B); 35. (A); 36. (B)**

Myxedema and Addison's disease are endocrine deficiency syndromes caused by hypofunction of the thyroid and the adrenal cortex, respectively. Both have profound systemic effects, some of which are similar in the two diseases.

**(30)** Both myxedema and Addison's disease are usually the result of an organ-specific autoimmune process. The most common cause of hypothyroidism in the United States is so-called idiopathic primary hypothyroidism, a process now known to be linked to HLA-DR3 and HLA-B8 haplotypes and to be caused by production of autoantibodies to the thyroid-stimulating hormone receptor. Hashimoto's thyroiditis, another prototypic organ-specific autoimmune disease, is the most common cause of goitrous hypothyroidism in regions having a sufficiency of iodine. Most cases of Addison's disease (60 to 70%) are caused by autoimmune adrenalitis. In the past, tuberculosis was the most common cause, but it now accounts for only about 10% of cases. As part of a polyglandular autoimmune syndrome, myxedema and Addison's may be associated with one another or with other autoimmune disorders such as pernicious anemia or diabetes mellitus.

**(31)** Certain clinical manifestations, such as fatigability and constipation, are common in both diseases. **(32)** Hypertension, however, is a feature of neither myxedema nor Addison's disease. On the contrary, virtually all patients with Addison's disease are hypotensive. Similarly, systolic pressures also are reduced in myxedema, because the disease causes a characteristic cardiomyopathy that results in an enlarged, flabby heart. However, diastolic pressures are elevated in myxedema secondary to increased peripheral vascular resistance. **(33)** Those with full-blown myxedema usually develop congestive heart failure. The term "myxedema heart" or hypothyroid cardiomyopathy is given to this distinctive cardiac disease, which is characterized histologically by interstitial mucopolysaccharide deposition and swelling of myofibers with loss of striations.

**(34)** Hyperpigmentation is a distinguishing feature of Addison's disease. It results from increased secretion of adrenocorticotrophic hormone (ACTH) as a result of lowered serum cortisol levels and reduced feedback inhibition to the hypothalamus and pituitary. Increased synthesis of both ACTH and melanotropin ensues, melanocytes are stimulated, and hyperpigmentation results.

**(35)** In contrast to cortisol insufficiency, lack of thyroid hormone produces a slowing of mental as well as physical processes. Thus, myxedema is associated with a reduction in intellectual function that is not seen in Addison's disease.

**(36)** Both myxedema and Addison's disease may be associated with other autoimmune diseases. It recently has become evident, however, that syndromes of multiple autoimmune disorders that include Addison's disease fall into distinct subsets. One type is characterized by at least two elements of the triad of Addison's disease, hypoparathyroidism, and mucocutaneous candidiasis. A second type, known as Schmidt's syndrome, is characterized by Addison's disease, autoimmune thyroid disease, and/or insulin-dependent diabetes mellitus without hypoparathyroidism or candidiasis. *(pp. 1124–1125; 1126–1127; 1158–1160)*

**37. (C); 38. (D); 39. (B); 40. (B); 41. (B)**

Pheochromocytoma and neuroblastoma constitute the two most significant disease processes of the adrenal medulla. Pheochromocytomas originate from the adrenal medullary chromaffin cells, whereas neuroblastoma are derived from autonomic ganglion cell precursors known as neuroblasts.

**(37)** Both of these tumors characteristically elaborate catecholamines, predominantly norepinephrine in both cases. **(38)** Occurrence in young adults would be relatively unusual for either tumor type. Approximately 80% of neuroblastomas occur in children under the age of 5, and sporadically occurring pheochromocytoma arises most commonly in adults ages 40 to 60 years. **(39)** In sharp contrast to pheochromocytomas, which are usually benign, neuroblastomas are virtually always malignant and are usually metastatic by the time the diagnosis is made.

**(40)** Only about 5% of pheochromocytomas occurring in the adrenal are malignant. They have a better prognosis than their extra-adrenal counterparts, which are much more likely to be malignant. Neuroblastomas, although invariably malignant, carry a poorer prognosis when arising in the adrenal than when occurring in extra-adrenal sites.

**(41)** Deletion of the short arm of chromosome 1 distal to band p32 is the most characteristic karyotypic abnormality in neuroblastoma. It correlates with loss of a suppressor gene for neuroblastoma and a poor prognosis for the tumor. This abnormality is not seen in pheochromocytomas. *(pp. 459–461; 1162–1165)*

**42. (C); 43. (B); 44. (B); 45. (A); 46. (A); 47. (A); 48. (A); 49. (C); 50. (D); 51. (D)**

Diabetes mellitus is a chronic endocrine disorder characterized by an absolute or relative deficiency of insulin. Marked derangements in the metabolism of carbohydrate, fat, and protein are the result. The disease has two major variants: insulin-dependent diabetes mellitus (IDDM or type I diabetes), constituting about 10 to 20% of cases, and non–insulin-dependent diabetes mellitus (NIDDM) or type II diabetes), by far the more common of the two types.

**(42)** Although the two variants have numerous distinctive features, they have in common an inability to utilize glucose. **(43)** In contrast to IDDM, which is the result of injury to the beta cells of the pancreatic islets, producing an absolute and severe lack of insulin, only a relative lack of insulin is present in NIDDM. However, NIDDM has an additional pathogenetic feature: resistance of the peripheral tissues to respond to the action of insulin. Insulin resistance is the result of both a decrease in cellular insulin receptors and defects in the postreceptor intracellular signaling responses that usually are initiated by insulin binding to the cell surface receptor.

**(44)** In NIDDM (but not IDDM), obesity is an extremely common associated feature and an important diabetogenic influence. Even in the absence of diabetes, obesity alone will cause decreased insulin sensitivity of tissues. It is significant that about 80% of patients with NIDDM are obese and that weight loss in the overweight diabetic improves the metabolic derangement.

**(45)** In contrast to NIDDM, IDDM is believed to be an organ-specific (more accurately, a cell-specific) autoimmune disorder. Circulating islet cell autoantibodies are present in 90% of patients with IDDM. There is also evidence for a cellular immune response in the form of sensitized T cells reactive against beta cells. In animal models of type I diabetes, CD4+ T cells from diseased animals can transfer diabetes to normal animals. **(46)** In patients with recent-onset IDDM, lymphocytic infiltration of the pancreatic islets, a phenomenon known as "insulitis," is a characteristic histologic finding. Such infiltrates contain both CD4+ and CD8+ T cells and suggest that T-cell autoimmunity plays a primary role in the pathogenesis of the disease. Insulitis is not a feature of NIDDM, a fact that underscores the difference in pathogenesis of the two types of diabetes and the absence of T-cell autoimmunity in NIDDM.

**(47)** Although there are no specific genetic markers for either form of diabetes, it is certain that diabetes mellitus is at least in part a genetic disorder. Epidemiologic studies indicate that genetic factors play a much larger role in the induction of NIDDM than in that of IDDM. For example, the concordance rate for NIDDM in identical twins is 90 to 100%, as contrasted with a 50% concordance rate in IDDM. However, IDDM shows a strong association with specific alleles in the class II histocompatibility complex (HLA-D linked), whereas it has not been possible to demonstrate a relationship between NIDDM and specific human lymphocyte antigen (HLA) types. Genetic susceptibility to IDDM has been linked to HLA-DQ3.2 (associated with an eightfold increased risk of IDDM) and HLA-DR3 (which, in combination with HLA-DQ3.2, increases the risk of IDDM 20-fold). Conversely, the HLA-DQ1.2 haplotype decreases the risk of IDDM.

**(48)** There is also ample evidence that environmental factors may trigger the autoimmune response in genetically susceptible individuals in some cases of IDDM. Viral infections, chemical toxins, and food allergens (e.g., cow's milk) all have been implicated in the initiation of the disease. However, in the majority of cases of IDDM, no associated environmental factors are known. In NIDDM, no associations with environmental factors have been elucidated at all.

**(49)** Despite the major etiologic differences between IDDM and NIDDM, their major systemic pathologic manifestations are remarkably similar. One of the most common and characteristic pathologic features of diabetes, regardless of type, are the retinal vascular changes known collectively as diabetic retinopathy. It has been estimated that a patient with a 25-year history of diabetes mellitus has a 90% chance of developing this complication. **(50)** Unfortunately, both types of diabetes also have a shortened life expectancy and continue to be among the leading causes of death in the United States.

**(51)** Ketoacidosis rarely occurs in NIDDM, and it is no longer a major cause of death in the IDDM population. In fact, with proper insulin therapy, it has become rare as a cause of mortality. In contrast, atherosclerotic complications (e.g., myocardial infarction, cerebrovascular accidents, gangrene, renal insufficiency) are common causes of death in long-standing diabetes of either form. *(pp. 910–922)*

**52. (B); 53. (C); 54. (C); 55. (A); 56. (D); 57. (D)**

The endocrine system is composed of numerous unique and complex organs with diverse functions and embryologic origins. A knowledge of the embryologic source of each organ is useful in understanding their respective developmental pathologies.

**(52)** The thyroid gland develops from a tubular invagination at the root of the tongue called the foramen cecum. The tube, called the thyroglossal duct, elongates as the thyroid migrates to its final position in front of the trachea. Vestigial remnants of the thyroglossal duct may develop into midline cystic structures later in life and require surgical removal.

**(53)** Although at least one pair are intimately associated with the thyroid gland, the parathyroid glands originate from an altogether different embryologic source—the third (lower pair) and the fourth (upper pair) pharyngeal pouches. **(54)** The thymus gland also originates from the third and sometimes fourth pair of pharyngeal pouches, so one or two parathyroids occasionally become enclosed within the thymic capsule.

**(55)** The pituitary is actually a composite gland made up of an anterior, epithelium-derived portion and a neurally derived posterior portion. The anterior pituitary is derived from an evagination of the roof of the primitive oral canal called Rathke's pouch, whereas **(56)** the posterior pituitary arises from an outpouching of the floor of the third ventricle. Although in the course of normal development Rathke's pouch is detached from its origin by the growing sphenoid bone, rests of epithelial cells occasionally may be caught below the sphenoid and give rise to pharyngeal pituitary tissue.

**(57)** The pineal gland is a small structure located at the base of the brain that is derived from ependymal cells lining the third ventricle. Although its function is still somewhat obscure, the pineal gland is thought to play some role in maintaining diurnal awake-asleep rhythms and sexual cycles. *(pp. 1114; 1122–1123; 1143; 1165; 1168)*

**58. (E); 59. (C); 60. (A); 61. (D); 62. (E); 63. (B); 64. (A)**

Prolactin, growth hormone, corticotropin, and thyrotropin are all hormones produced in the anterior pituitary. **(58)** Hormones made in the hypothalamus but stored in the posterior pituitary include oxytocin and vasopressin. The hypothalamus also produces releasing factors for all six of the anterior pituitary hormones and release-inhibiting factors for at least two. **(59)** The corticotrophic cells of the anterior pituitary actually elaborate three separate hormones. Besides corticotrophin, they also make melanocyte-stimulating hormone and lipotrophin. All three hormones are generated from the same precursor molecule, pro-opiomelanocortin.

**(60)** For reasons that are poorly understood, the vast majority of functioning pituitary adenomas secrete either prolactin, growth hormone, or corticotropin. Prolactinomas are the most common form of pituitary tumor, and hyperprolactinemia is the most common pituitary tumor-related endocrinopathy. **(61)** Tumors secreting thyrotropin, luteinizing hormone, or follicle-stimulating hormone are all very uncommon. The rarest of these are the thyrotroph adenomas, estimated to constitute less than 1% of all pituitary adenomas. **(62)** In contrast to benign pituitary tumors, which are frequently secretory, pituitary carcinomas are not only exceedingly rare but only rarely elaborate hormones.

**(63)** Hypopituitarism usually arises from some destructive process involving the anterior pituitary and usually involves more than one hormone. Rarely, however, pituitary insufficiency may manifest itself as an isolated hormone deficiency. In such cases, it usually takes the form of a growth hormone deficit causing dwarfism (Questions 65 through 69).

**(64)** Overproduction of prolactin (prolactinomas) may induce hypogonadism in both the male and female and causes galactorrhea in the female. Other reproductive abnormalities associated with hyperprolactinemia include amenorrhea in the female and, in the male, impotence and infertility. *(pp. 1114–1119)*

**65. (C); 66. (B); 67. (C); 68. (B); 69. (C)**

A dwarf is an abnormally undersized person. Dwarfism is not a discrete disease entity but rather a retardation of growth that may occur as a result of a number of diverse underlying conditions. For example, hypopituitarism with growth hormone deficiency in the prepubertal child causes so-called pituitary dwarfism. Thyroid hypofunction in the infant causes a form of dwarfism known specifically as cretinism. Other causes include hypoadrenalism, renal osteodystrophy, partial combined immunodeficiency disorders, and end-organ insensitivity to growth hormone stimulation. Achondroplastic dwarfism is a relatively common form of dwarfism not known to be associated with an endocrinologic deficit.

**(65)** Achondroplasia is an inherited disorder with both autosomal dominant and autosomal recessive forms of transmission. The autosomal recessive form is more severe, and only the autosomal dominant form is compatible with normal longevity. Achondroplasia is characterized by a failure of cartilage cell proliferation and premature closure of the growth plates of bones preformed in cartilage. In neither form of achondroplasia are the exact pathogenetic mechanisms known. **(66)** Neither pituitary dwarfism nor achondroplastic dwarfism is associated with decreased intelligence. Cretinism, however, produces profound retardation of intellectual growth as well as physical growth.

**(67)** Achondroplastic dwarfism can be distinguished readily on the basis of its characteristic body habitus. Shortened proximal extremities, a trunk of relatively normal length and an enlarged head with a bulging forehead are characteristic. Head growth is not affected in this disorder, because many bones of the face and cranium are produced by membranous rather than endochondral bone formation.

**(68)** A broad, flat nose and a very large, protuberant tongue are characteristic features of cretinism and are not seen in dwarfism.

**(69)** Pituitary dwarfism and cretinism are the result of hormone deficiencies, so, if recognized early enough, they can be treated successfully by iatrogenic replacement of the missing hormonal elements. There is at present, however, no known effective therapy for achondroplasia. *(pp. 1119; 1125; 1218)*

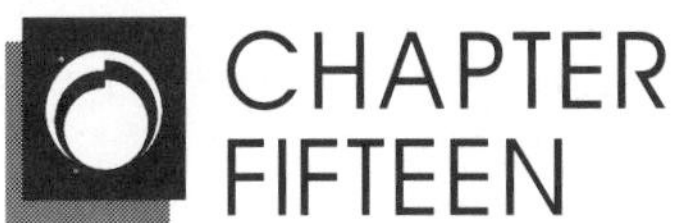

CHAPTER
FIFTEEN

# The Musculoskeletal System

**DIRECTIONS:** For Questions 1 through 13, choose the ONE BEST answer to each question.

**1.** All of the following statements about osteoblasts are true EXCEPT:

A. They are multinucleate cells.
B. They are precursors of osteocytes.
C. They synthesize the collagen component of osteoid matrix.
D. They synthesize osteocalcin.
E. They control parathormone-induced osteoclastic bone resorption.

**2.** All of the following statements about normal skeletal muscle are true EXCEPT:

A. Muscle fibers are syncytial cells with multiple nuclei.
B. The nuclei of muscle fibers are characteristically located in the cell periphery.
C. Muscle fibers are innervated by myelinated nerve fibers.
D. Each muscle fiber is innervated by a separate motor neuron.
E. The type of innervating motor neuron determines the functional type of the muscle fiber.

**3.** All of the following statements about myasthenia gravis are true EXCEPT:

A. Ocular muscles characteristically are weakened.
B. Muscle strength improves with administration of anticholinesterase agents.
C. Nerve conduction studies are typically normal.
D. The risk of developing autoimmune thyroid disease is increased.
E. Nearly all patients have underlying thymomas.

**4.** Pyogenic osteomyelitis is associated with all of the following complications EXCEPT:

A. Periostitis
B. Pott's disease
C. Sequestrum formation
D. Brodie's abscesses
E. Involucrum formation

**5.** A fracture that communicates with the skin surface is known as:

A. A pathologic fracture
B. A greenstick fracture
C. A complete fracture
D. A compound fracture
E. A comminuted fracture

**6.** All of the following features are associated with the bone disease pictured in Figure 15–1 EXCEPT:

A. Retroviral infection of bone
B. Radiologic findings of marked bony thickening
C. Markedly increased breaking strength of bones
D. High serum levels of alkaline phosphatase
E. Increased risk of developing osteosarcoma

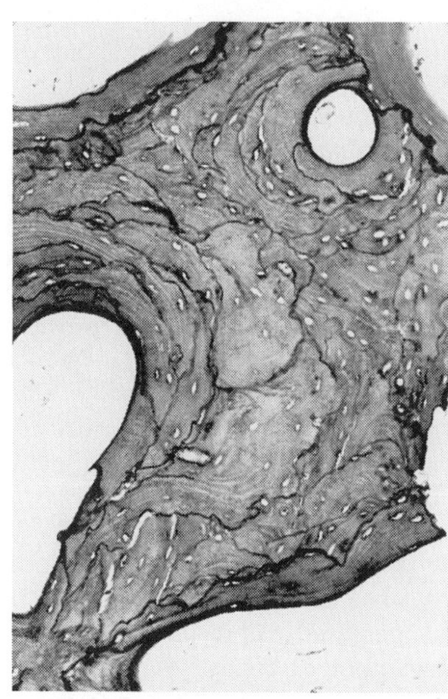

Figure 15–1

**7.** The disease most frequently associated with hypertrophic osteoarthropathy is:

A. Pleural mesothelioma
B. Bronchogenic carcinoma
C. Infective endocarditis
D. Congenital heart disease
E. Ulcerative colitis

**8.** Which of the following statements about giant cell tumors of bone is true?

A. Infants most often are affected by this neoplasm.
B. The giant cells in this tumor are osteoclasts.
C. Lesions typically appear osteoblastic on radiographs.
D. The bones about the knee are involved most commonly.
E. Metastases to the lung are common.

**9.** Pathologic features of osteoarthritis include all of the following EXCEPT:

A. Cartilage fibrillation
B. Pannus formation
C. Eburnation of bone
D. Heberden's node formation
E. Osteophyte formation

**10.** All of the following abnormalities are features of renal osteodystrophy EXCEPT:

A. Increased osteoclastic bone resorption
B. Osteomalacia
C. Osteoslcerosis
D. Osteoporosis
E. Osteonecrosis

**11.** All of the following statements about osteopetrosis are true EXCEPT:

A. All causes are hereditary.
B. The underlying abnormality is osteoclast dysfunction.
C. Affected bones are resistant to fracture.
D. Extramedullary hematopoiesis is a typical feature.
E. Bone marrow transplantation provides effective therapy.

**12.** An asymptomatic 13-year-old boy was discovered to have a single bone involved by the lesion pictured in Figure 15–2. The patient:

A. Most likely presented with severe localized pain
B. Most likely had this lesion in a rib
C. Is at increased risk of developing more of these lesions in other bones
D. Most likely has an underlying endocrine disorder
E. Has a 50% chance of developing an osteosarcoma

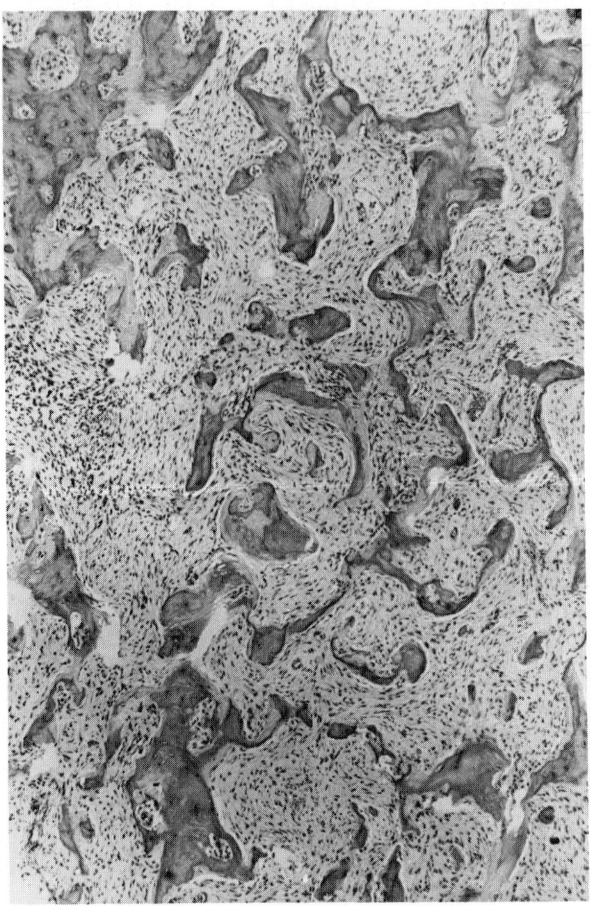

**Figure 15–2**

**13.** Characteristic features of Ewing's sarcoma include all of the following EXCEPT:

A. Occurrence primarily in childhood
B. Origin from the medullary cavity of bone
C. Derivation from lymphocytic cell line precursors
D. Periodic acid–Schiff positive cytoplasmic granules
E. High cure rate with current therapy

**DIRECTIONS:** For Questions 14 through 32, you are to decide whether EACH choice is TRUE or FALSE.

For each of the following statements about primary senile osteoporosis, choose whether it is TRUE or FALSE.

**14.** It is caused by impaired osteoid mineralization.
**15.** It seldom occurs in males.
**16.** Its development is related to decreased dietary calcium intake with age.
**17.** Its development is related to decreased physical activity with age.
**18.** The associated bony changes on plain radiographs are diagnostic.

For each of the following statements about rheumatoid arthritis, choose whether it is TRUE or FALSE.

**19.** The disease is associated with specific HLA-DR haplotypes.
**20.** Large joints of weight-bearing areas typically are involved.
**21.** Antibodies directed against immunoglobulin G are present in most cases.
**22.** Involvement of the skin produces rheumatoid nodules.
**23.** Involvement of the heart produces rheumatic heart disease.
**24.** Involvement of blood vessels produces systemic vasculitis.
**25.** It is the most common cause of reactive systemic amyloidosis.

For each of the following statements about gout, choose whether it is TRUE or FALSE.

**26.** Most individuals with hyperuricemia develop gout.
**27.** An underlying disease causing excessive cell breakdown usually is present.
**28.** Synthesis of uric acid is increased in most cases.
**29.** Acute arthritis of the great toe is the most common presentation.
**30.** Acute gouty arthritis is the result of urate crystal formation.
**31.** Chronic gouty arthritis is characterized by pannus formation.
**32.** The formation of tophi in the central nervous system is a debilitating complication.

**DIRECTIONS:** For Questions 33 through 51, the set of lettered headings is followed by a list of numbered words or phrases. For each numbered word or phrase choose:

A—if the item is associated with (A) only
B—if the item is associated with (B) only
C—if the item is associated with *both* (A) and (B)
D—if the item is associated with *neither* (A) nor (B)

For each of the characteristics listed below, choose whether it describes desmoids, nodular fasciitis, both, or neither.

A. Desmoid
B. Nodular fasciitis
C. Both
D. Neither

**33.** Is a true neoplasm
**34.** Is associated with pregnancy
**35.** Occurs commonly in extremities
**36.** Characteristically infiltrates surrounding soft tissues
**37.** Typically has a myxoid extracellular matrix on histologic examination
**38.** Tends to recur following incomplete surgical excision
**39.** Undergoes malignant transformation in 5 to 10% of cases

For each of the characteristics listed below, choose whether it describes osteochondromatosis, enchondromatosis, both, or neither.

A. Osteochondromatosis
B. Enchondromatosis
C. Both
D. Neither

**40.** Has an X-linked mode of hereditary transmission
**41.** Represents multiple true neoplasms
**42.** Is associated with colonic polyps in Gardner's syndrome
**43.** Is associated with cavernous hemangioma in Maffucci's syndrome
**44.** Is associated with an increased risk of developing chondrosarcoma

For each of the characteristics listed below, choose whether it describes osteosarcoma, chondrosarcoma, both, or neither.

A. Osteosarcoma
B. Chondrosarcoma
C. Both
D. Neither

**45.** Constitutes the most common form of primary cancer of bones
**46.** Occurs most frequently in children and adolescents
**47.** Arises *de novo* as a primary lesion in the majority of cases
**48.** Arises most commonly in the knee
**49.** Often contains both bone and cartilage
**50.** Rarely metastasizes to lymph nodes
**51.** Behaves predictably according to tumor grade

**DIRECTIONS:** Questions 52 through 72 are matching questions. For each numbered item, choose the most likely associated lettered item from those provided. Each numbered item has ONLY ONE answer. Within each group, each lettered item may be the answer to one, more than one, or none of the numbered items.

For each of the features listed below, choose whether it is characteristic of Duchenne muscular dystrophy, myotonic dystrophy, congenital myopathy, all of these, or none of these.

A. Duchenne muscular dystrophy
B. Myotonic dystrophy
C. Congenital myopathy
D. All of these
E. None of these

**52.** Occurs only in males
**53.** Is rarely associated with mental retardation
**54.** Is incompatible with long survival
**55.** Characteristically involves extramuscular systems
**56.** Characteristically produces involvement of a single myofiber type
**57.** Is characterized histologically by "ring fibers"
**58.** Is caused by a myotropic virus

For each of the characteristics listed below, choose whether it describes rhabdomyosarcoma, synovial sarcoma, malignant fibrous histiocytoma, liposarcoma, or none of these.

A. Rhabdomyosarcoma
B. Synovial sarcoma
C. Malignant fibrous histiocytoma
D. Liposarcoma
E. None of these

**59.** Commonly occurs in children
**60.** Most often has a myxoid appearance
**61.** Has an aggressive "alveolar" variant
**62.** Contains both epithelioid and spindle-shaped cells ("biphasic" growth)
**63.** Typically produces a storiform (pinwheel) growth pattern
**64.** Typically stains for desmin by immunohistochemistry
**65.** Often stains positively for keratin by immunohistochemistry

For each of the characteristics listed below, choose whether it describes osteogenesis imperfecta, osteopetrosis, achondroplasia, all of these, or none of these.

A. Osteogenesis imperfecta
B. Osteopetrosis
C. Achondroplasia
D. All of these
E. None of these

**66.** Is genetically transmitted
**67.** Represents a defect in type I collagen synthesis
**68.** Represents a defect in osteoclast function
**69.** Represents a defect in epiphyseal cartilage growth
**70.** Is associated with blue sclerae
**71.** Commonly is complicated by multiple exostoses
**72.** Commonly is complicated by anemia and hepatosplenomegaly

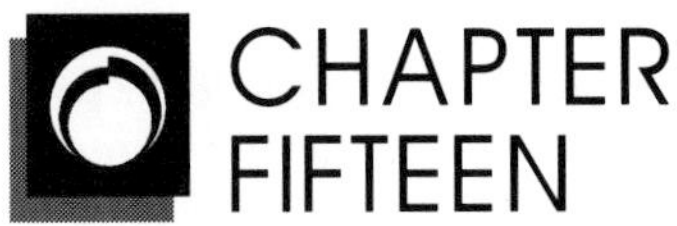

CHAPTER FIFTEEN

# The Musculoskeletal System

## ANSWERS

**1. (A)** Osteoblasts are bone-forming cells that synthesize the collagenous component of the osteoid matrix. They also initiate the process of bone mineralization through the elaboration of mineralization proteins (osteocalcin) and calcium-binding proteins (osteonectin and bone sialoprotein) required for the deposition of inorganic hydroxyapatite in the organic osteoid that they produce. Osteocalcin is a product of osteoblasts uniquely and is measurable in the serum. Thus, it is a sensitive and specific marker of osteoblast activity. When osteoblasts become enclosed within the matrix they produce, they are then termed osteocytes. Both osteoblasts and osteocytes are uninucleate and thus can be distinguished easily from osteoclasts, which are multinucleate cells.

Although the major function of osteoblasts is bone formation, they also control bone resorption in response to stimuli such as parathyroid hormone, interleukin-1, interleukin-6, and tumor necrosis factor-β. Although osteoblasts bear receptors for these hormones and are activated by them, osteoclasts are insensitive to them. The signal for bone resorption is transmitted to the osteoclasts from the activated osteoblasts through the release of a soluble mediator. Thus, without osteoblasts, parathormone-induced osteoclastic bone resorption does not occur. *(pp. 1213–1216)*

**2. (D)** Muscle fibers (myocytes) are composed of syncytia of numerous individual cells. Their multiple nuclei are characteristically located in the cell periphery, with internal nuclei comprising only about 3% of the total nuclear number. Increased numbers of internalized nuclei are distinctly pathologic and always indicate muscle disease or injury (e.g., denervation atrophy). Indeed, they are the most prominent pathologic feature in one form of congenital myopathy named for this finding: centronuclear myopathy.

Muscle fibers are innervated by myelinated nerve fibers that are the axons of motor neurons. Each muscle fiber is innervated by a separate axon, but one motor neuron typically supplies multiple muscle fibers. It is the type of innervating motor neuron that determines the functional type of the muscle fiber. Two types of muscle fibers exist: (1) slow-twitch fibers specialized for sustained force and weigh bearing, and (2) fast twitch fibers specialized for sudden movement and purposeful motion. Slow-twitch fibers have a red color and contain abundant lipid and scant glycogen. Fast-twitch fibers are white and contain scant lipid and abundant glycogen. The two types are readily differentiated on ATPase histochemical stains. *(pp. 1274–1277; 1288)*

**3. (E)** Myasthenia gravis (MG) is an autoimmune disorder characterized by autoantibodies to the acetylcholine receptors (AChRs) of postsynaptic membranes at the motor end plate. The circulating antibodies increase the degradation rate of AChRs, decreasing AChR numbers. These antibodies also appear to fix complement and produce direct injury of the postsynaptic membrane. Thus, transmission of neural impulses at the neuromuscular junction is abolished, and marked muscle weakness results. Characteristically, the first manifestation of MG is weakening of the eye muscles, with diplopia and dropping of the eyelids. Trunk and limb muscles frequently are affected later in the disease. A distinctive feature of MG that constitutes the basis of a diagnostic clinical test (Tensilon test) is the recovery of strength following administration of an anticholinesterase agent. Despite the abnormalities in neuromuscular function in MG, nerve conduction studies are typically normal, as are autonomic and sensory nerve function. Thus, MG can be distinguished easily from a peripheral neuropathy.

Individuals with MG and members of their family have an increased incidence of other autoimmune disorders, including thyroid disease, rheumatoid arthritis, systemic lupus erythmatosus, and pernicious anemia. The thymus appears to play a central role in the etiology of MG, but the underlying immunopathologic mechanisms are still unclear. Although the thymus is abnormal in nearly all patients with MG, thymomas are found in fewer than half of cases (15 to 40%). Conversely, however, 50% of all thymomas that come to clinical attention are related to MG. Thymic hyperplasia in MG is characteristically much more common and occurs in 65 to 75% of cases. *(pp. 183; 1166–1168; 1292)*

**4. (B)** Pyogenic osteomyelitis is almost always a bacterial (or rarely fungal) infection of bone. Almost any bacterium can be responsible, but the most common organisms involved in adult disease are *Staphylococcus aureus*, *Escherichia coli*, *Pseudomonas*, and *Klebsiella*. In neonates, *Haemophilus influenzae* and group B streptococci are common offenders. In 50% of cases, however, no organisms can be cultured for either technical (inadequate sampling or culture methods) or iatrogenic (prior antibiotic therapy) reasons. The infection most often appears to arise as a primary infection in a previously healthy individual and, in this setting, is thought to be produced by transient bacteremias from such trivial sources as injury to the intestinal mucosa, vigorous chewing of hard foods, or minor injury to the skin. Less often, the infection has a more obvious source and is the result of local trauma, metastatic seeding from a distant infection, or local spread of a contiguous soft tissue infection.

In hematogenous osteomyelitis, the inflammatory process typically begins in the marrow and progresses through the cortex into the periosteum (periostitis). Lifting of the periosteum impairs the blood supply to the bone, and a sequestrum (a large fragment of dead bone that detaches as a free body) may form as a combined result of both suppurative and ischemic injury. In turn, reactive woven or lamellar bone may be deposited around the devitalized bony sequestrum as a sleeve of living tissue known as an involucrum. If endogenous reactive/reparative processes succeed in walling off an area of bony infection, a localized intraosseous abscess may remain as a chronic nidus of infection known as a Brodie's abscess.

Pott's disease is tuberculous osteomyelitis of the spine. Unlike pyogenic osteomyelitis, which is typically an acute process, tuberculous osteomyelitis tends to be an insidious chronic infection that is characteristically more destructive and resistant to control. Thus, Pott's disease commonly results in compression fractures that produce serious spinal deformities. *(pp. 1230–1232)*

**5. (D)** Fractures of different types heal with different speeds, the repair process being affected by both the nature and the extent of the injury. A greenstick or incomplete fracture usually refers to long bone injuries in which the cortex snaps apart on one side and remains attached on the other. Complete fractures are through and through ruptures with total dissociation of the fractured edges. In a comminuted ("pulverized") fracture, the bone is shattered into splinters. In a closed or simple fracture, the overlying tissue is intact, but in compound fractures, the fracture site communicates with the skin surface. Pathologic fractures result less from trauma to the bone than from an underlying defect that greatly weakens the bone and renders it unusually susceptible to fracture (e.g., metastatic tumor or Paget's disease). Thus, pathologic fractures may occur in the absence of injury during everyday activities such as walking, sitting down or descending stairs. *(p. 1227)*

**6. (C)** The pathognomonic histologic feature of Paget's disease of bone (osteitis deformans), a mosaic pattern of bone formation, is illustrated in Figure 15–1. Paget's disease is characterized by excessive resorption of normal bone followed by excessive new bone formation in a haphazard arrangement. The newly formed units of lamellar bone are demarcated by prominent osteoid seams that form the histologic "mosaic." There is now strong evidence that Paget's disease is a slow virus infection caused by a paramyxovirus, with osteoblasts and osteoclasts being the target of infection. It is known that retroviruses such as paramyxovirus induce the secretion of cytokines such as interleukin-6 from infected cells. Interleukin-6 is a product of osteoblasts and is a potent stimulator of osteoclast recruitment and resorptive activity. Thus, it is plausible that much of the frenetic metabolic activity that characterizes Paget's disease may be cytokine driven.

Involved bones characteristically are greatly thickened, a feature readily seen on radiographs. The intense osteoblastic activity typically produces high serum alkaline phosphatase levels. In fact, the alkaline phosphatase levels in Paget's disease are generally greater than in any other bone disorder.

Although involved bones are thickened markedly, they are, nevertheless, extremely weak. They are composed largely of poorly mineralized osteoid matrix and vascular connective tissue and are usually light, soft, and porous. Thus, pagetic bones have a significantly *decreased* breaking strength and are prone to pathologic fractures, a common complication. The most ominous complication of Paget's disease is the development of a sarcoma in the involved bone, a consequence that occurs in about 5 to 10% of patients with severe polyostotic disease. *(pp. 1223–1225)*

**7. (B)** Hypertrophic osteoarthropathy is a disorder of unknown etiology characterized by periosteal inflammation at the ends of tubular bones with lifting of the periosteum, subjacent new bone formation, and arthritis of the adjacent joints. Clubbing of the digits is a common manifestation. Although it may occur in association with a wide variety of neoplastic and inflammatory disorders, the disease with which it occurs most frequently is bronchogenic carcinoma. No other single disease produces hypertrophic osteoarthropathy with as great a frequency (10% of cases) as bronchogenic carcinoma. Additional associated disorders include other intrathoracic tumors such as pleural mesothelioma, pulmonary metastases, or mediastinal Hodgkin's disease, chronic lung infection, or chronic liver disease. Clubbing alone, without distal long bone neo-osteogenesis or arthritis, may occur with cyanotic heart disease, infective endocarditis or aortitis, inflammatory bowel disease (ulcerative colitis or Crohn's disease), or cancer of the esophagus or colon. Hypertrophic osteoarthropathy sometimes precedes clinical manifestations of an underlying disease and can call attention to it. The arthropathy is usually reversible with surgical resection or medical correction of the underlying disorder. *(pp. 296–297)*

**8. (D)** Giant cell tumor of bone is a relatively uncommon benign (but locally aggressive) neoplasm characterized by large numbers of multinucleated, osteoclast-type tumor giant cells. These tumors inappropriately have been called "osteoclastomas," but the giant cells are not osteoclasts. They are believed to be of monocyte-macrophage lineage, the giant cells being the result of monocyte fusion. Giant cell tumors occur most commonly in adults ages 20 to 40 and are distinctly rare in skeletally immature individuals (children). Distinctively, the lesions almost always arise in the epiphyses of long bones, most commonly around the knee. Radiographically, giant cell tumors typically appear as large, purely lytic "soap bubble" lesions that are eccentrically located and erode into the subchondrial bone plate.

Most giant cell tumors are composed of well-differentiated cells with few, if any, mitoses and minimal atypicality. Yet, about 4% of giant cell tumors metastasize to the lung. Their unpredictable biologic behavior, not predicted from their histologic appearance, complicates clinical management. *(pp. 1245–1246)*

**9. (B)** Osteoarthritis (degenerative joint disease) is the most common form of arthritis. It is a destructive process, both deforming and debilitating, that may occur *de novo* in advanced age or at any age as a secondary consequence of congenital, structural, traumatic, metabolic, or inflammatory joint disease.

No matter what the underlying pathogenesis, the histologic changes of osteoarthritis are quite constant. Clefts appear in the surface of the articular cartilage and may extend to the underlying subchondral bone, a pathologic feature known as cartilage fibrillation. With progressive erosion of articular cartilage, focal areas of subchondral bone become denuded and sclerotic (eburnation). Bony spurs (osteophytes) arise from the margins of the articular cartilage and may project from opposing bones, causing pain and limitation of motion. Characteristic in women but not in men, osteophytic spurs arise from the base of the terminal phalanges; these are known as Heberden's nodes.

Pannus formation is a process characterized by intense inflammation of the synovial lining. A highly vascularized polypoid mass of inflammatory tissue arises from the synovium and often overgrows the articular surface, beginning at the joint margins. Pannus formation is highly characteristic of rheumatoid arthritis, although not pathognomonic. It also may occur in other inflammatory joint disease, such as that associated with psoriasis or gout. However, pannus formation is not a feature of osteoarthritis. *(pp. 1247–1249)*

**10. (E)** The term "renal osteodystrophy" is used to describe the spectrum of skeletal changes occurring in chronic renal disease of any etiology. These changes include: (1) increased osteoclastic bone resorption; (2) delayed matrix mineralization (osteomalacia); (3) osteosclerosis; (4) osteoporosis; and (5) growth retardation. These changes represent the effect of the numerous and complex pathophysiologic alterations in renal ion exchange, vitamin D metabolism, and secondary hyperparathyroidism that occur with renal failure. In addition, administration of aluminum-containing compounds, leading to aluminum deposition at sites of matrix mineralization, now is considered to be a major iatrogenic contribution to the genesis of osteodystrophy in chronic renal failure. Osteonecrosis is not included among the abnormalities associated with chronic renal failure. Bone death usually occurs only as a result of ischemic or destructive infectious processes and is rarely, if ever, associated with diseases causing metabolic derangements of bone homeostasis. *(p. 1227)*

**11. (C)** Osteopetrosis refers to a group of rare hereditary diseases characterized by osteoclast dysfunction that result in the formation of diffusely sclerotic bones lacking medullary cavities. Without osteoclast activity, bone cannot be remodeled in the course of osteogenesis and tends to be woven, rather than lamellar, in architecture. Although the name "osteopetrosis" suggests a stony hardness, the malformed bones are actually extremely brittle and break very easily. The lack of medullary cavities in the bones precludes normal hematopoietic marrow formation and all hematopoiesis occurs in extramedullary sites. Thus, anemia and infections are common as a result of the inadequacy of red and white cell production, respectively, under these circumstances. Bone marrow transplantation provides effective therapy because the graft supplies normally functioning osteoclasts (derived from marrow monocyte stem cells). *(pp. 1222–1223)*

**12. (B)** The bony lesion pictured in Figure 15–2 is a tumor-like condition of bone known as fibrous dysplasia. In essence, it represents a localized arrest in bone development. All of the elements of normal bone are present, but they fail to differentiate into mature structures. The result is haphazardly arranged trabeculae of woven bone within a background of cellular connective tissue. In about 70 to 75% of cases, the lesion is limited to a single bone and referred to as monostotic fibrous dysplasia. As in the case described, the condition typically becomes manifest in early adolescence. It is usually asymptomatic and often discovered as an incidental finding on radiographs. The rib is the most common location of monostotic fibrous dysplasia, followed by the femur, tibia, maxilla, mandible, calvarium, and humerus.

In about 30% of cases of fibrous dysplasia, multiple bones are involved. The polyostotic form of the disease usually appears at a slightly earlier age, is more likely to involve the craniofacial bones, and is less likely to involve the ribs than the monostotic form. In about 3% of polyostotic fibrous dysplasia cases, the condition is accompanied by skin pigmentation (café-au-lait spots) and a variety of endocrine disorders, including precocious sexual development, hyperthyroidism, Cushing's syndrome, and hyperparathyroidism. The association of fibrous dysplasia of bone with skin pigmentation and endocrinopathies is known as the McCune-Albright syndrome.

There is no known association between the monostotic and polyostotic forms of fibrous dysplasia; transition from the monostotic to the polystotic form has never been reported. Therefore, a patient with a single lesion such as the one described is not at increased risk of developing multiple lesions. Furthermore, there is little risk of malignant transformation. Fibrous dysplasia rarely undergoes sarcomatous change. The risk, such as it is, of developing an osteogenic sarcoma or malignant fibrous histiocytoma (estimated at less than 1% overall) is related primarily to the polyostotic forms of fibrous dysplasia. However, radiation of lesions may increase the risk of malignancy. *(pp. 1242–1243)*

**13. (C)** Ewing's sarcoma is a highly malignant primary bone tumor composed of small round cells with few differentiation characteristics. Thus, it bears a close histologic resemblance (but is not otherwise related) to other small round cell tumors such as lymphoma, rhabdomyosarcoma, neuroblastoma, and small-cell carcinoma. It is primarily a tumor of childhood, with 80% of patients being less than 20 years old and most being 10 to 15 years of age. It is second only to osteosarcoma as the most common primary bone sarcoma in children. It is believed to originate from a primitive neuroectodermal cell because it shares a unique and characteristic chromosomal abnormality (reciprocal translocation of long arms of chromosomes 11 and 22) with other neuroectodermal tumors and because the tumor cells can be induced to undergo neural differentiation in culture. Histologically, the tumor is composed of masses of small uniform cells with little cytologic pleomorphism. A helpful diagnostic feature of Ewing's sarcoma is the finding of characteristic periodic acid–Schiff positive granules in the cytoplasm of the tumor cells.

Ewing's sarcoma typically arises in the metaphyses of long tubular bones and virtually never originates in epiphyseal regions. It tends to perforate the bony cortex and penetrate adjacent soft tissues, often producing larger extraosseous than intraosseous masses. With combined surgery, chemotherapy, and radiation therapy, the 5-year survival rate for this tumor is about 75%, and 50% of treated cases are long-term cures. *(p. 1244)*

**14. (False); 15. (False); 16. (False); 17. (True); 18. (False)**

**(14)** Osteoporosis is a general term denoting increased porosity of the skeleton from a reduction in bone mass. It is characterized by reduction in both the mineral and matrix phases of structurally normal bone (not just impaired osteoid mineralization) as a result of accelerated bone loss along with some slowing of bone formation. It is an extremely common condition that in the majority of cases represents a primary process in the bone related either to aging (senile type) or estrogen deficiency in females (postmenopausal type) or both. However, osteoporosis also may occur as a secondary effect of a specific underlying disease (either endocrine, neoplastic, gastrointestinal, metabolic, rheumatologic, or drug-related in type), and then is classified as secondary osteoporosis. Pathologically, however, primary and secondary forms of osteoporosis are indistinguishable from one another.

**(15)** Senile osteoporosis affects both sexes equally but is more common in whites than in blacks (racial differences may be related to genetically determined differences in peak skeletal mass). The bone loss is greater in trabecular than in cortical bone. Therefore, fractures of bone composed predominantly of trabecular bone, such as vertebral bodies and the femoral necks, are common.

**(16)** Despite much attention given to this possibility, the pathogenesis of senile osteoporosis does not appear to be related to dietary deficiencies of calcium or vitamin D. However, dietary deficiency of calcium in adolescent females (not males) whose intake of calcium has been shown to be lower than recommended amounts during this period of rapid bone growth is suspected to contribute to the appearance of osteoporosis in later life.

**(17)** Although senile osteoporosis appears to be related in part to intrinsic age-related changes in bone cell metabolic activity and responsiveness to matrix-bound growth factors, its development also is linked to reduced physical activity, an important physiologic stimulus to the maintenance or increase of bone mass. Thus, weight-bearing exercise programs may prevent or slow development of senile osteoporosis.

**(18)** Unfortunately, senile osteoporosis is difficult to recognize until it is well advanced. It is asymptomatic until a complication ensues, and sensitive, specific diagnostic tests are lacking. Bony changes cannot be seen on plain radiographs (an insensitive, nonspecific method of detection) until 30 to 40% of bone mass has been lost, and, even when seen, cannot be differentiated from those of secondary osteoporosis. *(pp. 1219–1222)*

**19. (True); 20. (False); 21. (True); 22. (True); 23. (False); 24. (True); 25. (True)**

**(19)** Rheumatoid arthritis (RA) is a chronic systemic inflammatory disease that is autoimmune in nature and produces a progressive deforming arthritis as one of its primary manifestations. Genetic predisposition is an important risk factor for RA. There are well-defined associations with specific HLA-DR genotypes (i.e., HLA-DR4 or -DR1 or both are found in 60 to 85% of patients). **(20)** In contrast to osteoarthritis, which tends to involve weight-bearing joints, RA typically affects the small joints of the hands and feet in a symmetrical distribution. **(21)** About 80% of patients with RA have antibodies directed against the Fc fragment of autologous immunoglobulin G. These autoantibodies (usually immunoglobulin M in type), called rheumatoid factor, form complement-activating immune complexes that contribute to the inflammatory manifestations of RA.

**(22)** Although joints are the principal target of RA, many tissues and organs may be involved. Involvement of the skin occurs in about 25% of patients and produces what are known as rheumatoid nodules. These lesions are composed of dense collections of histiocytes surrounding central areas of fibrinoid necrosis and resemble caseating granulomas. The histiocytes tend to align themselves in a radial array around the necrotic center, a phenomenon known as "palisading." Rheumatoid nodules are not unique to skin but also may be seen in other organs involved by RA.

**(23)** Involvement of the heart produces rheumatoid heart disease, not to be confused with rheumatic heart disease. Rheumatoid heart disease usually produces a fibrinous pericarditis that may progress to dense adhesions. Rheumatic heart disease, the chronic sequelae of cardiac involvement by rheumatic fever (an immune response to β-hemolytic streptococcal infection with cross reactivity to endogenous tissue antigens), targets the heart valves. Although they have similar names, rheumatoid and rheumatic heart disease are completely unrelated processes. **(24)** Involvement of blood vessels in RA produces systemic vasculitis, a potentially catastrophic complication. It usually affects small and medium-sized arteries in multiple organs and may result in life-threatening visceral infarction.

**(25)** Rheumatoid arthritis is now the most common cause of reactive systemic (secondary) amyloidosis, although it is reported to occur in only 3% of patients with RA. Amyloidosis is a debilitating complication of long-standing disease and constitutes one of the contributing factors to the shortened life span of patients with RA. (*pp. 234; 547; 568–569; 1249–1253*)

**26. (False); 27. (False); 28. (True); 29. (True); 30. (True); 31. (True); 32. (False)**

Gout is a chronic disabling disease caused by the precipitation of monosodium urate crystals from supersaturated body fluids in patients with hyperuricemia. **(26)** Although hyperuricemia is very common (about 10% of the population of the Western world are hyperuricemic, the *sine qua non* of gout), it does not inevitably produce the disease. Only a small fraction (less than 5%) of individuals who are hyperuricemic develop gout. **(27)** Although gout may occur as a secondary phenomenon in any disease process causing hyperuricemia, the vast majority of cases (approximately 90%) occur in the absence of a defined metabolic defect and are referred to as "primary idiopathic gout." **(28)** In most cases of primary gout, the hyperuricemia is largely the result of increased uric acid synthesis rather than impaired excretion. However, underexcretion of uric acid with normal urate synthesis may occur in some cases.

**(29)** Acute gouty arthritis of the metatarsophalangeal joint of the great toe is the most common presentation of the disease. At least half of the initial attacks involve this joint. **(30)** The arthritis is evoked by the precipitation of monosodium urate crystals into the joint fluid. It is characterized by sudden development of swelling, redness, warmth, and excruciating pain in the involved joint that can be mistaken for suppurative arthritis. **(31)** Chronic gouty arthritis is the result of multiple recurrent attacks of acute arthritis leading to inflammatory synovial pannus formation. The pannus, in turn, progressively destroys the underlying articular cartilage and ultimately causes structural deformation and disabling disease.

**(32)** Tophi, the pathognomonic lesions of gout, are composed of masses of crystalline or amorphous urates surrounded by an intense inflammatory and foreign body giant cell reaction. Because urates do not penetrate the blood-brain barrier, tophi do not develop in the central nervous system. (*pp. 1255–1258*)

**33. (D); 34. (A); 35. (B); 36. (C); 37. (B); 38. (A); 39. (D)**

**(33)** Desmoids and nodular fasciitis both are considered to be reactive pseudosarcomatous proliferations (fibromatoses). They are exuberant tumor-like fibrous tissue growths that are more aggressive than common reactive proliferations but are not clearly neoplastic. Desmoids (aggressive fibromatoses) form tumorous masses that can be quite large (up to 15 cm in diameter) and may be difficult to differentiate from a sarcoma. Nodular fasciitis is somewhat of a misnomer because it does not always arise in fascia (it most commonly occurs in subcutaneous tissues) and does not represent an inflammatory process. Like desmoids, nodular fasciitis commonly is mistaken clinically for a neoplasm.

**(34)** Some desmoids appear to be hormonally responsive lesions. Abdominal wall desmoids have a striking female predominance, generally arise during or after pregnancy, and have been found to contain estrogen receptors. Intra-abdominal desmoids have no sexual associations, but they often occur in patients with Gardner's syndrome. Nodular fasciitis occurs with equal frequency in both sexes and has no association with pregnancy.

**(35)** In contrast to desmoids, which rarely exist in extremities, nodular fasciitis has a predilection for the extremities (the forearm is the most common site). **(36)** Both desmoids and nodular fasciitis tend to be unifocal lesions with irregular, poorly demarcated borders that characteristically infiltrate the surrounding soft tissues. **(37)** Histologically, the extracellular matrix of a desmoid typically is collagenized heavily, whereas the matrix of nodular fasciitis is usually myxoid.

**(38)** Both desmoid tumors and nodular fasciitis can be cured by surgical resection. However, incompletely excised desmoids tend to recur locally, whereas postoperative recurrence of nodular fasciitis, even when incompletely resected, is exceedingly rare. **(39)** Neither of these lesions has a propensity for neoplastic transformation. The rare reports of metastatic dissemination of a desmoid are believed to represent misdiagnoses of low-grade fibrosarcoma. (*pp. 1263–1264; 1265*)

**40. (D); 41. (B); 42. (A); 43. (B); 44. (C)**

**(40)** Osteochondromatosis and enchondromatosis are syndromes characterized by multiple osteochondromas and enchondromas, respectively—lesions that are most commonly solitary and sporadic in occurrence. Osteochondromas are cartilage-capped bony projections growing from the lateral contours of endochondral bones. They are developmental aberrations rather than true neoplasms and also are known as exostoses. The syndrome of osteochondromatosis is an autosomal dominant rather than a sex-linked disorder, but it does affect males three times more often than females. **(42)** Multiple osteochondromas also may occur as a part of another hereditary disorder known as Gardner's syndrome (see Chapter 8, Questions 1 and 12), which also includes desmoid tumors, sebaceous cysts, and adenomatous polyps of the colon. The latter pose a significantly increased risk of colonic adenocarcinoma.

**(41)** Enchondromas are true benign neoplasms composed of mature hyaline cartilage arising in the interior of a bone. **(43)** Enchondromatosis (also known as Ollier's disease) usually develops at a younger age than osteochondromatosis and typically is discovered early in childhood, but there is no clear evidence of hereditary transmission in this disease. However, it may occur as part of a familial syndrome that also includes multiple cavernous hemangiomas, known as Maffucci's syndrome.

**(44)** Both osteochondromatosis and enchondromatosis are associated with an increased incidence of chondrosarcoma, with the rate of malignant transformation in Ollier's disease and Maffucci's syndrome being particularly high (30 to 50%). (*pp. 814; 1237–1238*)

**45. (A); 46. (A); 47. (C); 48. (A); 49. (C); 50. (C); 51. (B)**

Malignancies arising from the cell types in bone are much less common than those arising from marrow elements (myeloma and leukemia). Infrequent though they may be, however, primary bone tumors are among the most biologically aggressive neoplasms in humans. **(45)** Osteosarcoma is the most common cancer of bone, and **(46)** most commonly occurs in children and adolescents. Chondrosarcoma occurs half as often as osteosarcoma, but, even so, it is second only to osteosarcoma in frequency. It tends to arise in middle age to later life. **(47)** Like chondrosarcomas, osteosarcomas arise *de novo* ("primary" osteosarcomas) in the majority of cases. Less frequently, they develop in a background of pre-existing bone disease ("secondary" osteosarcomas) such as Paget's disease, enchondromatosis, osteochondromatosis chronic osteomyelitis, fibrous dysplasia, infarcts, or fractures of bone.

**(48)** Osteosarcoma most commonly arises about the knee (60% of cases), whereas chondrosarcomas originate most frequently from bones of the central portions of the skeleton (e.g., pelvis, shoulder, ribs). **(49)** Histologically, both osteosarcomas and chondrosarcomas often contain both bony and cartilaginous elements. Their specific diagnosis depends on the identification of frankly malignant, anaplastic cells in association primarily with either osteoid matrix (osteosarcoma) or chondroid matrix (chondrosarcoma). In chondrosarcomas with ossification, the bone formation occurs within cartilage (endochondral ossification), whereas, in osteosarcomas, the neo-osteogenesis arises out of the background of anaplastic, osteoblastic cells.

**(50)** It is rare for either osteosarcoma or chondrosarcoma to metastasize to lymph nodes. Hematogenous dissemination is the major mode of metastasis for both of these tumors. **(51)** In contrast to the experience with osteosarcoma, in which there is little correlation between histologic grade and patient survival, there is an excellent correlation between the histopathology of chondrosarcomas and tumor behavior. Obviously, then, histologic grading of chondrosarcoma is of great clinical significance. (*pp. 1234–1236; 1240–1241*)

**52. (A); 53. (C); 54. (A); 55. (B); 56. (E); 57. (B); 58. (E)**

Muscular dystrophies and congenital myopathies are inherited primary disorders of muscle fibers that produce muscle weakness, atrophy, and loss of tendon reflexes. Although the different types of muscular dystrophy (MD) tend to have distinctive clinical features, they produce the same basic morphologic changes in the involved muscles, and they typically become apparent in early childhood. Congenital myopathies, in contrast, are not clinically distinctive but produce fairly specific morphologic changes. Most congenital myopathies present at birth as a "floppy infant" syndrome.

**(52)** The two major types of MD, the Duchenne MD and Becker MD, and a mild uncommon type, Emery-Dreifuss MD, are inherited as sex-linked conditions and occur only in males. Congenital myopathies, with only one rare exception, are not X-linked.

**(53)** Both Duchenne MD and myotonic dystrophy, the most severe and the most prevalent dystrophies, respectively, are associated with decreased intelligence. Although mild reduction in intelligence is common among individuals with Duchenne MD, frank mental retardation is present only in about 30%. The majority of individuals with myotonic dystrophy, however, manifest frank mental retardation or even dementia. Congenital myopathies, in contrast, rarely are associated with mental retardation.

**(54)** The Duchenne MD is incompatible with long survival; it is a progressive disease that usually leads to death by age 20. Although myotonic dystrophy is also a progressive disease, muscle involvement generally proceeds far more slowly and is neither totally incapacitating nor incompatible with long survival. In contrast to the MDs, the congenital myopathies are not progressive and are compatible with a normal life span and normal activity.

**(55)** Unlike the other forms of muscular dystrophy and the congenital myopathies, myotonic dystrophy characteristically involves many extramuscular systems. Thus, in addition to weakness and myotonia of the distal muscles, frontal baldness, cataracts, and testicular atrophy are major clinical features.

**(56)** In all forms of MD, there is a loss of histochemical differentiation between type I and type II myofibers, but neither fiber type is spared. Several of the congenital myopathies tend to involve one fiber type more than the other, but in no case is the damage limited to a single fiber type. **(57)** "Ring fibers" represent single myofibers transversely encircling other myofibers in the same bundle. They are a distinctive histologic feature of myotonic dystrophy and, when present, provide the opportunity to identify this form of dystrophy morphologically. **(58)** The MDs and congenital myopathies are hereditary disorders of muscle fibers and are not known to be related to any acquired disease, such as viral infection. (*pp. 1285–1288*)

**59. (A); 60. (D); 61. (A); 62. (B); 63. (C); 64. (A); 65. (B)**

**(59)** Most soft tissue sarcomas are adult tumors. Rhabdomyosarcoma is the exception, occurring most commonly in children. Aside from the pleomorphic variant (a rarity), rhabdomyosarcomas are uncommon in adults, and 90% occur before the age of 20. Overall, rhabdomyosarcoma is the most common sarcoma of childhood and adolescence. **(61)** In contrast to other soft tissue sarcomas, rhabdomyosarcoma has an "alveolar" variant characterized by interlacing strands of fibrovascular stroma enclosing spaces filled with loose or solid clusters of small tumor cells. Cytogenetic studies have shown a translocation between chromosomes 2 and 13 in this type of rhabdomyosarcoma.

**(60)** Most soft tissue sarcomas manifest a variety of histologic growth patterns. Unfortunately, many of these histologic variants overlap, making specific diagnosis of soft tissue sarcomas a challenging endeavor. The myxoid histologic variant is the most common form of liposarcoma. However, a myxoid variant is also common in malignant fibrous histiocytoma and is second only to the typical storiform-pleomorphic variant (see Question 63) in frequency. **(62)** Uniquely, synovial sarcoma is characterized by a biphasic histologic pattern; it is composed of both epitheloid and spindle-shaped cells recapitulating the derivation of cuboidal synovial lining cells from primitive mesenchymal cells.

**(63)** Storiform or pinwheel patterns of growth are highly characteristic of, even unique to, malignant fibrous histiocytoma. **(64)** Immunohistochemical staining techniques sometimes can be helpful in differentiating the soft tissue sarcomas. Desmin is an intermediate filament specific for neoplasms showing muscle (either striated or smooth) differentiation. Thus, among the tumors mentioned, only rhabosarcoma expresses desmin. **(65)** Immunoperoxidase staining for keratin (the major intermediate filament of epithelial cells) is unusual for sarcomas but often can be seen in the epithelium-like components of synovial sarcomas. (*pp. 299; 1262–1263; 1267–1268; 1269*)

**66. (D); 67. (A); 68. (B); 69. (C); 70. (A); 71. (E); 72. (B)**

**(66)** Osteogenesis imperfecta, osteopetrosis, and achondroplasia are hereditary disorders of bone with varying morbidity and mortality. **(67)** Although there are four variants with different modes of inheritance and different clinical features, the basic defect in all forms of osteogenesis imperfecta is some biochemical abnormality in the synthesis of type I collagen. **(68)** In osteopetrosis, the underlying defect in both hereditary subsets is one of osteoclast function resulting in overgrowth and sclerosis of bone (see Question 11). **(69)** In achondroplasia (a form of dwarfism), a defect in epiphyseal cartilage growth results in premature ossification at the osteochondral junction and truncated growth of long bones.

**(70)** One of the most distinctive clinical features of osteogenesis imperfecta is the appearance of the sclerae. They are translucent and look blue because of the visualization of the underlying choroid plexus.

**(71)** Exostoses are not associated with any of these three hereditary conditions but rather constitute a separate and unrelated hereditary condition of bone known as osteochondromatosis (see Questions 40 through 44).

**(72)** Anemia and hepatosplenomegaly are common complications of osteopetrosis. In this condition, the marked overgrowth of bone narrows the marrow cavity and, in advanced cases, may obliterate it altogether. In such cases, hepatosplenomegaly results from extramedullary hematopoiesis. (*pp. 1218–1219; 1222–1223*)

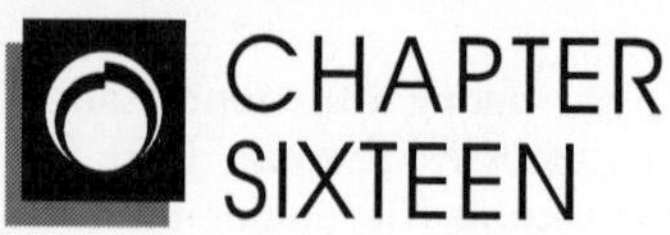

# The Nervous System

**DIRECTIONS:** For Questions 1 through 16, choose the ONE BEST answer to each question.

**1.** All of the following conditions cause increased intracranial pressure EXCEPT:

A. Alzheimer's disease
B. Metastatic tumor
C. Cerebral infarction
D. Lead encephalopathy
E. Water intoxication

**2.** A disorder of the central nervous system that is almost exclusively iatrogenic is:

A. Aseptic meningitis
B. Progressive supranuclear palsy
C. Leigh's disease
D. Central pontine myelinolysis
E. Metachromatic leukodystrophy

**3.** All of the following features describe progressive multifocal leukoencephalopathy EXCEPT:

A. Caused by a virus
B. Affects oligodendrocytes exclusively
C. Causes demyelination of white matter throughout the brain
D. Occurs only in immunosuppressed individuals
E. Produces no *specific* histologic changes

**4.** Which of the following statements about Creutzfeldt-Jakob disease (subacute spongiform encephalopathy) is correct?

A. The causative agent is visible only with the electron microscope.
B. The affected brain is typically markedly atrophic.
C. The usual mode of transmission is person-to-person via aerosolized droplet exposure.
D. A brisk cellular immune response without granuloma formation is characteristic.
E. The disease typically causes a rapidly progressive dementia.

**5.** Which of the following statements about epidural hematoma is correct?

A. It is almost always accompanied by a skull fracture.
B. The bleeding is usually of venous origin.
C. The onset of symptoms is typically delayed for many hours after the vascular rupture.
D. The major symptom is a fluctuating level of consciousness.
E. It occasionally occurs as a result of rupture of a berry aneurysm.

**6.** Each of the following histopathologic features represents a specific type of neuronal injury EXCEPT:

A. Rosenthal fibers
B. Negri bodies
C. Lewy bodies
D. Cowdry A bodies
E. Red neurons

**7.** All of the following pathologic features are characteristic of Alzheimer's disease EXCEPT:

A. Amyloid angiopathy
B. Neuritic plaques
C. Neurofibrillary tangles
D. Pick bodies
E. Granulovacuolar degeneration of neurons

**8.** Subdural empyema is associated with:

A. Bacterial meningitis
B. Skull fracture
C. Brain abscess
D. Sinusitis
E. Acute bacterial endocarditis

**9.** Nervous system infection by herpes simplex viruses causes all of the following disorders EXCEPT:

A. Acquired immunodeficiency syndrome–related necrotizing encephalitis
B. Neonatal panencephalitis
C. Postherpetic neuralgia
D. Viral meningitis
E. Cold sores

**10.** Berry aneurysms are described correctly as:

A. The most common cause of subarchnoid hemorrhage
B. Virtually always solitary
D. Typically fusiform in shape
D. Usually atherosclerotic in origin
E. Most commonly located in the basilar artery

**11.** Human immunodeficiency virus 1 infection of the central nervous system directly causes all of the following disorders EXCEPT:

A. Acute aseptic meningitis
B. Peripheral neuropathy
C. Vacuolar myelopathy
D. Cranial neuropathy
E. Subacute encephalitis

**12.** Which one of the following statements correctly describes central nervous system (CNS) responses to ischemia?

A. Oxygen reserves in the brain are depleted after 1 minute of ischemia.
B. Glucose reserves in the brain are depleted after 3 minutes of ischemia.
C. Normal cerebral function can continue for only 2 to 4 minutes after cerebral ischemia.
D. Irreversible damage occurs after 6 to 10 minutes of ischemia.
E. Glial cells are the CNS cells most susceptible to ischemia.

**13.** Meningiomas commonly are associated with all of the following pathologic features EXCEPT:

A. Irregular infiltrative borders
B. Penetration of the adjacent bone
C. Psammoma bodies
D. Expression of progesterone receptors
E. Expression of epithelial membrane antigen

**14.** The most typical pathologic feature of idiopathic Parkinson's disease is:

A. Neurofibrillary tangles
B. Striking atrophy of the caudate nucleus
C. Severe neuronal loss in the putamen
D. Depigmentation of the substantia nigra
E. Hirano bodies

**15.** Amyotrophic lateral sclerosis is characterized by all of the following features EXCEPT:

A. Degeneration of the upper motor neurons in all cases
B. Degeneration of the lower motor neurons in all cases
C. Mutation of the superoxide dismutase gene in familial cases
D. Association with infection by an enterovirus in nonfamilial cases
E. An inevitably fatal course in all cases

**16.** All of the following statements correctly describe plexiform neurofibromas EXCEPT:

A. They arise only from cutaneous peripheral nerve sheaths.
B. It is not possible to separate the lesion from the associated nerve.
C. They are diagnostic of neurofibromatosis type 1.
D. They do not occur as sporadic lesions.
E. They have significant potential for malignant transformation.

**DIRECTIONS:** For Questions 17 through 32, you are to decide whether EACH choice is TRUE or FALSE.

For each of the following statements about vascular disease of the central nervous system, choose whether it is TRUE or FALSE.

**17.** Ischemic encephalopathy most commonly is associated with inadequate cardiopulmonary resuscitation following cardiac arrest.
**18.** Thrombotic occlusion of intracranial vessels is more common than embolic occlusion.
**19.** The majority of thrombotic occlusions are due to atherosclerosis.
**20.** Hemorrhagic infarction typically is associated with embolic events.
**21.** Nonhemorrhagic infarction typically is associated with thrombosis.
**22.** Cerebral hemorrhage is caused most often by hypertensive vascular disease.
**23.** Hypertensive vascular disease characteristically produces lacunar infarcts.
**24.** Hypertensive encephalopathy is characterized by cortical demyelination.
**25.** The most common cause of vascular injury in the spinal cord is hypertensive vascular disease.

For each of the following statements about multiple sclerosis, choose whether it is TRUE or FALSE.

**26.** The primary pathologic process is generalized central nervous system demyelination.
**27.** Most cases occur in children.
**28.** Intellectual deterioration is an early manifestation of the disease.
**29.** The cerebrospinal fluid typically contains increased immunoglobulins.
**30.** Onset usually occurs shortly after a viral infection.
**31.** Perivascular collections of multinucleated macrophages (globoid cells) are a characteristic histologic feature.
**32.** Long-term corticosteroid treatment prevents progression of the disease.

**DIRECTIONS:** For Questions 33 through 49, the set of lettered headings is followed by a list of numbered words or phrases. For each numbered word or phrase choose:

A—if the item is associated with (A) only
B—if the item is associated with (B) only
C—if the item is associated with *both* (A) and (B)
D—if the item is associated with *neither* (A) nor (B)

For each of the features listed below, choose whether it describes communicating hydrocephalus, noncommunicating hydrocephalus, both of these, or neither of these.

A. Communicating hydrocephalus
B. Noncommunicating hydrocephalus
C. Both of these
D. Neither of these

**33.** Often fails to produce ventricular distention
**34.** Is associated with postmeningitic states
**35.** Is associated with neoplasms
**36.** Is associated with thrombosis of the dural sinuses
**37.** Is associated with the Dandy-Walker syndrome

For each of the features listed below, choose whether it describes rabies, poliomyelitis, both of these, or neither of these.

A. Rabies
B. Poliomyelitis
C. Both of these
D. Neither of these

**38.** A primary infection elsewhere precedes nervous system disease.
**39.** Diagnostic inclusions are seen in infected cells.
**40.** The causative viral agent affects only dorsal root ganglion cells.
**41.** Lower motor neuron paralysis is produced.
**42.** The most common cause of death is failure of the brain stem respiratory center.

For each of the features listed below, choose whether it describes Huntington's disease, Friederich's ataxia, both of these, or neither of these.

A. Huntington's disease
B. Friederich's ataxia
C. Both of these
D. Neither of these

**43.** The disorder typically presents in infancy.
**44.** Onset usually is preceded by a viral infection.
**45.** The disease involves the spinal cord.
**46.** The motor disorder sometimes is accompanied by a sensory deficit.
**47.** Diabetes mellitus frequently occurs as an associated condition.
**48.** Cardiac disease frequently occurs as an associated condition.
**49.** Recovery without neurologic impairment is the rule.

**DIRECTIONS:** Questions 50 through 81 are matching questions. For each numbered item, choose the most likely associated lettered item from those provided. Each numbered item has ONLY ONE answer. Within each group, each lettered item may be the answer to one, more than one, or none of the numbered items.

For each of the characteristics of central nervous system (CNS) cells listed below, choose whether it describes astrocytes, oligodendrocytes, ependymal cells, all of these, or none of these.

A. Astrocytes
B. Oligodendrocytes
C. Ependymal cells
D. All of these
E. None of these

**50.** Are defined as neuroglial cells
**51.** Function as macrophages
**52.** Provide physical (structural) support for neurons
**53.** Form glial scars following CNS injury
**54.** Maintain CNS myelin
**55.** Produce cerebrospinal fluid
**56.** Resorb cerebrospinal fluid

For each of the features listed below, choose whether it describes meningococcal meningitis, mumps meningitis, tuberculous meningitis, all of these, or none of these.

A. Meningococcal meningitis
B. Mumps meningitis
C. Tuberculosis meningitis
D. All of these
E. None of these

**57.** The cerebrospinal fluid (CSF) sugar content is usually normal.
**58.** The CSF protein content usually is elevated.
**59.** Neutrophils characteristically are found in the CSF.
**60.** Photophobia and stiff neck are *not* commonly present.
**61.** Obliterative endarteritis is an associated complication.

For each of the characteristics listed below, choose whether it describes astrocytoma, oligodendroglioma, ependymoma, or none of these.

A. Astrocytoma
B. Oligodendroglioma
C. Ependymoma
D. None of these

**62.** It constitutes the most common brain tumor in adults.
**63.** It rarely occurs in children.
**64.** It is the most common type of glial tumor of the spinal cord.
**65.** High-grade lesions are known as glioblastoma multiforme.
**66.** Calcifications within the tumor tissue are characteristic.
**67.** Tumor cell rosettes are a typical histologic feature.
**68.** Tumor cell pseudorosettes are a typical histologic feature.
**69.** Metastases to bone occur commonly.
**70.** Dramatic responses to chemotherapy are common.

For each of the statements below, choose whether it describes metachromatic leukodystrophy, Krabbe's disease (globoid cell leukodystrophy), adrenoleukodystrophy, or none of these.

A. Metachromatic leukodystrophy
B. Krabbe's disease (globoid cell leukodystrophy)
C. Adrenoleukodystrophy
D. None of these

**71.** It usually becomes manifest clinically after age 10.
**72.** It is produced by a deficiency of arylsulfatase A.
**73.** It is produced by a deficiency of galactocerebroside β-galactosidase.
**74.** It is characterized histologically by multinucleate histiocytic cells in the white matter.
**75.** It is characterized histologically by diagnostic inclusion bodies in Schwann cells.

For each of the causes of peripheral neuropathies listed below, decide whether it is usually associated with a pattern of ascending motor paralysis, symmetrical polyneuropathy, asymmetrical polyneuropathy, or none of these.

A. Ascending motor paralysis
B. Symmetrical polyneuropathy
C. Asymmetrical polyneuropathy
D. None of these

**76.** Diabetic neuropathy
**77.** Alcoholic neuropathy
**78.** Guillain-Barré syndrome
**79.** Diphtheritic neuropathy
**80.** Polyarteritis nodosa neuropathy
**81.** Lead neuropathy

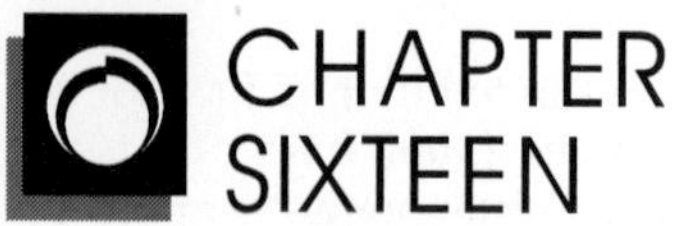

CHAPTER SIXTEEN

# The Nervous System

## ANSWERS

**1. (A)** Increased intracranial pressure is the end result of any pathologic condition that expands the volume of the intracranial contents beyond the limits set by its bony confines. It is the common consequence of numerous central nervous systems disorders. Processes that are characterized by cellular swelling, interstitial edema, space-occupying lesions (e.g., tumors, hematomas, dilated ventricles) or a combination of these all will produce increased intracranial pressure. Metastatic tumor, in addition to being a space-occupying mass, also causes local damage to capillary endothelial cells and/or induces new capillary formation. Damaged capillaries that have lost their permeability barrier function or new capillaries that have not yet acquired it leak fluid into the intercellular space, a process known as vasogenic cerebral edema. Transduction of fluid from the ventricular system across the ependymal lining (interstitial edema) also may contribute to the volume expansion. Similar mechanisms of vascular injury producing vasogenic edema occur in association with infarction, lead encephalopathy (cytotoxic edema), abscesses, and contusions. Water intoxication leads to cytotoxic edema by producing an acute hypo-osmolar state in the plasma with a resultant shift of water into the cerebral cells to maintain osmotic equilibrium.

Alzheimer's disease, a degenerative disease of the cerebral cortex (see Question 7), is not associated with increased intracranial pressure. On the contrary, brain volume is reduced as a result of severe atrophy. Enlargement of the ventricular system occurs as a compensatory change secondary to the loss of parenchyma (hydrocephalus *ex vacuo*), not as a result of increased pressure in the ventricular system. It should not be confused with obstructive or communicating hydrocephalus, in which expansion of the ventricles is caused by increased cerebrospinal fluid volume and intracranial pressure is increased. *(pp. 1298–1330; 1329)*

**2. (D)** Central pontine myelinolysis is an iatrogenic disease characterized by demyelination in the midportion of the pons. Although small foci of involvement may be asymptomatic, large lesions produce a flaccid quadriplegia. The disorder is produced by rapid rises in serum sodium concentrations, most frequently associated with intravenous administration of sodium-containing solutions (i.e., rapid correction of hyponatremia). The extent of demyelination also correlates with the duration of the preceding hyponatremia.

"Aseptic" meningitis is a nonbacterial process, but it usually is caused by viral infection (therefore, not really aseptic at all). In 70% of cases a viral pathogen can be identified, most commonly an enterovirus (e.g., echoviruses, coxsackievirus, or nonparalytic poliovirus). Some cases may be the result of chemical injury (e.g., rupture of an epidermoid cyst into the arachnoid space) and are truly "aseptic." The histologic picture is the same, however, with a lymphocytic infiltrate of the leptomeninges.

Progressive supranuclear palsy is an idiopathic (noniatrogenic) degenerative disease of the basal ganglia and brain stem that produces movement disorders and sometimes progressive dementia. Widespread neuronal loss and neurofibrillary tangles are found in the globus pallidus, substantia nigra, colliculi, and dentate nucleus of the cerebellum.

Leigh's disease (subacute necrotizing encephalomyelopathy) is an autosomal-recessive inborn error of metabolism resulting in mitochondrial defects such as cytochrome oxidase C deficiency. It produces bilateral symmetrical necrosis in the thalamus, midbrain, pons, medulla, and spinal cord.

Metachromatic leukodystrophy is also an autosomal recessive disorder that produces a deficiency of arylsulfatase A, accumulation of sulfatides, and consequent demyelination in both the central and peripheral nervous system. It has no iatrogenic component. *(pp. 1316; 1329; 1333; 1338).*

**3. (E)** Progressive multifocal leukoencephalopathy (PML) is a viral infection of oligodendrocytes by JC papovavirus.

The infection is restricted to oligodendrocytes (the myelin-producing cells of the central nervous system) because the JC virus promotor and enhancer DNA sequences upstream from the viral genes are active in glial cells but not in neurons or endothelial cells. However, the disease is expressed only in immunosuppressed individuals (e.g., those with lympho- or myeloproliferative disorders or acquired immunodeficiency syndrome; those receiving immunosuppressive chemotherapy). About 65% of normal individuals have serologic evidence of exposure to the JC virus by age 14 but develop no disease. Thus, it is unknown whether PML results from primary infection or secondary reactivation of old infection in the immunosuppressed patient. The disease results in widespread patchy destruction of white matter throughout the brain and, occasionally, the spinal cord. Histologically, specific changes in areas of demyelination include markedly enlarged oligodendrocytes with glassy intranuclear viral inclusions accompanied by characteristically bizarre giant (often multinucleated) astrocytes. Viral particles can be identified specifically by immunohistochemistry, *in situ* hybridization, or electron microscopy. *(pp. 315; 1322–1323)*

**4. (E)** Creutzfeldt-Jakob disease is a well-characterized form of spongiform encephalopathy. The spongiform encephalopathies are a group of diseases that produce a characteristic vacuolization (spongiform change) of the gray matter, lead rapidly to dementia, and are caused by a transmissible agent. The transmissible agent is not a microorganism but rather a mutated cellular protein known as a prion. The gene for the normal 30-kDa protein is on chromosome 20. Mutations in the prion gene are believed to lead to the production of prions that undergo an abnormal conformational change (at variable rates). These abnormal prions are capable both of facilitating comparable structural transformation of other prion molecules in the same individual and of corrupting the integrity of normal prions in other individuals to whom they are transmitted. Thus, abnormal prions are "infectious." Prions cannot be visualized by any method, including electron microscopic examination. Documented cases of person-to-person transmission have occurred via a parenteral route, but most disease is sporadic. The disease is characterized pathologically by neuronal loss and marked gliosis in the absence of inflammation. Intracytoplasmic membrane-bound vacuoles in neuronal and glial processes that appear grossly as spongiform change are pathognomonic. Clinically, a rapidly progressive dementia is the rule, and death usually ensues following an average survival of 7 months. *(pp. 1323–1324)*

**5. (A)** An epidural hematoma results from bleeding into the potential space between the skull and the dura matter. Unlike subdural hematomas, which often result from blunt trauma without skull fractures, epidural hematomas almost always occur in association with an overlying skull fracture. The bleeding is usually of arterial origin (the middle meningeal artery that runs within the dura is especially vulnerable to injury), so the rise in intracranial pressure and the onset of symptoms are typically rapid, usually developing within minutes to a few hours after the trauma. Typically, the patient is lucid for several hours after the initial trauma before descending into a progressively deepening coma. Prompt neurosurgical drainage of the hematoma is required. A delayed onset of symptoms (1 to 2 days) and a fluctuating level of consciousness is suggestive instead of a subdural hematoma, which is a venous hemorrhage that expands more slowly. Epidural hematomas are almost always due to trauma; other causes are distinctly uncommon. Ruptured berry aneurysms typically produce subarachnoid hemorrhage, not epidural hematoma. *(pp. 1306–1307; 1312)*

**6. (A)** Neurons in the central nervous system (CNS) sometimes display distinctive patterns of injury in response to specific disease processes. The recognition of these patterns is often key to establishing a tissue diagnosis. Indeed, some of these changes are pathognomonic for the causative disorder. Intraneuronal inclusions are a particularly distinctive feature of a few viral diseases that either target or commonly affect the CNS. Rabies infection, in particular, produces pathognomonic eosinophilic cytoplasmic inclusions called Negri bodies in the pyramidal neurons of the hypocampus and the Purkinje cells of the cerebellum. Cytomegalovirus and herpes virus infections of the CNS produce large pink inclusions surrounded by clear halos called Cowdry A bodies in the nuclei of neurons (glial cells also are affected). In idiopathic Parkinson's disease, large eosinophilic cytoplasmic inclusions with denser pink central cores called Lewy bodies are pathognomonic findings in neurons of the substantia nigra and locus ceruleus. Red neurons refer to neurons that have undergone coagulative necrosis in response to ischemic injury. Red neurons are shrunken in size and have intensely eosinophilic cytoplasm and pyknotic nuclei.

Rosenthal fibers are thick, elongated eosinophilic inclusions found in the cytoplasm of astrocytes (not neurons) in processes characterized by long-standing gliosis. *(pp. 1296–1297; 1319–1320; 1332)*

**7. (D)** Alzheimer's disease (AD) is a degenerative disease of the gray matter of the cerebral cortex that ultimately leads to dementia. Alzheimer's disease is associated with several distinctive histopathologic changes in the cerebral cortex: neuritic plaques, neurofibrillary tangles, amyloid angiopathy, and granulovacuolar degeneration of neurons. Neuritic plaques are focal collections of dilated, tortuous neuritic processes (dystrophic neurites) surrounding a central amyloid core. The major component of the amyloid is a small protein known as $A\beta_2$, which is derived from a much larger transmembrane glycoprotein known as amyloid precursor protein (APP). Amyloid angiopathy, a virtually invariable feature of AD, is characterized by the deposition of $A\beta_2$ amyloid in the walls of the intracortical and small subarachnoid blood vessels (but may even be found in vessels outside of the central nervous system). Neurofibrillary tangles (bundles of neurofilaments in the cytoplasm of neurons) that typically encircle the nucleus and denote neuronal degeneration, are most notably, but not exclusively, associated with Alzheimer's disease. An abnormally hyperphosphorylated form of the axonal protein known as tau (important in microtubule assembly) is a major component of neurofibrillary tangles, but A$\beta_2$ protein is also a recognized component. Granulovacuolar degeneration of neurons refers to the formation of small intraneuronal cytoplasmic vacuoles, each of which contains an argyrophilic granule of unknown composition. This form of neuronal degeneration is particularly characteristic of AD. Although the pathogenesis of AD is unknown, attention has been focused on the possible etiologic roles of A$\beta_2$ protein and its precursor, APP. In some familial forms of AD, point mutations in the gene encoding APP (on chromosome 21) have been identified, some of which are associated with increased rates of generation of the amyloidogenic A$\beta_2$ protein. The toxic effects of A$\beta_2$ protein on neurons have been demonstrated in tissue culture studies.

Pick bodies are cytoplasmic inclusions of neurofilaments, endoplasmic, reticulum, and paired helical filaments (also found in the neurofibrillary tangles of AD) in neurons of the atrophic frontal and temporal lobes of patients with Pick's disease. In contrast to the neurofibrillary tangles of AD, Pick bodies do not survive the death of the involved neuron and do not remain as markers of the disease. Like AD, Pick's disease is a degenerative disease of the cerebral cortex that produces profound dementia but typically involves only the frontal and temporal lobes. Unlike AD, it conspicuously spares the posterior two thirds of the superior temporal gyrus and only rarely affects either the parietal or occipital lobes. *(pp. 232; 1329–1331)*

**8. (D)** A subdural empyema is an infection (most frequently bacterial) of the skull bones, middle ear, mastoid, and paranasal sinuses (50% of cases) that has penetrated into the subdural space by direct extension. Thus, most patients with a subdural empyema also have sinusitis and fever. Usually, the process remains localized, and the underlying arachnoid mater and subarachnoid space are uninvolved. Injury to the brain may occur by indirect means (such as secondary thrombophlebitis of central veins crossing the subdural space with venous infarction of the brain) or by direct compression (such as a mass effect from the collection of subdural pus), but brain abscesses neither typically produce nor result from subdural empyema.

Bacterial meningitis is acquired by hematogenous spread of pathogens (usually from the nasopharynx) to the cerebrospinal fluid, where they come in contact with the meninges and brain. Skull fracture often results in epidural, subdural, subarchnoid, or intraparenchymal hemorrhage. Acute bacterial endocarditis produces septic embolism of the cerebral arterial vessels, most often resulting in brain abscess or meningitis. However, none of these processes typically is associated with subdural empyema (either as a cause or as an effect), with the rare exception of secondary infection of an undrained subdural hematoma, producing a subdural empyema. *(pp. 552; 1306–1307; 1316–1317)*

**9. (C)** Human infection by herpes simplex virus (HSV), either type 1 (HSV-1) or type 2 (HVS-2 or genital herpes), most commonly involves either epithelial cells, cells of the (central or peripheral) nervous system, or both. The most common and least morbid form of neural infection involves the sensory nerve ganglia innervating infected skin or mucosa. Reactivation of latent infection in these cells results in periodic re-eruption of mucocutaneous vesicles known as "cold sores" or "fever blisters" that may be uncomfortable but are not dangerous. A less common but far more serious consequence of nervous system infection by HSV is encephalitis. Both HSV-1 and HSV-2 produce encephalitis and may do so either in the immunocompetent or in the immunosuppressed individual. Severe neonatal encephalitis results from infection acquired during vaginal delivery in as many as 50% of infants born to mothers with active HSV-2 infection. Beyond the neonatal period, HSV-1 is the more common causative agent. In AIDS patients, HSV-2 may produce an acute hemorrhagic, necrotizing form of encephalitis. HSV-2 is also responsible for most cases of herpetic viral meningitis.

Postherpetic neuralgia, however, refers to the pain associated with reactivation of latent herpes zoster (not herpes simplex) infection, a condition commonly known as "shingles" (see Question 40). *(pp. 340–341; 1319)*

**10. (A)** Berry aneurysms are developmental arterial defects (often called "congenital" but not present at birth) that are the most common cause of subarchnoid hemorrhage in the central nervous system. They are typically saccular in shape and are believed to result from congenital defects of the media of the involved vessels. They occur most commonly at the junction of the anterior cerebral and anterior communicating arteries (40%), the major bifurcation of the middle cerebral artery in the Sylvian fissure (34%), and the junction of the internal carotid and posterior communicating arteries (20%). Only 4% involve the basilar artery. Although they are often solitary, more than one aneurysm is found in up to 30% of cases. The probability of rupture increases with the size of the lesion (50% risk with lesions >10 mm in diameter). Rupture has a high mortality rate. About 25 to 50% of patients die with initial rupture, and rebleeding is common in the survivors. *(pp. 1312–1313)*

**11. (C)** The human immunodeficiency virus 1 (HIV-1) directly infects the central nervous system and produces at least three different neuropathologic syndromes: (1) subacute encephalitis (most common), designated clinically as the acquired immunodeficiency syndrome (AIDS)–dementia complex; (2) acute aseptic meningitis (a self-limited process occurring at the time of seroconversion); and (3) a variety of cranial and peripheral neuropathies. In addition, of course, HIV-1 infection also significantly increases the risk of opportunistic central nervous system (CNS) infections, especially from agents such as cytomegalovirus, varicella zoster, herpes simplex, *Cryptococcus neoformans*, and *Toxoplasma gondii*, and increases the risk of primary CNS lymphoma.

Vacuolar myelopathy, a subacute degenerative disease of the white matter of the posterior and lateral columns of the spinal cord, is found in 20 to 30% of AIDS patients but does not appear to be related directly to HIV-1 infection. The HIV virus cannot be found in many lesions, and the disorder also occurs in immunosuppressed patients who do not have AIDS. *(pp. 230; 1321–1322; 1348)*

**12. (D)** A constant supply of oxygen and glucose are critical for brain function, and, without them, cerebral injury quickly ensues. The brain is a highly aerobic tissue, but there are no oxygen reserves in the tissue. Normal cerebral function can continue for only 8 to 10 *seconds* after cerebral ischemia, and irreversible damage occurs after 6 to 10 minutes of ischemia. Neurons are the central nervous system cells most susceptible to ischemia, but they vary in their susceptibility according to their location in the brain, a fact that primarily reflects differences in regional blood flow. Cessation of the oxygen supply is a more critical insult to neurons than the cessation of the glucose supply. Glucose stores in the brain are sufficient to sustain function for 30 to 60 minutes in the absence of a continuing supply.

It is important to differentiate the separate contributions of hypoxia and reduced blood flow to neurologic dysfunction. Pure hypoxia (deprivation of oxygen) with maintenance of normal blood flow, as might occur on exposure to reduced atmospheric pressures, is tolerable to neurons for much longer periods of time than ischemia (reduced or interrupted blood flow). This is because cessation of blood flow is accompanied by pH changes and an accumulation of metabolic products that to not occur with anoxia alone. Typically, however, severe hypoxia is followed quickly by hypotension and cardiac arrest, making ischemia the final common pathway of anoxia of any cause. Evidence from experimental studies suggests that neurons can tolerate pure hypoxia for as long as 25 minutes, whereas ischemia produces permanent neuronal damage after about 6 minutes. *(p. 1308)*

**13. (A)** Meningiomas are primary tumors of the meningothelial cells of the arachnoid that are most frequently slow-growing, benign tumors associated with a good prognosis. Only rarely do the anaplastic and papillary variants of this tumor behave in a malignant fashion and invade the brain or even metastasize. They are typically rounded, well-circumscribed masses with smooth encapsulated borders. Nevertheless, extension into the underlying bone is not unusual. A common characteristic of meningiomas, especially the transitional variant (having histologic characteristics intermediate between the syncytial and fibroblastic types), is the presence of psammoma bodies, basophilic concretions that look like little bull's-eyes. These concentrically laminated spheroids of calcium salts give the tumor a gritty texture on gross examination and may appear as stippling on radiologic images. Immunohistochemical studies have shown that meningiomas express epithelial markers such as carcinoembryonic antigen (CEA), epithelial membrane antigen, and, focally in some tumors, keratin. These tumors also express progesterone receptors and, thus, may undergo rapid growth during pregnancy. *(p. 1349)*

**14. (C)** Idiopathic Parkinson's disease (IPD) is a progressive disturbance of motor function characterized by damage to the nigrostriatal dopaminergic system. It typically results in reduced facial expression, stooped posture, slowness of voluntary movement, festinating gait (short rapid steps), rigidity, and a characteristic "pill-rolling" tremor. These clinical features also are seen in a number of different conditions besides IPD, including drug/toxin injuries, postencephalitic parkinsonism, striatonigral degeneration, Shy-Drager syndrome, and progressive nuclear palsy, all of which affect the striatonigral dopaminergic system. However, in IPD, the syndrome occurs in the absence of a toxin or other known etiology.

Histologically, the disease is characterized by the presence of Lewy bodies (targetoid eosinophilic intracytoplasmic inclusion bodies containing neurofilament proteins) in the neurons of the substantia nigra and locus ceruleus. In addition, the melanin-containing neurons in these regions of the brain typically are depigmented. Lewy bodies are not to be confused with Hirano bodies, the elongated glassy neuronal inclusions composed primarily of actin that are found in Alzheimer's disease.

Neurofibrillary tangles are seen in the affected neurons of postencephalitic parkinsonism and progressive supranuclear palsy but are not seen in IPD. Severe neuronal loss in the putamen and caudate is a characteristic of striatonigral degeneration, another degenerative disease of the basal ganglia that is clinically similar to IPD but pathologically different. In striatonigral degeneration, neither Lewy bodies nor neurofibrillary tangles are present. Diagnostic differentiation of striatonigral degeneration from IPD is important because only the latter is responsive to levodopa treatment. *(pp. 1332–1334)*

**15. (D)** Amyotrophic lateral sclerosis (ALS) is the most common disorder among the group of degenerative diseases of motor neurons. In ALS, degeneration of both the upper motor neurons (in the motor cortex) and lower motor neurons (in the cranial motor nuclei and anterior horns of the spinal cord) occurs. The disease has an invariably fatal outcome (death usually results from respiratory complications) after a variable 2- to 6-year course.

Unlike poliomyelitis, a disease of lower motor neurons caused by an enterovirus, ALS is not known to be associated with a viral agent. The pathogenesis is unknown at present, but missense mutations of a Cu/Zn-binding superoxide dismutase gene have been identified in familial cases of ALS. Certain human lymphocyte antigen (HLA) associations have been defined (HLA-A3 and -B12 haplotypes), suggesting a genetically determined susceptibility factor, yet other evidence from animal models has suggested the possibility of a neurotoxic etiology. *(pp. 1336–1337)*

**16. (A)** Plexiform neurofibromas are the peripheral nerve tumors that are the defining lesions of neurofibromatosis type 1 (NF1), an autosomal dominant disorder. NF1 is caused by mutation of a tumor suppressor gene on chromosome 17q11.2 that encodes a *ras* oncogene regulatory protein known as neurofibromin. Unlike common, solitary neurofibromas, which occur only in the skin or peripheral nerve, plexiform neurofibromas may occur in any site in the body (internal or external) and also may involve the cranial nerves. Plexiform neurofibromas do not occur as sporadic lesions and, thus, are diagnostic of NF1. In neurofibromas, nerve fibers are found scattered throughout the tumor mass, which appears as a bulbous expansion of the entire nerve fascicle. Thus, in contrast to schwannomas, which are located eccentrically on the side of the nerve and can be excised surgically, neurofibromas cannot be resected without removing the involved nerve. In contrast to solitary sporadic neurofibromas, plexiform neurofibromas have a significant propensity to undergo malignant transformation. *(pp. 148–149; 1352–1353)*

**17. (True); 18. (False); 19. (True); 20. (True); 21. (True); 22. (True); 23. (True); 24. (False); 25. (False)**

As a group, vascular disorders of the central nervous system are the most common cause of neurologic problems encountered among hospitalized patients and constitute the third leading cause of death in the United States (after heart disease and cancer). **(17)** Overall, ischemic encephalopathy is most commonly associated with inadequate cardiopulmonary resuscitation following cardiac arrest.

**(18)** Cerebral infarction ("stroke") is caused by arterial occlusion that may be either thrombotic or embolic in origin. In general, embolic occlusion of intracranial vessels is more common than thrombotic occlusion. In the extracerebral carotid system, thrombotic occlusion is more common. **(19)** Wherever their site of occurrence, however, thrombotic occlusions are most often due to atherosclerosis of the involved vessel. Causes such as vasculitis and trauma are much less common.

**(20)** Hemorrhagic infarction typically is associated with embolism. Infarction from arterial occlusion does not overlap the territorial distribution of the involved vessel, so hemorrhagic infarction often can be differentiated from a cerebral hemorrhage (i.e., bleeding into tumors, hypertensive intracerebral hemorrhage, etc.), which would not necessarily cause a pattern of involvement corresponding to a given vascular distribution. **(21)** In contrast, nonhemorrhagic infarction typically is associated with thrombosis. The distinction is important because anticoagulant therapy is contraindicated in hemorrhagic infarction.

**(22)** Cerebral hemorrhage (bleeding into the brain substance) most commonly is caused by hypertensive vascular disease. In this disorder, bleeding is thought to occur from rupture of microaneurysms (Charcot-Buchard aneurysms) that form at bifurcations of intraparenchymal arteries. **(23)** Hypertensive vascular disease characteristically produces lacunar infarcts. Lacunar infarcts are small infarcts in the deep portions of the brain (especially the thalamus, putamen, and internal capsule) that, owing to their small size and variable location, can produce a variety of ischemic syndromes or may even be asymptomatic. **(24)** Hypertensive encephalopathy is characterized by vascular necrosis, cerebral edema, and petechial hemorrhages. It is associated only with acute malignant hypertension (e.g., eclampsia, acute nephritis). In contrast, chronic stable hypertension sometimes produces a syndrome of diffuse loss of deep hemispheric white matter, with demyelination and gliosis, known as subcortical leukoencephalopathy or Binswanger's disease.

**(25)** Unlike the brain, the spinal cord most often sustains vascular injury from disruption of the spinal arteries secondary to dissecting aortic aneurysms. *(pp. 1309–1311; 1314)*

**26. (True); 27. (False); 28. (False); 29. (True); 30. (False); 31. (False); 32. (False)**

**(26)** Multiple sclerosis (MS) is a disease of undetermined etiology that causes diffuse primary (having no other known underlying cause) demyelination in the central nervous system. However, it is defined by its clinical manifestations, rather than its tissue pathology. It produces distinct episodes of neurologic deficits, separated in time, that are attributable to white matter lesions that are separated in space. **(27)** MS usually affects adults between 20 and 40 years of age and is rare before puberty or after age 55. **(28)** The disease typically begins with diplopia (involvement of the optic nerve is a common initial event), paresthesias, or cerebellar incoordination, but intellectual deterioration is not an early manifestation. **(29)** The cerebrospinal fluid (CSF) typically contains an increased immunoglobulin content, and immunoelectrophoretic analysis demonstrates oligoclonal bands that are not present in the serum. The antigenic targets of the CSF immunoglobulins in MS are widely variable and, apparently, myelin is not among them. In fact, there is no evidence that the disease is mediated through antibody-dependent mechanisms.

**(30)** MS is not associated with antecedent infection of any kind. This contrasts with acute disseminated encephalomyelitis (ADEM), another form of demyelinating disease, which typically occurs after a viral infection or, rarely, a viral immunization. ADEM has an acute course ending either in death (25%) or full recovery, and, in further contrast to MS, an acute autoimmune reaction to myelin is suspected (but not proven) in this disease.

**(31)** Histologically, MS is characterized by lesions called active plaques. These consist of multiple, small, sharply defined foci of myelin breakdown associated with perivascular lymphocytic and monocytic inflammation. As the active plaques become quiescent, the inflammatory infiltrate diminishes, myelin disappears from the center of the plaque, and gliosis becomes evident. Perivascular collections of multinucleated macrophages (globoid cells) are not a feature of MS, but instead accompany the process of demyelination in an inherited leukodystrophy known as Krabbes' disease (see Questions 71 through 75). **(32)** At present, there is no truly effective treatment for this disease. During relapses, however, patients are often treated with corticosteroids, adrenocorticotrophic hormone, or other immunosuppressive agents with some temporary benefit, but immunosuppression does not alter the long-term course of the disease. *(pp. 1326–1329)*

**33. (D); 34. (C); 35. (B); 36. (A); 37. (B)**

Distention of the ventricles with an associated increase in the volume of cerebrospinal fluid (CSF) is known as hydrocephalus. Although it rarely may be caused by overproduction of fluid, decreased absorption of CSF is the most common cause. Decreased CSF absorption may, in turn, result either from decreased transfer of CSF to the venous system by the arachnoid villi (communicating hydrocephalus) or from decreased flow through the CSF as a result of obstruction anywhere along the ventricular system (noncommunicating hydrocephalus). **(33)** Both types produce ventricular distention. **(34)** Either type may occur following acute pyogenic meningitis, depending on the nature and extent of the injury and the location of the subsequent fibrosis. (In general, acute pyogenic meningitis often causes adhesions between the meninges and the brain.) Severe bacterial meningitis may lead to communicating hydrocephalus secondary to arachnoid fibrosis and obliteration of the subarachnoid space. Intra-arachnoid adhesions around the brain stem may occlude the foramina of Magendie and Luschka, producing noncommunicating hydrocephalus.

**(35)** Obstructive (noncommunicating) hydrocephalus characteristically is seen in association with neoplasms that invade or compress the foramina in the CSF pathway. **(36)** Thrombosis of the dural sinuses interferes with transport of CSF into the venous system and typically produces communicating hydrocephalus. **(37)** The Dandy-Walker syndrome is a congenital malformation of the cerebellum in which the cerebellar vermis fails to develop. Consequently, occlusion or obliteration of the foramina of Magendie and Luschka occurs and noncommunicating hydrocephalus is produced. *(pp. 1300; 1302–1303)*

**38. (B); 39. (A); 40. (D); 41. (B); 42. (A)**

Rabies and poliomyelitis are both viral diseases of the central nervous system (CNS) that end in paralysis. **(38)** As typically occurs with most viral diseases of the CNS, poliomyelitis is preceded by a primary infection elsewhere, in this case the gastrointestinal tract. Rabies is a noteworthy exception to this rule because the virus is inoculated directly into the peripheral nerves (from a cutaneous wound) and ascends promptly to the brain. **(39)** In rabies, diagnostic cytoplasmic inclusions called Negri bodies are found in the pyramidal neurons of the hippocampus and the Purkinje cells of the cerebellum. Negri bodies are eosinophilic, round, oval, or bullet shaped, and often multiple. They are composed of viral nucleocapsid proteins. In poliomyelitis, viral infection of the neurons does not produce intracellular inclusions.

**(40)** Although rabies virus does affect the dorsal root ganglia, it also typically involves the neurons of Ammon's horn in the temporal lobe, as well as the Purkinje cells of the cerebellum and the spinal cord. The principal target of poliovirus is the anterior horn cell of the spinal cord, although the posterior horn may be affected in very fulminant cases. The viral agent that shows specific and exclusive tropism for the dorsal root ganglion cells is herpes zoster. Following acute infection by herpes zoster (chickenpox), the virus remains latent for long periods of time within the dorsal root ganglia. Reactivation of the latent virus, commonly called "shingles," may occur with immunosuppression or advancing age.

**(41)** Rabies characteristically produces a severe encephalitis with flaccid paralysis in the late stage of the disease. In contrast, poliomyelitis, with its specifically targeted injury, characteristically causes a lower motor neuron paralysis. **(42)** Although the most common cause of death in both of these diseases is respiratory failure, it occurs on the basis of respiratory center failure in rabies and from paralysis of the respiratory muscles in polio. *(pp. 349–350; 1320)*

**43. (D); 44. (D); 45. (B); 46. (B); 47. (B); 48. (B); 49. (D)**

Huntington's disease (HD) and Friederich's ataxia (FA) are both severe motor disorders characterized by relentless progression. **(44)** They are both genetically determined diseases with an autosomal dominant inheritance pattern in all cases of HD and some cases of FA (autosomal recessive inheritance is more common in FA). Neither disease is related to infection.

**(43 and 45)** HD is a disease of the brain characterized by degeneration of the striatal neurons of the caudate nucleus and disruption of the circuitry of the basal ganglia. The spinal cord is not involved. HD produces choreiform (jerky, hyperkinetic) movements affecting all parts of the body without sensory dysfunction. It usually presents in persons between 20 and 50 years of age.

**(43, 45, and 46)** In contrast, FA is a disease of the brain and spinal cord and is characterized by degeneration of neurons in the dorsal root ganglia, Clarke's column, cranial nerves VIII, X, and XII, the dentate nucleus, and the superior vermis. The average age at onset is 11 years. Initially, gait ataxia predominates, but dysarthria, loss of deep tendon reflexes, and loss of sensory function (e.g., perception of vibration, joint position, temperature, and pain) also are seen. **(47 and 48)** There is a high incidence of both diabetes mellitus and cardiac disease (with arrhythmias and congestive heart failure) in patients with FA.

**(49)** Both diseases have predictably dire outcomes. In FA, most patients progress to paralysis within 20 years. In HD, with progression of disease, parkinsonism and rigidity may replace chorea as the predominant clinical manifestations. Death usually occurs within 15 years of the onset of disease. *(pp. 1334–1335)*

**50. (D); 51. (E); 52. (A); 53. (A); 54. (B); 55. (E); 56. (E)**

Although the neuron is the basic parenchymal element of the central nervous system (CNS), numerous specialized supportive and protective interstitial cells are necessary for normal neuronal functioning. **(50)** These supportive elements, called neuroglial cells, consist of astrocytes, oligodendrocytes, ependymal cells (all derived from neuroectoderm), and microglial cells (derived from bone marrow). **(51)** It is the microglial cells that represent the fixed macrophage system of the CNS. They are CD4+, and, when activated, these cells resemble macrophages in both their cytoplasmic histochemical profiles and their phagocytic activity.

**(52 and 53)** Astrocytes (star-shaped cells found in both gray and white matter) form an extensive cellular plexus that serves as the structural framework for the all-important neurons. They are also thought to provide nutrients, to act as metabolic buffers or detoxifiers, and to provide electrical insulation for neighboring neurons. Following injury, astrocytes are responsible for the CNS equivalent of scar formation, a process known as gliosis. In contrast to fibrosis, gliosis does not lead to the production of collagen. Rather, defects are filled by "glial fibers," which are actually cellular processes of astrocytes containing abundant intermediate filaments made up of vimentin and glial fibrillary acidic protein.

**(54)** Oligodendrocytes, so called because they have fewer and shorter dendrites than astrocytes, are the main cellular constituents of the white matter and are responsible for the production and maintenance of CNS myelin. In contrast to the Schwann cell, the myelin-forming cell of the peripheral nervous system, each oligodendrocyte contributes segments of myelin sheaths to multiple axons. In demyelinating diseases of the CNS, oligodendrocytes sustain most of the injury.

**(55 and 56)** Although ependymal cells line the ventricles of the brain, they are not responsible for the production of the cerebrospinal fluid contained within, nor are they responsible for its resorption. The cells of the choroid plexus produce cerebrospinal fluid, which, after traversing the ventricles and entering the subarachnoid space, is resorbed by the cells of the arachnoid villi. (*pp. 1296–1297; 1300*)

**57. (B); 58. (D); 59. (A); 60. (C); 61. (C)**

Meningitis refers to inflammation limited to the leptomeninges in the subarachnoid space and most often is caused by infection. The nature of the inflammatory process largely is determined by the causal organism. Acute pyogenic meningitis is usually bacterial in origin, and meningococcal meningitis is a common example. Acute aseptic meningitis, usually virally induced, is exemplified by mumps meningitis. Chronic meningitis, a more slowly evolving process, is associated with infection by bacteria or fungi. Tuberculosis meningitis is a prototypic example. **(57)** Only in acute aseptic meningitis is the sugar content of the cerebrospinal fluid (CSF) almost invariably normal. Pyogenic meningitis causes a strikingly reduced CSF sugar content (bacteria metabolize this substrate), whereas chronic meningitis is associated with a variably reduced sugar content. **(58)** In contrast, all forms of meningitis usually produce elevations in the protein content of the CSF. These vary only in magnitude.

**(59)** Large numbers of neutrophils in the CSF are characteristic of acute pyogenic meningitis, such as that of meningococcal origin. In mumps meningitis, the CSF pleocytosis consists mainly of lymphocytes, and, in tuberculosis meningitis, it is composed largely of mononuclear cells. **(60)** Only the acute forms of meningitis, either pyogenic or lymphocytic, are associated clinically with signs of meningeal irritation: a stiff neck, headache, photophobia, irritability, and clouding of consciousness. Chronic meningitis (such as tuberculosis meningitis) presents with more generalized neurologic symptoms, including headache, malaise, mental confusion, and vomiting, rather than a stiff neck. **(61)** Obliterative endarteritis is a complication of chronic meningitis caused by the continuing inflammatory reaction around the vessels. Infarctions in the underlying brain may result. Thus, obliterative endarteritis is one of the most dire complications of chronic tuberculosis meningitis. (*pp. 1315–1317*)

**62. (A); 63. (D); 64. (C); 65. (A); 66. (B); 67. (C); 68. (C); 69. (D); 70. (D)**

Astrocytomas, oligodendrogliomas, and ependymomas are all glial tumors, but each has distinctive characteristics. **(62)** Astrocytomas are the most common type of primary brain tumor in adults, accounting for about 80% of all cases. **(65)** High-grade astrocytomas are known as glioblastoma multiforme. They are the most anaplastic of all gliomas and are associated with a very poor prognosis. **(63)** All types of glial tumors occur in the pediatric age group as well as adults. In childhood, tumors of the central nervous system account for as many as 20% of all cancers.

**(64)** In the spinal cord, the most common type of glial tumor is the ependymoma. Ependymomas constitute about 63% of intraspinal gliomas but only 5 to 6% of all intracranial gliomas. **(67 and 68)** Histologic features that are particularly characteristic of ependymomas are rosette and pseudorosette formation. A rosette is a small circle of tumor cells arranged around a central space that may contain neuroglial fibers. In a pseudorosette, the tumor cells are arranged around a central blood vessel.

**(66)** Among the neuroglial tumors, oligodendrogliomas are distinctive in their tendency to calcify. Calcification occurs in about 90% of these tumors. This feature serves as a diagnostic aid, because oligodendrogliomas characteristically appear stippled with calcifications on radiographs and computerized tomography (CT) scans.

**(69)** Extraneural metastases from any primary intracranial tumor are distinctly uncommon. When they do occur, they are most likely to be from a glioblastoma or a medulloblastoma. **(70)** Another characteristic shared by all neuroglial tumors is their resistance to chemotherapy. Depending on the feasibility of surgical resection, excision and radiotherapy thus far have provided the most successful therapeutic approaches to this family of tumors. Even with therapy, however, the average survival for patients with astrocytomas is less than a year. For oligodendrogliomas and ependymomas, average survival is 5 to 10 years and 4 years, respectively. (*pp. 1342–1346*)

**71. (C); 72. (A); 73. (B); 74. (B); 75. (C)**

The leukodystrophies are diseases of the white matter resulting from biochemical defects in the pathway of myelin metabolism. Mixed motor and sensory neuropathies are produced. **(71)** Krabbe's disease typically becomes manifest in early childhood as symmetrical, global disorders of myelinization and leads rapidly to death before the age of 2 years. Metachromatic leukodystrophy most commonly presents in late infancy, but congenital, juvenile, and adult presentations may occur. In contrast, the clinical manifestations of adrenoleukodystrophy are delayed. The onset of symptoms in males typically occurs earlier (ages 10 to 20 years) than in females (ages 20 to 40 years).

**(72)** Metachromatic leukodystrophy is an autosomal recessive disorder of sphingomyelin metabolism produced by a deficiency of arylsulfatase A (cerebroside sulfatase). It usually presents as a progressive motor impairment with mental deterioration and can be diagnosed by measuring urinary arylsulfatase A.

**(73)** Also an autosomal recessive disorder, Krabbe's disease results from a deficiency of galactocerebroside β-galactosidase and the accumulation of galactocerebroside. **(74)** In addition to demyelination, a characteristic histologic feature is the presence of multinucleate histiocytic cells called globoid cells.

**(75)** Adrenoleukodystropy is a familial, X-linked recessive disease leading to the accumulation of long-chain fatty acid esters of cholesterol, the result of a defect in fatty acyl–coenzyme A ligase (a peroxisomal transporter enzyme). It produces adrenal failure as well as segmental demyelination and axonal degeneration in the central nervous system. By electron microscopy, specific cytoplasmic inclusions composed of dense, long, thin leaflets enclosing an electron-lucent space are seen in the cerebral macrophages, adrenocortical cells, testicular Leydig cells, and Schwann cells. *(pp. 1281; 1337–1338)*

**76. (C); 77. (B); 78. (A); 79. (A); 80. (C); 81. (B)**

Peripheral neuropathies develop whenever axonal degeneration, demyelination, or a combination of these occurs in the peripheral nervous system. They may occur in association with a large number of diseases and produce varied clinical syndromes, depending on the size and the type (sensory, motor, or autonomic) of the axons principally involved. It is with variable predictability that most major causes of peripheral neuropathy produce specific patterns of injury and specific corresponding clinical syndromes.

**(76, 77, 80, and 81)** Diseases that produce focal patchy lesions rather than generalized diffuse injury tend to produce asymmetrical neuropathy. They affect single individual nerves and produce a mononeuritis or, if more than one nerve is affected, a mononeuritis multiplex. Processes that are associated with diffuse injury, however, tend to produce symmetrical polyneuropathies. Polyarteritis nodosa, diabetes, and sarcoidosis are examples of processes that are typically focal and cause neuropathies that are usually asymmetrical. Alcohol and lead both have diffuse systemic toxic effects and are associated with symmetrical sensorimotor polyneuropathies.

**(78 and 79)** Diseases that cause acute demyelination without significant axonal injury or associated acute ascending motor paralysis include the Guillain-Barré syndrome (acute inflammatory demyelinating polyradiculoneuropathy) and diphtheria. In the Guillain-Barré syndrome, the injury is believed to be due to a T-cell–mediated immune response to peripheral nerve myelin. In contrast, diphtheritic peripheral neuritis is the direct result of the action of diphtheria toxin on the peripheral nerve. In diphtheria, demyelination is limited to the dorsal root ganglia and the adjacent motor and sensory roots, because there is a naturally occurring defect in the blood barrier at these points that allows penetration of the toxin. *(pp. 351; 494; 1279–1280; 1282–1284)*